Varcarolis' MANUAL of PSYCHIATRIC NURSING CARE PLANNING

An Interprofessional Approach

6 EDITION

Varcarolis' MANUAL of PSYCHIATRIC NURSING CARE PLANNING

An Interprofessional Approach

Margaret Jordan Halter, PhD, APRN

Cleveland Clinic Akron General
The Ohio State University College of Nursing

ELSEVIER

ELSEVIER

3251 Riverport Lane
St. Louis, Missouri 63043

Varcarolis' Manual of Psychiatric Nursing Care Planning, Edition 6

ISBN: 978-0-323-47949-3

Notices

Previous editions copyrighted 2015, 2011, 2006, 2004, 2000

International Standard Book Number: 978-0-323-47949-3

Senior Content Strategist: Yvonne Alexopoulos
Content Development Manager: Lisa Newton
Senior Content Development Specialist: Danielle M. Frazier
Publishing Services Manager: Julie Eddy
Project Manager: Mike Sheets
Design Direction: Patrick Ferguson

Printed in the United States of America

Last digit is the print number:
9 8 7 6 5 4 3 2

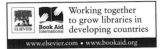

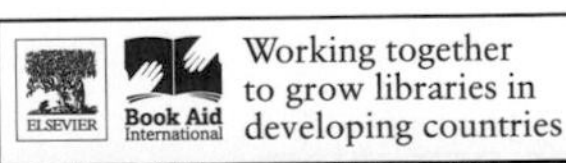

This book is dedicated to people who are living with and recovering from mental illness and to the nursing students and registered nurses who focus on supporting this recovery.

Reviewers

Leslie A. Folds Ed D.; PMHCNS-BC; CNE
Associate Professor of Nursing
School of Nursing
Belmont University
Nashville, TN

Phyllis M. Jacobs, RN, MSN
Assistant Professor Emeritus
School of Nursing
Wichita State University
Wichita, Kansas

Susan Justice MSN, RN, CNS
Clinical Assistant Professor
College of Nursing
University of Texas at Arlington College of Nursing and Health Innovation
Arlington, Texas

Chris Paxos, PharmD, BCPP, BCPS, BCGP
Pharmacotherapy Specialist
Department of Pharmacy
Cleveland Clinic Akron General
Akron, Ohio
Associate Professor of Pharmacy Practice
Department of Pharmacy Practice
Northeast Ohio Medical University, College of Pharmacy
Rootstown, Ohio
Associate Professor of Psychiatry
Department of Psychiatry
Northeast Ohio Medical University, College of Medicine
Rootstown, Ohio

Preface

As with previous editions, the sixth edition of the *Varcarolis' Manual of Psychiatric Nursing Care Planning* supports students and practitioners in planning realistic, evidence-based, and individualized nursing care for their patients. This thoroughly updated edition of the *Manual* provides readers with a foundation for clinical work in contemporary psychiatric settings. The chapters are logically and intuitively arranged in five parts:

- Part I provides a snapshot of basic psychiatric concepts and tools. These chapters focus on the nursing process, therapeutic relationships, and therapeutic communication.
- Part II explores specific diagnostic groups, an overview of major disorders within these groups, and guidelines for developing and providing psychiatric nursing care.
- Part III discusses psychiatric crises such as suicide and family violence and outlines the nursing process as it pertains to these crises.
- Part IV is devoted to psychopharmacology. Eight chapters provide essential information regarding specific classifications of drugs such as antipsychotics and antidepressants.
- Part V provides a summary of nonpharmacological approaches. Whereas psychotherapeutic models are mentioned in the clinical chapters, Chapter 29 provides an overview of evidence-based therapies such as cognitive–behavioral therapy. Chapter 30 introduces the increasingly common brain stimulation therapies, such as electroconvulsive therapy and vagus nerve stimulation.

Overall, the format of the *Manual* has been streamlined and blank space reduced. The organization of the clinical chapters now mirrors the *Diagnostic and Statistical Manual of Mental Disorders, Fifth Edition (DSM-5).* Although some classical references remain, citations are thoroughly updated.

In this edition, we have moved toward a terminology that more accurately reflects the way healthcare professionals describe patient problems in the real world. This move eliminates the use of NANDA-I nursing diagnoses, which requires nurses to learn a second language in addition to the primary terms that are used by other healthcare providers. We hope that this approach will promote and support interprofessional collaboration for nursing students and nurses.

Acknowledgments

Thanks to my Elsevier family for coordinating and completing another successful project. Kudos go out to Yvonne Alexopoulos, senior content strategist, for providing feedback and supporting my ideas for this sixth edition. Yvonne is a brilliant person with thought-provoking comments along with a humorous take on thorny issues. As always, cheers go out to Lisa Newton, our content development manager. This is a woman who responds to emails within an hour, sends positive greetings, and adds a personal touch to nearly all of our communications.

As a senior content development specialist, Danielle Frazier moved the publishing process along while tirelessly re-uploading files to the electronic management system. Big thanks to Mike Sheets, project manager, for pulling all the details together, ensuring consistency, and producing a reader-friendly edition for students and clinical nurses.

Moving from NANDA-I based nursing care plans to a patient problem approach was a big move. Other nurse editors have pioneered and already adopted this method in their popular textbooks. I am especially grateful to editors Donna Ignatavicius and Pamela Swearingen for taking the lead in this endeavor and helping me through the process.

Finally, I'd like to acknowledge Elizabeth (Betsy - the real wizard) Varcarolis. Betsy developed a leading undergraduate psychiatric nursing textbook, *Foundations of Psychiatric-Mental Health Nursing*, and later added the *Manual of Psychiatric Nursing Care Planning*. Together, Betsy and I went on to introduce the popular *Essentials of Psychiatric Mental Health Nursing*, a more condensed version of *Foundations*. Countless psychiatric nursing students have read her words and been prepared for the NCLEX based on her knowledge of this discipline. I am sincerely grateful to have been (and still am) Betsy's apprentice. I will always be indebted to her.

Peggy Halter

PART I
Foundations for Psychiatric Nursing Care

CHAPTER 1

The Nursing Process

The basis of psychiatric–mental health nursing is the therapeutic relationship. It is within this relationship that care is provided to address healthcare problems, both actual or potential. These problems occur in the context of or as the result of psychiatric disorders, also known as *mental illness* or *mental disorders.* A common language for nurses, physicians, social workers, psychologists, and other professionals who work in the mental health system facilitates patient care.

The *Diagnostic and Statistical Manual of Mental Disorders (DSM)* is the official publication of the American Psychiatric Association (APA) for categorizing medical diagnoses in the United States. The *DSM* provides clinicians, researchers, insurance companies, pharmaceutical firms, and policy makers with standard criteria for the classification of psychiatric disorders. Clinicians use this publication as a guide for planning care and evaluating patients' treatments.

First published in 1952, the current manual is the *Diagnostic and Statistical Manual of Mental Disorders,* fifth edition *(DSM-5)* (APA, 2013). The *Manual of Psychiatric-Mental Health Nursing Care Planning* uses the *DSM-5* for organizing the order of clinical chapters and for describing psychiatric disorders.

THE NURSING PROCESS

The nursing process is a problem-solving process. It is the basic framework for nursing practice with patients who are experiencing psychiatric disorders or conditions. The

National Council of State Boards of Nursing ([NCSBN] 2015, p. 3) defines the nursing process as "a scientific, clinical reasoning approach to client care that includes assessment, analysis, planning, implementation and evaluation." The nursing process is fundamental to patient care and is the basis for this textbook.

Safety and quality care for patients are also prime directives for nurses and nursing education. The national initiative that is centered on patient safety and quality of care is known as *Quality and Safety Education for Nurses (QSEN)*. QSEN competencies are integrated throughout this manual, and specific examples are highlighted along with each standard of practice. Box 1.1 provides a summary of the competencies.

Box 1.1 **Quality and Safety Education for Nurses (QSEN) Competencies**

Patient-centered care: Recognize the patient or designee as the source of control and full partner in providing compassionate and coordinated care based on respect for the patient's preferences, values, and needs.

Teamwork and collaboration: Function effectively within nursing and interprofessional teams, fostering open communication, mutual respect, and shared decision making to achieve quality patient care.

Evidence-based practice: Integrate best current evidence with clinical expertise and patient/family preferences and values for delivery of optimal health care.

Quality improvement: Use data to monitor the outcomes of care processes and use improvement methods to design and test changes to continuously improve the quality and safety of health care systems.

Safety: Minimizes risk of harm to patients and providers through both system effectiveness and individual performance.

Informatics: Use information and technology to communicate, manage knowledge, mitigate error, and support decision-making.

QSEN Institute. (n.d.). QSEN competencies. Retrieved from http://qsen.org/competencies/pre-licensure-ksas

ASSESSMENT

Psychiatric–mental health registered nurses collect information that guides the plan of care. Assessment is an essential initial activity and it is also ongoing. The focus and type of information that is gathered is based on the patient's specific condition and by anticipating future needs.

QUALITY AND SAFETY STANDARDS (QSEN) RELATED TO ASSESSMENT

- Patient-centered care: Elicit preferences, values, and expressed needs as part of the clinical interview.
- Informatics: Identify essential information that must be available in a common database to support patient care.

Patients with psychiatric disorders are not only found on behavioral health units. Symptoms such as depression, suicidal thoughts, anger, disorientation, delusions, and hallucinations are encountered in all settings. These settings include medical-surgical wards, obstetrical units, intensive care units, outpatient settings, extended-care facilities, emergency departments, and community centers. Psychiatric symptoms can also be the result of chemical imbalances, substance use, and disease. The assessment helps to identify and clearly articulate specific problems in the individual's life that are causing distress.

The assessment has several primary goals:

- Establish rapport.
- Elicit the patient's chief complaint (i.e., the perception of the problem in the patient's own words).
- Review physical status and obtain baseline vital signs.
- Determine the impact of the disorder and symptoms on the patient's life (self-esteem, loss of intimacy, role functioning, change in family dynamics, lifestyle change, and employment issues).
- Identify risk factors that may affect safety (e.g., confusion, suicidal thoughts, or homicidal thoughts).
- Gather information related to previous illnesses, treatment, and hospitalizations.
- Identify psychosocial status (family relationships, social patterns, interests and abilities, stress factors, substance use, social supports).
- Complete a mental status examination.

It is helpful if the patient's family members, friends, and relatives participate during the data collection whenever possible. If a law enforcement agent brought the patient into the emergency department or crisis intervention unit, it is important for the nurse to understand what situation warranted police intervention.

Past medical and psychiatric history can supply valuable information. This is particularly important if the patient is experiencing psychosis, is withdrawn and mute, or is too agitated to provide a history. Charts from previous hospitalizations or electronic medical records are extremely helpful. Laboratory reports also provide important information.

The use of a standardized nursing assessment tool facilitates the assessment process. Appendix A contains a patient-centered assessment tool. Most healthcare facilities provide patient assessments in either paper or electronic form. Although these tools are integral for gathering essential data, they can feel impersonal. With practice, nurses become proficient in gathering information in a less formal fashion, with the nurse clarifying, focusing, and exploring pertinent data with the patient. This method allows patients to state their perceptions in their own words and enables the nurse to observe a wide range of nonverbal behaviors. A personal style of interviewing congruent with the nurse's personality develops as comfort and experience increase. Box 1.2 presents the factors that are typically assessed.

Issues for Which Referral May Be Indicated

Patients may be referred to social services and might need further investigation when planning long-term care. This is especially important in the case of severe mental illness, if any of the following issues are noted:

- Problems with primary support (death, illness, divorce, sexual or physical abuse, neglect of a child, discord with siblings, birth of a sibling)
- Problems related to the social environment (death or loss of friends, inadequate social support, living alone, difficulty with acculturation, discrimination, adjustment to life-cycle transition [e.g., retirement])
- Educational problems (illiteracy, academic concerns, conflict with teachers or classmates, inadequate school environment)
- Occupational problems (unemployment, threat of job loss, stressful work schedule, difficult work conditions,

Box 1.2 Common Assessment Areas

Previous psychiatric treatment
Educational background
Occupational background
- Employed? Where? How long?
- Special skills

Social patterns
- Describe family.
- Describe friends.
- With whom does the patient live?
- To whom does the patient go in times of crisis?
- Describe a typical day.

Sexual patterns
- Sexually active? Practices safe sex? Practices birth control?
- Sexual orientation
- Sexual difficulties

Interests and abilities
- What does the patient do in his or her spare time?
- What sport, hobby, or leisure activity is the patient good at?

Medications
- What medications does the patient take? How often? How much?
- What herbal or over-the-counter drugs does the patient take? How often? How much?
- What psychotropic drugs does the patient take or use? How often? How much?
- How many drinks of alcohol does the patient take per day? Per week?
- What recreational drugs does the patient take or use? How often? How much?
- Does the patient identify the use of drugs as a problem?

Coping abilities
- What does the patient do when he or she gets upset?
- To whom can the patient talk?
- What usually helps to relieve stress?
- What did the patient try this time?

job dissatisfaction, job change, discord with boss or co-workers)
- Economic problems (poverty, inadequate finances, insufficient welfare support)
- Problems with access to healthcare services (inadequate healthcare services, transportation to healthcare facilities unavailable, inadequate health insurance)
- Problems related to interaction with the legal system or crime (arrest, incarceration, litigation, victim of crime)

Cultural and Social Assessment

Healthcare providers work with an increasingly culturally diverse population. Providing effective care necessitates an awareness of and appreciation for an individual's cultural background. All healthcare professionals, especially mental health professionals, need to continually expand their knowledge and understanding of the complexity of the cultural and social factors that influence health and illness. It is especially important to broaden one's understanding of how health and illness are influenced by cultural and social factors.

Spiritual and Religious Assessment

The importance of spirituality and religious beliefs is an often-overlooked element of patient care. Spirituality and religious beliefs have the potential to exert an influence on how people understand meaning and purpose in their lives and how they use critical judgment to solve problems. Box 1.3 offers suggestions for eliciting information to better adapt a plan of care to an individual patient's needs.

After the Assessment

After the initial assessment, it is useful to summarize the data with the patient. This summary provides patients with assurance that they have been heard. It also allows the patient the opportunity to clarify potential misinformation.

The patient should be told what will happen next. For example, if the initial assessment takes place in the hospital, the nurse should tell the patient what other clinicians he or she will be seeing. If a psychiatric nurse in a mental health clinic conducts the initial assessment, the nurse should let the patient know when and how often they will meet. If the nurse thinks a referral is necessary (e.g., to a psychiatrist,

Box 1.3 **Brief Cultural, Social, and Spiritual and Religious Assessment**

Cultural Assessment

Language

What is your primary spoken language?

How would you rate your fluency in English?

Would you like an interpreter?

Communication style

Observe nonverbal communication (gesture, posture, eye movement).

What are your feelings about touch?

Observe how much eye contact the patient is comfortable with.

How much or little do people make eye contact in your culture?

Family group

Describe the members of your family.

Who makes the decisions in your family?

Which family members can you confide in?

Health and illness beliefs

When you become ill, what is the first thing you do to take care of the illness?

How is this condition (medical or mental) viewed by your culture?

Are there special health care practices within your culture that address your medical or mental problem?

Are there any restrictions on diet or medical interventions within your religious, spiritual, or cultural beliefs?

What are the attitudes of mental illness in your culture?

Social Supports

Are there people outside the family (friends, neighbors) that you are close to and feel free to confide in?

Is there a place where you can go for support (church, school, work, club)?

Spiritual and Religious Beliefs and Practices

What importance does religion or spirituality have in the patient's life?

Do the patient's religious or spiritual beliefs relate to the way the patient takes care of himself or herself or of the patient's illness? How?

Does the patient's faith help the patient in stressful situations?

Whom does the patient see when he or she is medically ill? Mentally upset?

Continued

Box 1.3 Brief Cultural, Religious and Spiritual, and Social Assessment—cont'd

Are there special healthcare practices within the patient's culture that address his or her particular mental problems?

Would you like to have someone from your church/synagogue/temple or a spiritual advisor be informed or visit?

social worker, or medical personnel), this should be discussed with the patient.

Non–English-Speaking Patients

If a nurse does not speak the patient's language, data gathering may be inaccurate, incomplete, and extremely difficult to obtain. The Americans with Disabilities Act established federal standards to ensure that communication does not interfere with equal access to healthcare for everyone. All healthcare organizations must provide language interpreters, interpreters trained in sign language, telecommunication devices for the deaf (TDDs), closed-caption decoders for televisions, and amplifiers on phones. Translators should be available to provide documents written in the patient's own language.

Using family members, friends, or neighbors to act as interpreters could have significant drawbacks. For example, a family interpreter might want to protect the patient and filter out information given to the patient. Conversely, the family member might want to filter out information about a problem or crisis in the family. Using a nonprofessional interpreter increases the risk of wrong procedures, medications errors, and other adverse events. Almost 9% of the U.S. population has difficulty communicating in English and is at risk (Agency for Healthcare Research and Quality, 2012).

Several guidelines should be followed when working with an interpreter:

- Address the patient directly rather than speaking to the interpreter.
- Maintain eye contact with the patient to ensure patient involvement and strengthen personal connection.
- Avoid interrupting the patient and interpreter.
- Ask the interpreter to give you verbatim translations.

- Avoid using medical jargon the interpreter or the patient might not understand.
- Avoid talking or commenting to the interpreter at length. The patient might feel left out and distrustful.
- Ask for permission to discuss intimate or emotionally charged topics first, and prepare the interpreter for the content of the interview.
- Asking intimate or emotionally charged questions might be difficult for the patient as well as for the interpreter. Lead up to these questions slowly.
- If possible, arrange for the interpreter and the patient to meet each other ahead of time to establish some rapport.
- Aim for consistency by using the same interpreter for subsequent interactions.

When an interpreter is not immediately available, aids such as picture charts or flash cards can help the nurse and patient communicate important basic information about the patient's immediate needs (e.g., degree of pain or need for elimination). Because of cultural norms or because they want to be helpful, some patients with limited English might seem agreeable and nod "yes" even though they do not understand. Asking questions that require more than a yes or no answer can provide a better idea of the patient's level of understanding.

ANALYSIS

Based on a comprehensive assessment, psychiatric–mental health registered nurses analyze the data to determine patient problems and potential problems.

QUALITY AND SAFETY STANDARDS (QSEN) RELATED TO ANALYSIS

Patient-centered care: Integrate understanding of multiple dimensions of patient-centered care, including the patient's needs, preferences, and values, within their cultural parameters.

The term *patient* can be replaced with the words *family, group,* or *community.* A well-chosen and well-stated patient problem is the basis for selecting therapeutic goals and interventions. A problem statement is usually composed of the problem and probable cause.

Patient Problems

Problems, or unmet needs, are within the nurse's domain to treat. An example of a nursing patient problem is *potential for self-mutilation*. In the case of this patient problem, the nurse identified several characteristics during the assessment that puts the patient at risk for this behavior.

Probable Cause (Due to)

The probable cause includes factors that contribute to or are related to the development or maintenance of a patient problem. The probable cause tell us what needs to be addressed to bring about change and identifies what needs to be targeted through nursing interventions. In the case of potential for self-mutilation, the addition of a second part of the patient problem results in:

Potential for self-mutilation due to an altered body image

This statement indicates that the nurse and health-care team should initiate interventions that increase the patient's self-esteem and support an accurate perception of the patient's appearance. Altered body image can also be improved by increasing the patient's ability to express tensions verbally rather than act them out physically.

Consider the difference in a plan of care for someone with the same patient problem, but with a different probable cause. For example, *potential for self-mutilation due to command hallucinations* indicates that the patient is experiencing auditory hallucinations that tell the patient to engage in self-harm. In this case the self-injury may relieve anxiety because the voices are commanding him or her to do so. Interventions should be aimed at lowering the patient's anxiety, finding a calmer environment, evaluating the need for as needed or programmed medication, and teaching distraction techniques (reading out loud, singing).

Types of Patient Problems

Problem-Focused Statements

For problem-focused statements, the nurse makes a judgment about undesirable human responses to a health condition or life process. An example of a problem-focused statement is:

Anxiety due to losing employment and financial burdens.

Potential Problem Statements

Potential problem statements indicate a vulnerability that carries a high probability of developing negative responses. Problems in this category include preventable occurrences such as falls, self-injury, pressure ulcers, and infection. This type of problem always begins with the phrase "potential for" followed by the problem.

An example of a potential problem statement is:

Potential for self-mutilation due to impulsivity, inadequate coping, isolation, and unstable self-esteem.

OUTCOMES

As a basis for evaluation, overall desired outcomes are formulated. In the case of a patient who self-mutilates a desired outcome would be for the patient to use adaptive strategies for dealing with anxiety. Another essential and obvious outcome would be for the patient to free from self-harm.

QUALITY AND SAFETY STANDARDS (QSEN) RELATED TO OUTCOMES

- Patient-centered care: Integrate understanding of multiple dimensions of patient-centered care.
- Patient-centered care: Engage patients or designated surrogates (e.g., family members) in active partnerships that promote health, safety, well-being, and self-management.
- Quality improvement: Seek information about outcomes of care for populations served in care setting.

Outcome criteria are ideal outcomes that reflect the maximum level of health that the patient can realistically achieve through nursing interventions. In this clinical companion, overall desired outcome criteria are provided.

Nurses and nursing students may also identify outcomes as short- and long-term goals. Short- and long-term goals are stated in behavioral and measurable terms and might have time factors such as "in 1 week," "by discharge," or "within 2 days." These goals should also identify end results or desired results. The goals can be evaluated and revised as the patient progresses or does not progress. Goals are always patient-centered rather than staff-centered.

The short-term goals for each patient problem can include several steps that lead to the final outcome criteria. The amount of time needed to attain some of these goals will vary.

A patient with bipolar disorder may be extremely agitated and have hyperactive motor activity. In this case the patient problem might be:

Potential for injury due to extreme agitation, hyperactivity, fewer than 2 hours rest a night, poor skin turgor, and abrasions on hands and arms

Possible short-term goals might include the following:

- Patient will sleep 3 to 4 hours per night with the aid of medication (by time/date).
- Patient will drink 8 oz of fluid (juice, milk, milkshake) every hour.
- Patient's skin turgor will be within normal limits within 24 hours as evidenced by raised area disappearing in less than 4 seconds when skin over the sternum is pinched and released.
- Patient will spend 10 minutes in a quiet, non-stimulating area with a nurse each hour during the day.

Possible long-term goals might include the following:

- Within 1 week, patient will sleep 6 to 8 hours per night.
- Patient will maintain adequate diet (1500–2000 calories/day) and sufficient daily fluid intake by (date).
- Patient will be free from infections and abrasions and wounds will be in final healing stages by (time or date).

Moorhead and colleagues (2013) compile a standardized list of nursing outcomes in *Nursing Outcomes Classification (NOC)*. This resource provides standardized terminology along with definitions and measurement scales that help to track changes over time.

PLANNING

QUALITY AND SAFETY STANDARDS (QSEN) RELATED TO PLANNING

- Patient-centered care: Respect patient preferences for degree of active engagement in care process toward helping the patient meet his or her needs and goals.

- Evidence-based practice: Base the individualized care plan on the patient's values, clinical expertise, and evidence.
- Informatics: Document and plan patient care in an electronic health record.

Once you have completed an assessment and formulated patient problems, the problems must be prioritized. Maslow's Hierarchy of Needs (Fig. 1.1) provides a useful framework for doing so. Physiological needs and safety always come first because they have the potential for the most serious harm. Then the higher order needs can be addressed, including love and belonging and self-esteem. For each problem statement, desired outcomes are developed and interventions for achieving the outcomes are selected.

The nurse considers the following specific principles when planning interventions:

- *Safe:* Interventions must be safe for the patient, as well as for other patients, staff, and family.

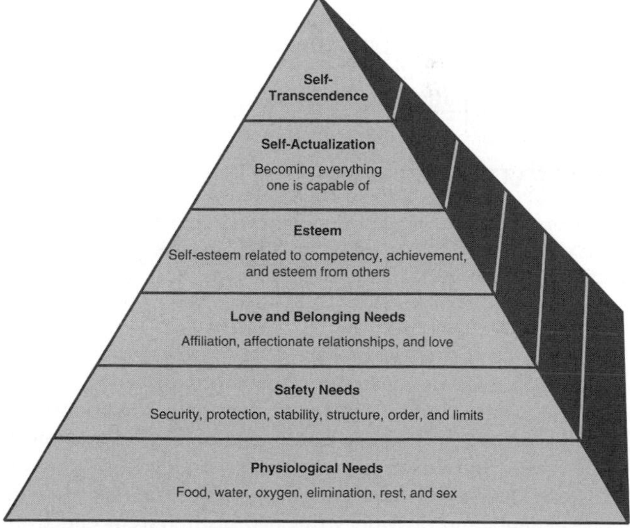

Fig. 1.1 Maslow's hierarchy of needs. (Adapted from Maslow, A. H. [1972]. *The farther reaches of human nature*. New York, NY: Viking.)

- *Compatible and appropriate:* Interventions must be compatible with other therapies and with the patient's personal goals and cultural values, as well as with institutional rules.
- *Realistic and individualized:* Interventions should be (1) within the patient's capabilities, given the patient's age, physical strength, condition, and willingness to change; (2) based on the availability of support staff (3) reflective of the actual available community resources; and (4) within the student's or nurse's capabilities.
- *Evidence-based:* Interventions should be based on scientific evidence and principles when available.

Evidence-based interventions and treatment is the gold standard in healthcare. Evidence-based practice for nurses is a combination of clinical skill and the use of clinically relevant research in the delivery of effective patient-centered care. Using the best available research, incorporating patient preferences, and making sound clinical judgment and skills provides an optimal patient-centered nurse–patient relationship.

The *Nursing Interventions Classification (NIC)* (Bulechek et al., 2013) is a research-based, standardized list of interventions. These interventions are linked to NOC outcomes. This evidence-based approach to care is consistent with QSEN standards. Nurses in all settings can use NIC to support quality patient care and incorporate evidence-based nursing actions.

IMPLEMENTATION

QUALITY AND SAFETY STANDARDS (QSEN) RELATED TO IMPLEMENTATION

- Patient-centered care:
  - Provide patient-centered care with sensitivity and respect for the diversity of human experience.
  - Recognize the boundaries of therapeutic relationships.
  - Participate in building consensus or resolving conflict in the context of patient care.
- Safety: During the interventions minimize the risk of harm to patients and providers through both system effectiveness and individual performance.
- Teamwork and collaboration:
  - Initiate requests for help when appropriate to the situation.

- Integrate the contributions of others who play a role in helping the patient or family achieve health goals to ensure quality patient care.

Implementation is the action the nursing staff takes to carry out the nursing measures identified in the care plan to achieve the expected outcome criteria. Nursing interventions might be called actions, approaches, or nursing orders. When carrying out the nursing interventions, additional data might be gathered, and further refinements of the care plan can be made.

The psychiatric–mental health registered nurse implements the plan with evidence-based interventions whenever possible, using community resources, and collaborating with the interprofessional team. According to the American Nurses Association, American Psychiatric Nurses Association, & the International Society of Psychiatric-Mental Health Nurses (2014), basic-level interventions include the following:

1. Coordination of care
2. Health teaching and health promotion
3. Pharmacological, biological, and integrative therapies
4. Milieu therapy
5. Therapeutic relationship and counseling

In addition to these five interventions, psychiatric–mental health advanced practice registered nurses are qualified to provide three higher level interventions:

5. Consultation
6. Prescriptive authority and treatment
7. Psychotherapy

EVALUATION

QUALITY AND SAFETY STANDARDS (QSEN) RELATED TO IMPLEMENTATION

Quality improvement: Seek information about outcomes for populations served in the care setting.

Evaluation is an ongoing process that includes evaluating the effectiveness of plans and strategies and documenting the results. Evaluation is often the most neglected part of the nursing process. Desired outcome evaluation occurs in the context of the entire plan of care and represents a comprehensive approach to determining the success of the plan.

In addition to addressing the success of desired outcomes, nursing students often include short- and long-term goals. These goals can have three possible outcomes: The goal is met, not met, or partially met. Using a previous example for the patient problem:

Potential for injury due to extreme agitation, hyperactivity, fewer than 2 hours rest at night, poor skin turgor, and abrasions on hands and arms, the following can be determined:

1. Short-term goal:
   Patient will drink 8 oz of fluid (juice, milk, milkshake) every hour.
   For evaluation the nurse might chart:
   Goal met: Patient takes frequent sips of fluid provided in cups with lids equaling 8 oz an hour during the hours of 9 a.m. to 4 p.m., with reminders from nursing staff.
2. Short-term goal:
   Patient will spend 10 minutes in a quiet, non-stimulating area with a nurse each hour during the day.
   For evaluation the nurse might chart:
   Goal partially met: After 2 days, patient continues restless and purposeless pacing; only able to stay quiet with nurse for 4 to 6 minutes per hour.
3. Short-term goal:
   Patient's skin turgor will be within normal limits within 24 hours as evidenced by raised area disappearing in less than 4 seconds when skin over the sternum is pinched and released.
   For evaluation the nurse might chart:
   Goal not met: At 8:00 a.m. patient's skin turgor still poor. Raised area from pinched skin over sternum disappeared 4 seconds after release. Evaluate need for increasing daytime fluids from 9 a.m. to 9 p.m.

As mentioned previously, *NOC* (Moorhead et al., 2013) provides a standardized method to evaluate the effect of nursing interventions. Each outcome has an associated group of indicators used to determine patient status in relation to the outcome. *NOC* provides indicators for the outcome of *suicide self-restraint* such as "expresses feelings," "verbalizes suicidal ideas," and " plans for future." These indicators are then evaluated on a Likert scale that quantifies the achievement from 1 (never demonstrated) to 5 (consistently demonstrated).

IN THE CHAPTERS THAT FOLLOW

This clinical reference guide is intended to help nurses formulate patient problems and develop a patient-centered plan of care. The chapters in Parts II and III of this book present specific *DSM-5* psychiatric disorders and psychiatric crises that might require nursing interventions. For each disorder or phenomenon, the most common patient problems are presented. Suggested outcomes are offered for each patient problem and specific nursing assessments and actions are suggested with supporting rationales. Students and nurses must identify those interventions that are appropriate for their patients.

The chapters that follow support nursing care through an overview of treatment methods. Part IV is devoted to psychopharmacology such as antidepressants and antianxiety agents. Part V focuses on nonpharmacological approaches such as psychotherapy (talk therapy) and brain stimulation therapies.

CHAPTER 2

Therapeutic Relationships

Psychiatric–mental health nursing is based on principles of *science.* Knowledge of anatomy, physiology, and chemistry is the basis for providing safe and effective biological treatments. Knowledge of pharmacology—a medication's mechanism of action, indications for use, and adverse effects based on evidence-based studies and trials—is vital to nursing practice. However, it is the caring relationship and the development of the interpersonal skills needed to enhance and maintain such a relationship that make up the *art* of psychiatric nursing. This art comes to life through the therapeutic relationship where caring and healing can occur.

NURSE–PATIENT RELATIONSHIP

The nurse–patient relationship is the basis of all psychiatric–mental health nursing treatment approaches, regardless of the specific goals. We all have distinct gifts—unique personality traits and talents—that we can learn to use creatively to form positive bonds with others. The use of these gifts to promote healing in others is referred to as the *therapeutic use of self.* A positive therapeutic alliance, which is collaborative and respectful, is one of the best predictors of positive outcomes in therapy (Gordon & Beresin, 2016).

Importance of Talk Therapy

A formalized approach to talk therapy that is based on theoretical models is called *psychotherapy.* Health care providers with advanced training, such as psychiatric–mental health advanced practice registered nurses, psychiatrists, and psychologists, are licensed to practice psychotherapy. Evidence suggests that psychotherapy within a therapeutic partnership actually changes brain chemistry in much the same way as medication. Thus the best treatment for most psychiatric problems is a combination of medication and psychotherapy.

Basic-level psychiatric–mental health nurses do not practice psychotherapy. They do, however, use counseling techniques in the context of the therapeutic relationship. Counseling is a supportive face-to-face process that helps individuals problem solve, resolve personal conflicts, and feel supported. Education and learning are also included under the counseling umbrella.

Goals and Functions

A therapeutic nurse–patient relationship has specific goals and functions, including the following:

- Facilitating communication of distressing thoughts and feelings
- Assisting with problem solving to help facilitate activities of daily living
- Exploring self-defeating behaviors and testing alternatives
- Promoting self-care and independence
- Providing education about medications and symptom management
- Promoting recovery

SOCIAL VERSUS THERAPEUTIC RELATIONSHIPS

Throughout life, we meet people in a variety of settings and share a variety of experiences. With some individuals, we develop long-term relationships. With others, the relationship lasts only a short time. Naturally, the kinds of relationships we enter vary from person to person and from situation to situation.

Social Relationships

A social relationship is a relationship that is initiated for the purpose of friendship, socialization, enjoyment, or accomplishment of a task. Mutual needs are met during social interaction. People may give advice and sometimes help meet basic needs such as lending money. During social interactions, roles may shift. For example, one day you may be the listener, and one day you may be listened to. Within a social relationship, there is little emphasis on the evaluation of the interaction (although we sometimes reflect on what we have said or done). In the following example, notice the casual friend-like tone of the nurse:

Patient: "Oh, I just hate to be alone. It's getting me down, and sometimes it hurts so much."

Nurse: "I know how you feel. I don't like being alone either. Getting on Facebook might help you, it does me."(In this response, the nurse is minimizing the patient's feelings and giving advice prematurely.)

Therapeutic Relationships

In a therapeutic relationship, the nurse uses communication skills, understanding of human behaviors, and personal strengths to enhance the patient's growth. Patients more easily engage in the relationship when the clinician addresses their concerns, respects patients as partners in decision making, and uses straightforward language. The focus of the relationship is on the patient's ideas, experiences, and feelings. The nurse and the patient identify areas that need exploration and periodically evaluate the degree of the patient's progress.

Although the nurse may assume a variety of roles (e.g., teacher, counselor, socializing agent, liaison), the relationship is consistently focused on the patient's problem and needs. The nurse's needs are met outside the relationship.

Nursing students have the opportunity to develop therapeutic nurse-patient relationships with the support of both clinical faculty and nursing staff. This clinical supervision is a mentoring relationship characterized by feedback and evaluation. Typically, students experience a gradual increase in autonomy and responsibility.

Like staff nurses, nursing students may struggle with the boundaries between social and therapeutic relationships, because there is a fine line between the two. In fact, students often feel more comfortable being a friend because it is a more familiar role, especially with patients close to their own age. When this occurs, students need to make it clear (to themselves and the patient) that the relationship is a therapeutic one.

A therapeutic relationship does *not* mean that the nurse is not friendly. Talking about everyday topics (e.g., television, weather, and children's pictures) is not forbidden. In fact, a small amount of self-disclosure on the nurse's part may strengthen the therapeutic relationship. For example, your patient is your age and asks you about nursing school. Briefly sharing your views on nursing school will increase the trust in the relationship. Can you imagine saying, "We won't be talking about me"? On the other hand, multiple questions about such topics as your dating life should result in redirection and clarification of roles.

In a therapeutic relationship, the patient's problems and concerns are explored. Consider the response of the nurse in this situation compared with the previous example of the nurse suggesting Facebook as a response to loneliness:

Patient: "Oh, I just hate to be alone. It's getting me down, and sometimes it hurts so much."

Nurse: "Loneliness can be painful. What is going on now that you are feeling so alone?"

Relationship Boundaries and Roles

Professional boundaries exist to protect patients. Boundaries are the expected and accepted social, physical, and psychological boundaries that separate nurses from patients. This separation is essential considering the power differential between the nurse and the patient. This differential also exists between the nursing student and patient, even if you do not feel powerful. You have read the patient's chart, you are there to help, you will soon be a registered nurse, and you are not a patient. These qualities put nursing students in a position of some authority, particularly from the patient's perspective.

Blurring of Boundaries

Boundaries are always at risk for becoming blurred. Two common circumstances in which boundaries are blurred are (1) when the relationship slips into a social context and (2) when the nurse's needs (for attention, affection, and emotional support) are met at the expense of the patient's needs.

Boundaries are necessary to protect the patient. The most extreme boundary violations are sexual. This type of violation results in high levels of malpractice actions and the loss of professional licensure on the part of the nurse. Other boundary issues are not as obvious.

Blurring of Roles

Blurring of roles in the nurse–patient relationship is often a result of unrecognized transference or countertransference. Transference occurs when the patient unconsciously transfers feelings and behaviors related to a significant other in the patient's past onto the nurse. The patient may even say, "You remind me of my [mother, sister, father, brother, etc.]." Transference seems to be intensified in relationships in which one person is in authority. This may occur because parental figures were the original figures of authority. Nurses, physicians, and social workers all are potential objects of transference.

If a patient is motivated to work with you, completes assignments between sessions, and shares feelings openly, it is likely the patient is experiencing positive transference. Positive transference does not need to be addressed with the patient. However, the nurse may need to explore negative transference that threatens the nurse–patient relationship. Common forms of transference include the desire for affection or respect and the gratification of dependency needs. Other transferential feelings are hostility, jealousy, competitiveness, and love.

Countertransference is transference in reverse. It occurs when the nurse unconsciously displaces feelings related to significant figures in the nurse's past onto the patient. Commonly, the intense emotions of transference on the part of the patient bring out countertransference in the nurse. For example, you remind your patient of his much-loved older sister and he works very hard to please you. In response to this idealization and caring, you experience feelings of tenderness toward the patient and spend extra time with him each day.

Countertransference often results in overinvolvement and impairs the therapeutic relationship. Patients are experienced not as individuals but rather as extensions of ourselves, such as in the following example:

Patient: "Well I decided not to go to that dumb group. 'Hi, I'm so-and-so, and I'm an alcoholic.' Who cares?"(The patient sits slumped in a chair chewing gum, and nonchalantly looking around.)

Nurse (in an impassioned tone): "You seem to always sabotage your chances at getting better. You need AA to get in control of your life. Last week you were going to go, and now you've disappointed everyone."

In this case, the patient reminds the nurse of her mother, who was an alcoholic. The nurse sorts her feelings out and realizes the feelings of disappointment and failure belonged with her mother and not the patient. She starts out the next session with the following approach:

Nurse: "Look, I was thinking about yesterday, and I realize the decision to go to AA or find other help is solely up to you. Let's talk about what happened to change your mind about going to the meeting."

If the nurse feels a strongly positive or a strongly negative reaction to a patient, the feeling most often signals countertransference. One common sign is overidentification with the patient. In this situation, the nurse may have difficulty recognizing or objectively seeing patient problems that are similar to the nurse's own. For example, a nurse who is struggling with a depressed family member may feel disinterested, cold, or disgusted toward a depressed patient. Other indicators of countertransference are when the nurse gets involved in power struggles, competition, or arguments with the patient. Identifying and working through transference and countertransference issues are crucial in accomplishing professional growth and in helping the patient meet personal goals.

When Values and Beliefs Do Not Match

It is important for nurses to understand that our values and beliefs are not right for everyone. It is helpful to realize that our values and beliefs (1) reflect our own culture or subculture, (2) are derived from a range of choices, and (3) are those we have *chosen* for ourselves from a variety of influences and role models. Our values guide us in making decisions and taking actions that we hope will make our lives meaningful, rewarding, and fulfilled.

Working with others whose values and beliefs are different can be a challenge. Topics that cause controversy in society in general—including religion, politic ideology, gender roles, abortion, war, drugs, alcohol, and sex—also can cause conflict between nurses and patients. What happens when the nurse's values and beliefs are different from those of a patient? Consider the following examples of possible conflicts:

- The patient is planning to have an abortion, which is in opposition to the nurse's belief that life begins at conception.

- The nurse values cleanliness, whereas the patient believes that showering more than once a week wastes water and harms the environment.
- The nurse believes in feminism and values women's rights. She resents her female patient who wears a hijab (head covering) for religious reasons.

Self-awareness requires that we understand what we value and those beliefs that guide our behavior. Being self-aware helps us to accept the uniqueness and differences of others.

THE NURSE–PATIENT RELATIONSHIP ACCORDING TO PEPLAU

Hildegard Peplau introduced the concept of the nurse–patient relationship in 1952 in her groundbreaking book *Interpersonal Relations in Nursing*. This model of the nurse–patient relationship is well accepted as an important tool for all nursing practice. A professional nurse–patient relationship consists of a nurse who has skills and expertise and a patient who wants to alleviate suffering, find solutions to problems, explore different avenues to increased quality of life, or find an advocate.

Peplau (1999) described the nurse–patient relationship as evolving through three distinct interlocking and overlapping phases. An additional preorientation phase, during which the nurse prepares for the orientation phase, is also included:

1. Preorientation phase
2. Orientation phase
3. Working phase
4. Termination phase

Most likely, you will not have time to experience all the phases of the nurse–patient relationship in your often brief psychiatric–mental health nursing rotation. However, it is important to be aware of these phases to recognize, practice, and use them later.

Preorientation Phase

The preorientation phase begins with preparing for your assignment. The patient chart is a rich source of information including mental and physical evaluation, progress notes, and patient orders. You will probably be required to research your patient's condition, learn about prescribed medications, and understand laboratory results. Staff may be available to share more anecdotal information or provide tips on how to best interact with your patient.

Another task before meeting the patient is recognizing your own thoughts and feelings. Nursing students usually have many concerns and experience anxiety, especially on their first clinical day. These universal concerns include being afraid of those with psychiatric problems, of saying the wrong thing, and of not knowing what to do in response to certain patient behaviors. Table 2.1 identifies patient behaviors and gives examples of possible reactions and suggested responses.

Experienced faculty and staff monitor the unit atmosphere and have a sense for behaviors that indicate escalating tension. They are trained in crisis interventions, and formal security is often available on-site to give the staff support. Your instructor will set the ground rules for safety during the first clinical day. These rules may include not going into a patient's room alone, staying where others are around in an open area, and reporting signs and symptoms of escalating anxiety.

Orientation Phase

The orientation phase is the first time the nurse and the patient meet and is the phase in which the nurse conducts the initial interview. During the orientation phase, the patient may begin to express thoughts and feelings, identify problems, and discuss realistic goals. Specific tasks of the orientation phase follow.

Introductions

The first task of the orientation phase is introductions. The patient needs to know about the nurse (who the nurse is and the nurse's background) and the purpose of the meetings. For example, a student might supply the following information:

Student: "Hello, Ms. Chang, I am Bob Jacobs, I'm a registered nursing student from Fairlawn University. I am in my psychiatric rotation and will be coming here for the next six Thursdays. I would like to spend time with you until you are discharged. I'm here as a support person for you as you work on your treatment goals."

Table 2.1 **Patient Behaviors, Possible Reactions, and Useful Responses**

Possible Reactions	Useful Responses
If the patient threatens suicide	
The nurse may feel overwhelmed or responsible for "talking the patient out of it." The nurse may pick up some of the patient's feelings of hopelessness.	The nurse assesses whether the patient has a plan and the lethality of the plan. The nurse tells the patient that this is serious, that the nurse does not want harm to come to the patient, and that this information needs to be shared with other staff: "This is very serious, Mr. Lamb. I don't want any harm to come to you. I'll have to share this with the other staff." The nurse can then discuss with the patient the feelings and circumstances that led up to this decision.
If the patient asks the nurse to keep a secret	
The nurse may feel conflict because the nurse wants the patient to feel safe and accepted.	The nurse *cannot* make this promise. The information may be important to the health or safety of the patient or others: "I cannot make that promise. It might be important for me to share it with other staff." The patient then decides whether to share the information.
If the patient asks the nurse personal questions	
The nurse may think that it is rude not to answer. The nurse may feel put on the spot and want to leave the situation. Asking personal questions keeps the focus off the patient.	The nurse may or may not answer the patient's query. If the nurse chooses to answer a simple question, he or she answers in a word or two, then refocuses on the patient: **Patient:** "Are you married?" **Nurse:** "Yes, I am. How about you? Do you have a spouse?" **Patient:** "Do you have any children?" **Nurse:** "No. Let's focus on what is going on with you. Tell me about yourself."

Table 2.1 **Patient Behaviors, Possible Reactions, and Useful Responses—cont'd**

Possible Reactions	Useful Responses
If the patient makes sexual advances	
The nurse feels uncomfortable but may feel conflicted about "rejecting" the patient or making him or her feel "unattractive" or "not good enough."	The nurse sets clear limits: "I'm not comfortable with [name the behavior]. This is a professional relationship. We will focus on your problems and concerns." Frequently stating the nurse's role can help maintain boundaries. The nurse might say: "If you can't stop this behavior, I'll have to leave. I'll be back at [time] to spend time with you then." Leaving gives the patient time to gain control. The nurse returns at the stated time.
If the patient cries	
The nurse may feel uncomfortable and experience increased anxiety or feel somehow responsible for making the person cry.	The nurse should stay with the patient and let him or her know that it is alright to cry. "You are still upset about your brother's death." "What are you thinking right now?" The nurse offers tissues.
If the patient does not want to talk	
A nurse who is new to this situation may feel rejected, incompetent, or disappointed in the clinical experience.	At first, the nurse might say: "It's alright. I would like to spend time with you. We don't have to talk." The nurse might spend short, frequent periods (e.g., 5 minutes) with the patient throughout the day: "Our 5 minutes is up. I'll be back at 10 a.m. and stay with you 5 more minutes." This gives the patient the opportunity to understand that the nurse means what he or she says and is back on time consistently. It also gives the patient time to feel less threatened.

Continued

Table 2.1 **Patient Behaviors, Possible Reactions, and Useful Responses—cont'd**

Possible Reactions	Useful Responses
If the patient gives the nurse a present	
The nurse may feel uncomfortable when offered a gift.	Organizations often have guidelines that should be explored. General advice: If the gift is expensive or money, the only response is to graciously refuse. If it is inexpensive and given at the end of the treatment, graciously accept. A gift given at the beginning of the relationship may interfere. In this case graciously refuse and explore the meaning behind the present: "Thank you, but it is my job to care for my patients."
If a patient interrupts a conversation with another patient	
The nurse may feel a conflict. The nurse does not want to appear rude. Sometimes the nurse tries to engage both patients in conversation.	By maintaining a focus on the original patient, the nurse demonstrates that the session is important: "I am with Mr. Rob for the next 20 minutes. At 10 a.m. we can talk."

Knowing what the patient would like to be called is also essential—names and titles are meaningful to most people. In the previous example, the student began by using a formal title of Ms. Chang. After checking the patient's identification band and reading it out loud, "Dorothy Chang," the student should ask, "What would you like to be called?"

Establishing Rapport

A major emphasis during the first few encounters with the patient is on providing an atmosphere in which trust and understanding, or rapport, can grow. As in any relationship, you can nurture rapport by demonstrating genuineness, empathy, and unconditional positive regard. Being consistent, offering assistance in problem solving, and providing support are also essential aspects of establishing and maintaining rapport.

Specifying a Contract. A contract emphasizes the patient's participation and responsibility because it shows that the nurse does something *with* the patient rather than *for* the patient. The contract, either stated or written, contains the place, time, date, and duration of the meetings. You should also discuss termination of the relationship.

Student: "Ms. Chang, we will meet at 10 a.m. each Thursday in the common area. We have 45 minutes to discuss the feelings that you have identified. We will also discuss your diagnosis and symptom management, and review your medications. Like I said earlier, we will be able to work together until you are discharged."

Explaining Confidentiality

The patient has a right to know (1) who else will be given the information shared with the nurse and (2) that the information may be shared with specific people such as a clinical supervisor, the physician, the staff, or other students in conference. The patient also needs to know that the information will not be shared with relatives, friends, or others outside the treatment team, except in extreme situations. Extreme situations include child or elder abuse and threats of self-harm or harm to others.

Working Phase

A strong working relationship allows the patient to safely experience increased levels of anxiety and recognize dysfunctional responses. New and more adaptive coping behaviors can be practiced within the context of the working phase. Specific tasks for the nurse in this phase include the following:

- Gathering additional assessment data
- Identifying problem-solving skills and self-esteem
- Providing education about the psychiatric disorder or condition
- Promoting symptom management
- Providing medication education
- Evaluating progress

During the working phase, the nurse and patient identify and explore areas that are causing problems in the patient's life. A major focus is on recognizing ineffective ways of coping and replacing them with healthier methods of coping. Sometimes the patient's coping methods were developed to survive in a chaotic and dysfunctional family environment. Although coping methods may have worked for the patient at an earlier age, they may now interfere with the patient's healthy functioning and interpersonal relationships.

Another important aspect of this working relationship is patient education. To facilitate this education you need to become familiar with biological factors (e.g., genetic, biochemical) and psychological factors (e.g., cognitive distortions, learned helplessness) that may be the basis of a patient's psychiatric disorders. Understanding psychotropic medications, laboratory work and results, and other treatments is also essential. This knowledge prepares you to help your patients to learn, which in turn prepares them to take the lead role in their own care.

Termination Phase

The termination phase is the final phase of the nurse–patient relationship. The nursing student discusses termination during the first interview and again during the working stage at appropriate times. Termination may occur when the patient is discharged or when the student's clinical rotation ends. The tasks of termination include the following:

- Summarizing the goals and objectives achieved in the relationship
- Discussing ways for the patient to incorporate into daily life any new coping strategies learned
- Exchanging memories, which can help validate the experience for both nurse and patient and facilitate closure of that relationship
- Identifying future goals and plans

If a patient has unresolved feelings of abandonment, loneliness, or rejection, these feelings may be reawakened during the termination process. This process can be an opportunity for the patient to express these feelings, perhaps for the first time. If a nurse has been working with a patient for a while, it is important for the nurse to recognize that separation may be difficult for the patient. A general question—such as "How do you feel about being discharged?"—may provide the opening necessary for the patient to describe feelings.

Part of the termination process is to discuss the patient's plans for the future. If the termination is the result of a discharge, part of these plans have usually been discussed by the psychiatrist or advanced practice nurse, including follow-up care and referrals. Registered nurses generally reinforce those plans and emphasize understanding of medications and recognizing when symptoms are getting out of control. Self-help groups can also be encouraged.

FACTORS THAT PROMOTE A PATIENT'S GROWTH

Personal characteristics of the nurse that promote change and growth in patients are: (1) genuineness, (2) empathy, and (3) positive regard. These are some of the intangibles that are at the heart of the art of nursing and patient-centered care.

Genuineness

Genuineness refers to the nurse's ability to be open, honest, and authentic in interactions with patients. Being genuine is a key ingredient in building trust. When a person is genuine, others get the sense that what is displayed on the outside of the person is congruent with who the person is on the inside. Nurses convey genuineness by listening to and communicating clearly with patients. Being genuine in a therapeutic relationship implies the ability to use therapeutic communication tools in an appropriately spontaneous manner rather than rigidly or in a parrot-like fashion.

Empathy

Empathy occurs when the helping person attempts to understand the world from the patient's perspective. This understanding is in contrast to sympathy, which involves feeling pity or sorrow for others. Although these are considered nurturing human traits, they may not be particularly useful in a therapeutic relationship.

The following examples clarify the distinction between empathy and sympathy. A friend tells you that her mother was just diagnosed with inoperable cancer. Your friend then begins to cry and pounds the table with her fist.

Sympathetic response: "I feel so bad for you *(tearing up)*. I know how close you are to your mom. She is such an amazing person. Oh, I am so sorry." (You hug your friend.)

Empathetic response: "This must be devastating for you *(silence)*. It must seem so unfair. What thoughts and feelings are you having?" (You stay with your friend and listen.)

Empathy is not a technique but rather an attitude that conveys respect, acceptance, and validation of the patient's strengths. Empathy may be one of the most important qualities that a psychiatric–mental health nurse can possess.

Positive Regard

Positive regard implies respect. It is the ability to view another person as being worthy of caring about and as someone who has strengths and achievement potential. Positive regard is usually communicated indirectly by attitudes and actions rather than directly by words.

Attitudes

One attitude that might convey positive regard, or respect, is a positive attitude about working with the patient. The nurse takes the patient and the relationship seriously. The experience is viewed not as "a job," or "part of a course," but as an opportunity to work with patients to help them develop personal resources and actualize more of their potential in living.

Actions

Some actions that manifest positive regard are attending, suspending value judgments, and helping patients develop their own resources.

Attending. Attending behavior is the foundation of a therapeutic relationship. To succeed, nurses must pay attention to their patients in culturally and individually appropriate ways. *Attending* is a special kind of listening that refers to an intensity of presence or being with the patient. At times, simply being with another person during a painful time can make a difference.

Suspending Value Judgments. As previously discussed, everyone has values and beliefs. Using our personal value system to judge patients' thoughts, feelings, or behaviors is not helpful or productive. For example, if a patient is taking drugs or is involved in risky sexual behavior, the nurse recognizes that these behaviors are unhealthy. However, labeling these activities as bad or good is not useful. Rather, the nurse should help the patient explore the thoughts and feelings that influence this behavior. Judgment on the part of the nurse will most likely interfere with further exploration.

The first steps in eliminating judgmental thinking and behaviors are to (1) recognize their presence, (2) identify how or where you learned these responses, and (3) construct alternative ways to view the patient's thinking and behavior. Denying judgmental thinking will only compound the problem.

Patient: "I guess you could consider me an addictive personality. I love to gamble when I have money and spend most of my time in the casino. It seems like I'm hooking up with a different woman every time I'm there, and it always ends in sex."

A judgmental response would be:

Nurse A: "So your compulsive gambling and promiscuous sexual behaviors really haven't brought you much happiness, have they? You're running away from your problems and could be financially ruined and end up with an STD."

A more helpful response would be:

Nurse B: "So your sexual and gambling activities are part of the picture also. How do these activities affect your life?"

In this example, Nurse B focuses on the patient's behaviors and how they affect his life. Nurse B does not introduce personal value statements or prejudices regarding the promiscuous behaviors, unlike Nurse A.

Helping Patients Develop Resources. It is important that patients remain as independent as possible to develop new resources for problem solving. The nurse does not do the work the patient should be doing unless it is absolutely necessary and then only as a step toward helping the patient act on his or her own. The following are examples of helping a patient to develop independence:

Patient: "This medication makes my mouth so dry. Could you get me something to drink?"

Nurse: "There is juice in the refrigerator. I'll wait here for you until you get back." *or* "I'll walk with you while you get some juice from the refrigerator."

Patient: "Could you ask the doctor to let me have a pass for the weekend?"

Nurse: "Your doctor will be on the unit this afternoon. I'll let her know that you want to speak with her."

Consistently encouraging patients to use their own resources helps minimize their feelings of helplessness and dependency. It also validates their ability to bring about change.

CHAPTER 3

Therapeutic Communication

Humans have an innate need to relate to others. Our advanced ability to communicate with others gives substance and meaning to our lives. All our actions, words, and facial expressions convey meaning to others. We cannot *not* communicate. Even silence can convey acceptance, anger, or thoughtfulness. Strong communication is the foundation for happy and productive relationships. On the other hand, ineffective communication within a relationship often results in stress and negative feelings.

In the provision of nursing care, communication takes on a new emphasis. Just as social relationships are different from therapeutic relationships, *basic communication* is different from patient-centered, goal-directed, and scientifically based *therapeutic communication.*

The ability to form patient-centered therapeutic relationships is fundamental to effective nursing care. *Patient-centered* refers to the patient as a full partner in care whose values, preferences, and needs are respected (Quality and Safety Education for Nurses, 2012). Therapeutic communication is crucial to the formation of patient-centered therapeutic relationships. Determining levels of pain in a postoperative patient; listening as parents express feelings of fear concerning their child's diagnosis; or understanding, without words, the needs of an intubated patient in the intensive care unit are essential skills in providing quality nursing care.

Ideally, therapeutic communication is a professional ability you learn and practice early in the nursing curriculum. In psychiatric–mental health nursing, communication skills take on a different and new emphasis. Psychiatric disorders cause physical symptoms (e.g., fatigue, loss of appetite, insomnia) and emotional symptoms (e.g., sadness, anger, hopelessness, euphoria) that affect a patient's ability to relate to others.

It is often during the psychiatric clinical rotation that students appreciate the usefulness of therapeutic communication. They begin to rely on techniques that may have once seemed artificial. For example, restating sounds so simplistic, the student may hesitate to use this technique:

Patient: "At the moment they told me my daughter would never be able to walk like her twin sister, I felt like I couldn't go on."

Student: *(restates the patient's words after a short silence)* "You felt like you couldn't go on."

The technique, and the empathy it conveys, is supportive in such a situation. Developing therapeutic communication skills takes time, and with continued practice, you will find your own style and rhythm. Eventually, these techniques will become a part of the way you instinctively communicate with others in the clinical setting.

Saying the Wrong Thing

Nursing students are often concerned that they may say the wrong thing, especially when learning to apply therapeutic techniques. Will you say the "wrong thing"? Yes, you probably will. That is how we all learn to find more useful and effective ways of helping individuals reach their goals.

Will saying the wrong thing be harmful to the patient? Consider that symptoms of psychiatric disorders—irritability, agitation, negativity, little communication, or being hypertalkative—often frustrate and alienate friends and family. It is likely that the interactions the patient had been having were not always pleasant. Patients tend to appreciate a well-meaning person who conveys genuine acceptance, respect, and concern for their situation. Even if you make mistakes in communication there is little chance that the comments will do actual harm.

VERBAL AND NONVERBAL COMMUNICATION

Verbal Communication

Verbal communication consists of all the words a person speaks. We live in a society of symbols, and our main social symbols are words. Words are the symbols for emotions and mental images. Talking is our link to one another and the primary instrument of instruction. Talking is a need, an art, and one of the most personal aspects of our private lives.

Nonverbal Communication

Have you heard, "It's not what you say but how you say it"? While this expression is not 100% true, it is the nonverbal behaviors that may be sending much of the real message through. The tone of voice, emphasis on certain words, and the manner in which a person paces speech are examples of nonverbal communication. Other common examples of nonverbal communication are physical appearance, body posture, eye contact, hand gestures, sighs, fidgeting, and yawning. Table 3.1 identifies examples of nonverbal behaviors.

Interaction of Verbal and Nonverbal Communication

Spoken words represent our public selves. They can be straightforward or used to distort, conceal, or disguise true feelings. Nonverbal behaviors include a wide range of human activities, from body movements to facial expressions to physical responses to messages received from others. How a person listens, uses silence, and uses the sense of touch may also convey important information about the private self that is not available from conversation alone.

Messages are not always simple. They can appear to be one thing when in fact they are another. Often, people have greater conscious awareness of their verbal messages than their nonverbal behaviors. The verbal message is sometimes referred to as the *content* of the message (what is said), and the nonverbal behavior is called the *process* of the message (nonverbal cues a person gives to substantiate or contradict the verbal message).

When the content is congruent with the process, the communication is more clearly understood and is considered healthy. For example, if a student says, "It's important that I get good grades in this class," that is *content*. If the student has bought the books, takes thorough notes, and has a study buddy, that is *process*. In this case the content

Table 3.1 **Nonverbal Behaviors**

Behavior	Nonverbal Cues	Example
Body behaviors	Posture, body movements, gestures, gait	The patient is slumped in a chair, puts her face in her hands, and occasionally taps her right foot.
Facial expressions	Frowns, smiles, grimaces, raised eyebrows, pursed lips, licking of lips, tongue movements	The patient grimaces when speaking to the nurse; when alone, he smiles and giggles to himself.
Eye expression and gaze behavior	Lowering brows, intimidating gaze	The patient's eyes harden with suspicion.
Voice-related behaviors	Tone, pitch, level, intensity, inflection, stuttering, pauses, silences, fluency	The patient talks in a loud sing-song voice.
Observable autonomic physiological responses	Increase in respirations, diaphoresis, pupil dilation, blushing, paleness	When the patient mentions discharge, she becomes pale, her respirations increase, and her face becomes diaphoretic.
Personal appearance	Grooming, dress, hygiene	The patient is dressed in a wrinkled shirt, his pants are stained, his socks are dirty, and he is unshaven.
Physical characteristics	Height, weight, physique, complexion	The patient is overweight and his posture is poor.

and process are congruent and straightforward, and there is a healthy message. If, however, the verbal message is not reinforced or is in fact contradicted by the nonverbal behavior, the message is confusing. If a student says, "It's important that I get good grades in this class" and does not have the books, skips classes, and does not study, the content and process do not match. The student's verbal and nonverbal behaviors are incongruent.

COMMUNICATION SKILLS FOR NURSES

Therapeutic Communication Techniques

Once you have established a therapeutic relationship, you and your patient can identify specific needs and problems. You can then begin to work with the patient on increasing problem-solving skills, learning new coping behaviors, and experiencing more appropriate and satisfying ways of relating to others. Strong communication skills will facilitate your work. These skills are called *therapeutic communication techniques* and include words and actions that help to achieve health-related goals. Some useful techniques for nurses when communicating with their patients are (1) silence, (2) active listening, (3) clarifying techniques, and (4) questions.

Using Silence

Students and practicing nurses alike may find that when the flow of words stops, they become uncomfortable. They may rush to fill the void with questions or idle conversation. These responses may cut off important thoughts and feelings the patient might be taking time to think about before speaking.

Although there is no specific rule concerning how much silence is too much, silence is worthwhile only as long as it is serving some function and not frightening the patient. Knowing when to speak largely depends on the nurse's perception about what is being conveyed through the silence. Icy silence may be an expression of anger and hostility.

Silence may provide meaningful moments of reflection for both participants. It provides an opportunity to contemplate thoughtfully what has been said and felt, weigh alternatives, formulate new ideas, and gain a new perspective. If the nurse waits to speak and allows the patient to break the silence, the patient may share thoughts and feelings that would otherwise have been withheld.

Some psychiatric disorders, such as major depression and schizophrenia, and medications may cause a slowing of thought processes. Patience and gentle prompting can help patients gather their thoughts. For example, "You were saying that you are worried about the side effects of the new antidepressant."

Active Listening

People want more than just a physical presence in human communication. In active listening, nurses fully concentrate, understand, respond, and remember what the patient is saying verbally and nonverbally. By giving the patient undivided attention, the nurse communicates that the patient is not alone. This kind of intervention enhances self-esteem and encourages the patient to direct energy toward finding ways to deal with problems. Serving as a sounding board, the nurse listens as the patient tests thoughts by voicing them aloud.

Clarifying Techniques

Understanding depends on clear communication, which is aided by verifying the nurse's interpretation of the patient's messages. The nurse can request feedback on the accuracy of the message received from verbal and nonverbal cues.

Paraphrasing. Paraphrasing occurs when you restate the basic content of a patient's message in different, usually fewer, words. Using simple, precise, and culturally relevant terms, the nurse may confirm an interpretation of the patient's message. Phrases such as "I'm not sure I understand" or "You seem to be saying…" help the nurse to interpret the message in what may be a bewildering mass of details. It also helps the patient to feel heard and may provide greater focus. The patient may confirm or deny the perceptions nonverbally by nodding or looking bewildered, or by direct responses: "Yes, that is what I was trying to say" or "No, I meant…"

Restating. Restating is an active listening strategy that helps the nurse to understand what the patient is saying. It also lets the patient know he or she is being heard. Restating differs from paraphrasing in that it involves repeating the same key words the patient has just spoken. If a patient remarks, "My life is empty… it has no meaning," additional information may be gained by restating, "Your life has no meaning?"

Although this is a valuable technique, it should be used sparingly. Patients may interpret frequent and indiscriminate use of restating as inattention or disinterest. Overuse makes restating sound mechanical. To avoid overuse of restating, the nurse can combine restatements with direct questions that encourage descriptions: "What sort of goals do you have for your evening?" "How is your family responding to your illness?"

Reflecting. Reflection assists patients to understand their own thoughts and feelings better. Reflecting may take the form of a question or a simple statement that conveys the nurse's observations of the patient. The nurse might briefly describe his or her interpretation of the patient's verbal and nonverbal behavior. For example, to reflect a patient's feelings about his or her life, a good beginning might be, "You sound as if you have had many disappointments."

When you reflect, you make the patient aware of inner feelings and encourage the patient to own them. For example, you may say to a patient, "You look sad." Perceiving your concern may allow the patient to spontaneously share feelings. The use of a question in response to the patient's question is another reflective technique (Arnold & Boggs, 2016). For example:

Patient: "Nurse, do you think I really need to be hospitalized?"

Nurse: "What do you think, Kelly?"

Patient: "I don't know. That's why I'm asking you."

Nurse: "I'll be willing to share my impression with you. However, you've probably thought about hospitalization and have some feelings about it. I wonder what they are."

Exploring. A technique that enables the nurse to examine important ideas, experiences, or relationships more fully is exploring. For example, if a patient tells you he does not get along well with his wife, you will want to further explore this area. Possible openers include the following:

"*Tell me more* about your relationship with your wife."

"*Give me an example* of how you and your wife don't get along."

Table 3.2 lists more examples of therapeutic communication techniques.

Questions

Open-Ended Questions. Open-ended questions encourage patients to share information about experiences, perceptions, or responses to a situation. The following are examples:

- "What are some of the stresses you are under right now?"

Text continued on p. 46

Table 3.2 **Therapeutic Communication Techniques**

Therapeutic Technique	Description	Example
Silence	Gives the person time to collect thoughts or think through a point.	Encouraging a person to talk by waiting for the answers
Accepting	Indicates that the person has been understood. An accepting statement does not necessarily indicate agreement but is nonjudgmental.	"Yes." "Uh-huh." "I follow what you say."
Giving recognition	Indicates awareness of change and personal efforts. Does not imply good or bad, right or wrong.	"Good morning, Mr. James." "I see you've eaten your whole lunch."
Offering self	Offers presence, interest, and a desire to understand. Is not offered to get the person to talk or behave in a specific way.	"I would like to spend time with you." "I'll stay here and sit with you awhile."
Offering general leads	Allows the other person to take direction in the discussion. Indicates that the nurse is interested in what comes next.	"Go on." "And then?" "Tell me about it."
Giving broad openings	Clarifies that the lead is to be taken by the patient. However, the nurse discourages pleasantries and small talk.	"Where would you like to begin?" "What are you thinking about?"
Placing the events in time or sequence	Puts events and actions in better perspective. Notes cause-and-effect relationships and identifies patterns of interpersonal difficulties.	"What happened before?" "When did this happen?"

Making observations	Calls attention to the person's behavior (e.g., trembling, nail biting, restless mannerisms). Encourages patient to notice the behavior and describe thoughts and feelings for mutual understanding.	"You appear tense." "I notice you're biting your lips." "You appear nervous whenever John enters the room."
Encouraging description of perception	Increases the nurse's understanding of the patient's perceptions. Talking about feelings and difficulties can lessen the need to act them out inappropriately.	"What do these voices seem to be saying?" "What is happening now?" "Tell me when you feel anxious."
Encouraging comparison	Brings out recurring themes in experiences or interpersonal relationships. Helps the person clarify similarities and differences.	"Has this ever happened before?" "Is this how you felt…?" "Was it something like…?"
Restating	Repeats the main idea expressed. Gives the patient an idea of what has been communicated. If the message has been misunderstood, the patient can clarify it.	**Patient:** "I can't sleep. I stay awake all night." **Nurse:** "You stay awake all night?"
Reflecting	Directs questions, feelings, and ideas back to the patient. Encourages the patient to accept his or her own ideas and feelings. Acknowledges the patient's right to have opinions and make decisions and encourages the patient to think of himself or herself as a capable person.	**Patient:** "What should I do about my husband's affair?" **Nurse:** "What do you think you should do?" *or* **Patient:** "My brother spends all of my money and then has the nerve to ask for more." **Nurse:** "You feel angry when this happens?"

Continued

Table 3.2 **Therapeutic Communication Techniques—cont'd**

Therapeutic Technique	Description	Example
Focusing	Concentrates attention on a single point. It is especially useful when the patient jumps from topic to topic. If a person is experiencing a severe or panic level of anxiety, the nurse should not persist until the anxiety lessens.	"This point you are making about leaving school seems worth looking at more closely." "You've mentioned many things. Let's go back to your thinking of 'ending it all.'"
Exploring	Examines certain ideas, experiences, or relationships more fully. If the patient chooses not to elaborate by answering "no," the nurse does not probe or pry. In such a case, the nurse respects the patient's wishes.	"Tell me more about that." "Would you describe it more fully?" "Could you talk about how it was that you learned your mom was dying of cancer?"
Giving information	Makes facts the person needs available. Supplies knowledge from which decisions can be made or conclusions drawn. Providing teaching.	"My purpose for being here is…" "This medication is for…" "The test will determine…"
Seeking clarification	Helps patients clarify their own thoughts and maximize mutual understanding between nurse and patient.	"I am not sure I follow you." "Give an example of a time you thought everyone hated you."
Presenting reality	Indicates what is real. The nurse does not argue or try to convince the patient, just describes personal perceptions or facts in the situation.	"That was Dr. Todd, not a man from the Mafia." "That was the sound of a car backfiring." "Your mother is not here; I am a nurse."

Voicing doubt	Expressing uncertainty regarding the reality of the patient's perceptions or conclusions, especially in hallucinations and delusions.	"Isn't that unusual?" "Really?" "That's hard to believe."
Verbalizing the implied	Puts into concrete terms what the patient implies, making the patient's communication more explicit.	**Patient:** "I can't talk to you or anyone else. It's a waste of time." **Nurse:** "Do you feel that no one understands?"
Summarizing	Brings together important points of discussion to enhance understanding.	"Have I got this straight?" "You said that…" "During the past hour, you and I have discussed…"
Translating words into feelings	Responds to the feeling expressed, not just the content.	**Patient:** "I am dead inside." **Nurse:** "Are you saying that you feel lifeless? That life seems meaningless?"
Formulating of a plan of action	Allows the patient to identify alternative actions for interpersonal situations the patient finds disturbing (e.g., when anger or anxiety is provoked).	"What could you do to let anger out harmlessly?" "What are some other ways you can approach your boss?"

Adapted from Hays JS, Larson K. *Interacting with patients.* New York, NY: Macmillan, 1963.

- "How would you describe your relationship with your wife?"

Because open-ended questions are not intrusive and do not put the patient on the defensive, they help the clinician elicit information. This technique is especially useful in the beginning of an interview or when a patient is guarded or resistant to answering questions. Open-ended questions are particularly useful when establishing rapport with a person.

Closed-Ended Questions. Nurses are usually urged to ask open-ended questions to elicit more than a "yes" or "no" response. However, closed-ended questions, when used sparingly, can give you specific and needed information. Closed-ended questions are most useful during an initial assessment or intake interview or to assess the patient's status, "Are the medications helping you?" "Are you hearing voices now?" "Did you seek therapy after your first suicide attempt?"

Nontherapeutic Communication Techniques

People often use "nontherapeutic" or ineffective communication. However, for nurses, using nontherapeutic communication can be particularly problematic because it impairs nurse–patient interaction. Table 3.3 describes nontherapeutic communication techniques and suggests more helpful responses.

Excessive Questioning

Excessive questioning—asking multiple questions (particularly closed-ended) consecutively or rapidly—casts the nurse in the role of interrogator who demands information without respect for the patient's willingness or readiness to respond. This approach conveys a lack of respect for and sensitivity to the patient's needs. Excessive questioning controls the range and nature of the responses, can easily result in a therapeutic stall, or may completely shut down an interview. It is a controlling tactic and may reflect the interviewer's lack of security in letting the patient tell his or her own story. It is better to ask more open-ended questions and follow the patient's lead. For example:

Excessive questioning: "Why did you leave your wife? Did you feel angry with her? What did she do to you? Are you going back to her?"

Table 3.3 **Nontherapeutic Communication Techniques**

Nontherapeutic Technique	Description	Example	More Helpful Response
Giving premature advice	Assumes the nurse knows best and the patient cannot think independently. Inhibits problem solving and fosters dependency.	"Get out of this situation immediately."	Encouraging problem solving: "What were some of the actions you thought you might take?" "What are some of the ways you have thought of to meet your goals?"
Minimizing feelings	The nurse seems unable to understand or empathize with the patient. Feelings or experiences are belittled, which can cause the patient to feel small or insignificant.	"Everyone gets down in the dumps." "Things get worse before they get better."	Empathizing and exploring: "You must be feeling very upset. Are you thinking of hurting yourself?"
Falsely reassuring	Attempting to provide comfort not based on fact or reality. Causes a person to feel unheard. May cause the patient to stop sharing feelings.	"I wouldn't worry about that." "Everything will be all right."	Clarifying the patient's message: "What specifically are you worried about?" "What are you concerned might happen?"
Making value judgments	Can make the patient feel guilty, angry, misunderstood, not supported, or anxious to leave.	"You smoke and your wife has lung cancer?"	Making observations: "I notice you are still smoking."
Asking "why" questions	Critically demands an explanation; often makes the patient feel defensive.	"Why did you stop taking your medication?"	Giving a broad opening: "Tell me some of the reasons that led up to quitting your medications."

Continued

Table 3.3 **Nontherapeutic Communication Techniques—cont'd**

Nontherapeutic Technique	Description	Example	More Helpful Response
Asking excessive questions	Results in the patient not knowing which question to answer and possibly being confused about what is being asked.	"How's your appetite? Are you losing weight? Are you eating enough?"	Clarifying: "Tell me about your eating habits since you've been depressed."
Giving approval, agreeing	Implies the patient is doing the *right* thing—and that not doing it is wrong. May lead the patient to focus on pleasing the nurse or clinician.	"I'm proud of you for applying for that job." "I agree with your decision."	Making observations: "I noticed that you applied for that job." Asking open-ended questions: "What led to that decision?"
Disapproving, disagreeing	Can make a person defensive.	"You really should have shown up for the medication group." "I disagree with that decision."	Exploring: "How did you decide not to come to your medication group?" "How did you arrive at that conclusion?"
Changing the subject	Invalidates the patient's feelings and needs. Leaves the patient feeling isolated and increases feelings of hopelessness.	**Patient:** "I'd like to die." **Nurse:** "Did you go to Alcoholics Anonymous like we discussed?"	Validating and exploring: "This sounds serious. Have you thought of harming yourself?"

Adapted from Hays JS, Larson K. *Interacting with patients.* New York, NY: Macmillan, 1963. Copyright © 1963 by Macmillan Publishing Company.

More therapeutic approach: "Tell me about the situation between you and your wife."

Giving Approval or Disapproval

We often give our friends and family approval when they do something well, but giving praise and approval becomes much more complex in a nurse–patient relationship. Saying, "That is an amazing mask you made in art therapy" is supportive and may, in fact, promote a dialogue about the emotional meaning of the mask. Contrast that comment with, "It makes me happy to see you sitting with Chelsea at lunch." When the patient is doing a behavior to please another person, it is not coming from the individual's own conviction. Thus the new response really is not a change in behavior as much as an act to win approval and acceptance from another.

Disapproval is the opposite side of the same coin. "I was disappointed that you showed up late for group therapy" or "You should quit smoking" are counterproductive for any therapeutic relationship. Statements such as these will cause negative feelings such as shame or resentment and undermine the patient's recovery process.

Giving Advice

We ask for and give advice all the time. In a way, nurses give advice when they teach (e.g., "You should take your medication with food."). The nontherapeutic form is when the advice becomes more personal in nature. "If I were you I would leave your husband" or even "You should find a new job" interferes with the patient's ability to make personal decisions. When a nurse offers the patient solutions, the patient eventually begins to think the nurse does not view him or her as capable of making effective decisions.

Asking "Why" Questions

"Why" demands an explanation and implies wrong-doing. Think of the last time someone asked you why: "Why didn't you go to the funeral?" or "Why did you pick *that* outfit?" Such questions imply criticism. We may ask our friends or family these questions, and in the context of a solid relationship, the *why* may be understood more as "What happened?" With people we do not know—especially those who may be anxious or overwhelmed—a *why* question from a person in authority (e.g., nurse, physician, or teacher) can be experienced as intrusive and judgmental, which serves only to make the person defensive.

THE COUNSELING SESSION

Ideally, the patient decides and leads the content and direction of the counseling session. The nurse uses communication skills and active listening to better understand the patient's situation.

Setting

Effective communication can take place almost anywhere. However, the quality of the interaction—whether in a clinic, a clinical unit, an office, or the patient's home—depends on the degree to which the nurse and patient feel safe. Establishing a setting that enhances feelings of security is important to the therapeutic relationship. A healthcare setting, a conference room, or a quiet part of the unit that has relative privacy but is within view of others is ideal, but when the communication takes place in the patient's home, it offers the nurse a valuable opportunity to assess the patient in the context of everyday life.

Seating

In all settings, arrange chairs so that conversation can take place in normal tones of voice and so that eye contact can be comfortably maintained or avoided. A nonthreatening physical environment for both nurse and patient would involve the following:

- Being the same height by both sitting or both standing.
- Avoiding a face-to-face arrangement when possible; a 90- to 120-degree angle or side-by-side position may be less intense, and the patient and nurse can look away from each other without discomfort.
- Providing safety and psychological comfort in terms of exiting the room. The patient should not be between the nurse and the door, nor should the nurse be positioned in such a way that the patient feels trapped in the room.
- Not having a desk barrier between the nurse and the patient.

Walking while talking may be an alternative to sitting. Some psychiatric disorders cause hyperactivity and agitation, making sitting extremely uncomfortable. Furthermore, activity reduces depressive symptoms and is healthier for both the patient and the nurse.

Introductions

Initially, the student tells the patient who he or she is, what the purpose of the meeting is, and how long and at what time they will be meeting with the patient. The issue of confidentiality should be addressed during the initial interview. The patient needs to know that whatever is discussed will stay confidential unless permission is given for it to be disclosed.

Ask the patient how he or she would like to be addressed. This question conveys respect and gives the patient direct control over an important ego issue. Some patients like to be called by their last name, whereas others prefer being on a first-name basis with the nurse.

Initiating the Session

After the introductions, you can encourage the patient to set the direction by using one of a number of open-ended questions or statements:

- "What are some of the stresses you have been coping with recently?"
- "Tell me a little about what has been happening in the past couple of weeks."
- "Perhaps you can begin by letting me know what some of your concerns have been recently."

You can facilitate communication by appropriately offering leads (e.g., "Go on"), making statements of acceptance (e.g., "Uh-huh"), or otherwise conveying interest.

Attending Behaviors

Engaging in attending behaviors and actively listening are two key principles of counseling on which almost everyone can agree. Positive attending behaviors serve to open up communication and encourage free expression, whereas negative attending behaviors are more likely to inhibit expression. All behaviors must be evaluated in terms of cultural patterns and past experiences of both the interviewer and the interviewee.

Eye Contact

Cultural and individual variations influence a patient's comfort with eye contact. For some patients and interviewers, sustained eye contact is normal and comfortable. For others, it may be more comfortable and natural to make brief eye contact but look away or down much of the time. A general rule of communication and eye contact is that it is appropriate for nurses to maintain more eye contact when the patient speaks and less constant eye contact when the nurse speaks.

Body Language

Facial expressions; eye contact or lack thereof; and the way a person holds the head, legs, and shoulders convey a multitude of messages. A person who slumps in a chair, rolls the eyes, and sits with arms crossed in front of the chest is generally perceived as resistant and unreceptive. On the other hand, a person who leans in slightly toward the speaker, maintains a relaxed and attentive posture, makes appropriate eye contact, and uses calm hand gestures will be perceived as open to and respectful of the communication.

The use of personal space is a significant variable when communicating with another person. Generally speaking, distance is based on the following in the United States:

- **Intimate distance** (0–18 inches) is reserved for those we trust most and with whom we feel most safe.
- **Personal distance** (18–40 inches) is for personal communications such as those with friends or colleagues.
- **Social distance** (4–12 feet) applies to strangers or acquaintances, often in public places or formal social gatherings.
- **Public distance** (12 feet or more) relates to public space (e.g., public speaking).

It is important to note that in individuals with some psychiatric conditions space should be altered. For example, if a person with schizophrenia is experiencing paranoia, personal and social distance should be increased. Likewise, during an episode of mania and agitation, space should also be increased.

Vocal Quality

Vocal quality, or paralinguistics, encompasses voice loudness, pitch, rate, and fluency. Speaking in soft and gentle tones is likely to encourage a person to share thoughts and feelings. Speaking in a rapid, high-pitched tone may convey anxiety and create it in the patient. Consider, for example, how drastically tonal quality and inflection can affect communication in a simple sentence like "I will see you tonight."

1. "*I* will see you tonight." (I will be the one who sees you tonight.)
2. "I *will* see you tonight." (No matter what happens, or whether you like it or not, I will see you tonight.)
3. "I will see *you* tonight." (Even though others are present, it is you I want to see.)
4. "I will see you *tonight*." (It is definite, tonight is the night we will meet.)

Clinical Debriefing

An increasingly popular method of providing clinical supervision is through debriefing. According to the National League for Nursing (2015), debriefing is such an excellent learning method that it should be incorporated into all clinical experiences. Debriefing refers to a critical conversation and reflection regarding an experience that results in growth and learning. Debriefing supports essential learning along a continuum of "knowing what" to "knowing how" and "knowing why."

Process Recordings

A good way to increase communication and interviewing skills is to review your clinical interactions exactly as they occur. Process recordings are written records of a segment of the nurse–patient session that reflect as closely as possible the verbal and nonverbal behaviors of both patient and nurse. Process recordings have some disadvantages because they rely on memory and are subject to distortions. However, you may find them to be useful in identifying communication patterns.

Communication Skills Evaluation

After you have had some introductory clinical experience, you may find the facilitative skills checklist in Table 3.4 is useful for evaluating your progress in developing interviewing skills. Note that some of the items might not be relevant for some of your patients (e.g., numbers 11–13 may not be possible when a patient is experiencing psychosis [disordered thought, delusions, and/or hallucinations]). Self-evaluation of clinical skills is a way to focus on therapeutic improvement. Role-playing can help prepare you for clinical experience and practice effective and professional communication skills.

Table 3.4 **Communication Self-Assessment Checklist**

Instructions: Periodically during your clinical experience, use this checklist to identify areas needed for growth and progress made. Think of your clinical patient experiences. Indicate the extent of your agreement with each of the following statements by marking the scale:

SA = strongly agree, A = agree, NS = not sure, D = disagree, SD = strongly disagree

1. I maintain appropriate eye contact.	SA	A	NS	D	SD
2. Most of my verbal comments follow the lead of the other person.	SA	A	NS	D	SD
3. I encourage others to talk about feelings.	SA	A	NS	D	SD
4. I ask open-ended questions.	SA	A	NS	D	SD
5. I restate and clarify the person's ideas.	SA	A	NS	D	SD
6. I paraphrase the person's nonverbal behaviors.	SA	A	NS	D	SD
7. I summarize in a few words the basic ideas of a long statement made by the person.	SA	A	NS	D	SD
8. I make statements that reflect the person's feelings.	SA	A	NS	D	SD
9. I share my feelings relevant to the discussion when appropriate to do so.	SA	A	NS	D	SD
10. I give feedback.	SA	A	NS	D	SD
11. At least 75% or more of my responses help enhance and facilitate communication.	SA	A	NS	D	SD
12. I assist the person in listing some available alternatives.	SA	A	NS	D	SD
13. I assist the person in identifying some specific and observable goals.	SA	A	NS	D	SD
14. I assist the person in specifying at least one next step that might be taken toward the goal.	SA	A	NS	D	SD

Myrick D, Erney T. *Caring and sharing.* Educational Media Corporation, 1984.

CHAPTER 4

Neurodevelopmental Disorders

During any given year 13% to 20% of children and adolescents living in the United States experience a mental disorder (Centers for Disease Control [CDC] and Prevention, 2013). If left untreated, all areas of the child's or adolescent's life can be tragically impeded, leaving young people socially isolated, stigmatized, and unable to live up to their potential and/or contribute to society. Problems first evidenced in infants, children, and adolescents often continue into adulthood.

Although many of the same techniques for working with adults apply to children and adolescents, there are some unique differences. Before turning attention to psychiatric disorders and associated nursing care, we will begin this chapter by exploring assessment techniques and therapeutic methods used with children and adolescents.

INITIAL ASSESSMENT

The observation and interaction part of a mental health assessment begins with a semistructured assessment. In this initial assessment, the child or adolescent is asked about life at home with parents and siblings and life at school with teachers and peers. Children and adolescents should be free to describe their current problems and provide information about their developmental history. Play activities, such as games, drawing, puppets, and free play are used for younger children who cannot respond to a more direct approach. An important part of the first interaction is observing communication between the child, caregiver, and siblings when possible.

Whenever possible, families should always be involved in therapy. They should be given support in parenting skills that are designed to help them provide nurturance and set consistent limits. They are the key players in carrying out the treatment plan. Parents can learn to use behavior modification techniques, monitor medication, collaborate with the school to encourage academic success, and make a home environment that promotes the achievement of normal developmental tasks. When families are abusive, use substances, or are chaotic, the child may require out-of-home placement.

Psychotherapeutic Approaches

Treatment of childhood and adolescent disorders usually requires a multimodal approach. Close work with schools, remediation services, and mental health professionals who provide behavior modification should all be part of the intervention.

Therapies include cognitive–behavioral therapies. Effective behavioral techniques for supporting desirable behaviors include the following:

- Positive reinforcement
- Time out
- Token economy—earning points for privileges or rewards
- Response costs—withdrawing privileges based on undesirable behavior

Other therapies, including social skills groups, family therapy, parent training in behavioral techniques, and individual therapy focused on esteem issues, have all been found to be useful. Skills training might focus on a variety of areas, depending on the child's or adolescent's presenting symptoms. For example, some children need to learn basic activities of daily living (ADLs), others have difficulty with their impulse control and frustration tolerance, and those with anxiety disorders might benefit from anxiety-reduction skills.

Children and adolescents benefit from learning a variety of social skills (problem solving, decision making, initiating and maintaining contacts with peers) that will help them negotiate satisfying and productive relationships and friendships in the outside world. Many young people suffer from severe symptoms of depression, and although medication might be immediately useful, family and individual therapies should be made a pivotal part of the patient's treatment. Rarely, if ever, is medication alone the ideal treatment.

Selected Childhood Disorders

Disorders most commonly seen in children and adolescents are discussed in this chapter. Disorders that result in disruptive behaviors are addressed first along with associated nursing care. These disruptive disorders include attention-deficit/hyperactivity disorder (ADHD), conduct disorder, and oppositional defiant disorder, a set of behavioral disorders that frequently occur together. This discussion is followed by an overview of the autism spectrum disorders and associated nursing care.

DISRUPTIVE BEHAVIOR DISORDERS

Attention-Deficit/Hyperactivity Disorder

Individuals with ADHD exhibit inattention, impulsiveness, and hyperactivity. Some children are inattentive but not hyperactive. In the absence of hyperactivity, the diagnosis is shortened to attention deficit disorder (ADD). To diagnose a child with ADHD symptoms must be present in at least two settings (e.g., at home and school) and occur before age 12 years. The disorder is most often detected when the child has difficulty adjusting to elementary school. Attention problems and hyperactivity contribute to low frustration tolerance, temper outbursts, labile moods, poor school performance, peer rejection, and low self-esteem.

Peer relationships are strained because of difficulty taking turns, poor social boundaries, intrusive behaviors, and interrupting others. Those with inattentive type of ADHD may exhibit high degrees of distractibility and disorganization. They may be unable to complete challenging or tedious tasks, become easily bored, lose things often, or require frequent prompts to complete tasks. Children with ADHD are also more likely than their peers to experience enuresis (bedwetting) with a similar trend for encopresis (fecal soiling).

Epidemiology

ADHD affects 10% of children and adolescents between the ages of 5 and 17. It affects about 14% of boys and about 6% of girls in that age range (CDC, 2013). Children in poor health are more than twice as likely to have ADHD (21% versus 8%). The median age of onset is 7 years, although some people may go undiagnosed until functional impairments become noticeable in adulthood. Adult ADHD occurs at a rate of about 5%.

Risk Factors

ADHD tends to run in families. The concordance rate for identical twins is between 51% and 58% (Ebert et al., 2016). Although certain genes are correlated with the disorder, there have been no absolute connections. Very low birth weight increases the risk of ADHD by three times. Maternal smoking and alcohol use, child abuse, neglect, neurotoxin exposure (e.g., lead), and infections (e.g., encephalitis) have also been implicated in subsequent ADHD.

Treatment

Treatment for ADHD includes behavior modification, special education programs for academic difficulties, and psychotherapy and play therapy for concurrent emotional problems. Psychostimulants are used to treat ADHD to improve the sluggish frontal lobe that is believed to cause the disorder. See Chapter 21 for medications used in this disorder.

Oppositional Defiant Disorder

Oppositional defiant disorder (ODD) is a persistent pattern of negativity, disobedience, defiance, and hostility directed toward authority figures. Almost all children at some time exhibit symptoms characteristic of ODD, such as having temper tantrums, being argumentative, or refusing to obey or do chores. However, to be diagnosed with ODD, these behaviors need to happen more persistently and more frequently than what would be considered within the range of normal behaviors.

Children with ODD exhibit persistent angry, irritable mood; stubbornness; argumentative, defiant behaviors;

and vindictive behaviors. These behaviors are evident at home but may not be present elsewhere. These children and adolescents do not see themselves as defiant; instead, they feel they are responding to unreasonable demands or situations.

Individuals with ODD who exhibit mostly angry and irritable symptoms tend to progress to mood disorders. Symptoms of defiance, argumentativeness, and vindictiveness increase the risk of subsequently developing conduct disorder.

Epidemiology

The average prevalence of ODD is about 3%. It is somewhat more common in males than in females (1.4 : 1) before adolescence. After adolescence the ratio of males to females evens off.

Risk Factors

Some biological markers such as lower heart rate, skin conductance, and abnormalities in the prefrontal cortex and amygdala have been associated with ODD. Problems related to emotional regulation (e.g., emotional reactivity, lack of frustration tolerance) may increase this disorder. Children from families with inconsistent parenting, harsh punishments, or neglect are overrepresented in this population

Treatment

Pharmacotherapy is generally not indicated for ODD. However, comorbid conditions that increase defiant symptoms such as ADHD or anxiety should be managed. Youths with ODD are generally treated as outpatients, with much of the focus on strengthening parenting ability. Parent-management training programs and family therapy to teach parents and other family members how to manage the child's behavior are helpful. Cognitive–behavioral therapy can help the individual manage responses more effectively, as can social skills programs.

Conduct Disorder

Conduct disorder is a serious behavioral and emotional condition characterized by a persistent pattern of behavior in which the rights of others and societal norms and rules are violated. This pattern typically begins during childhood and adolescence and occurs in all settings. Although conduct disorder itself can continue into adulthood, symptoms often become characteristic of antisocial personality disorder.

There is a subset of people with conduct disorder who are referred to as being callous and unemotional. Callousness is characterized by a lack of empathy, such as disregarding and being unconcerned about the feelings of others. Pyromania, or fire setting, and kleptomania, or stealing, are also associated with this disorder.

Childhood-onset conduct disorder can be evident as early as 2 years of age (irritable temperament, poor compliance, inattentiveness, impulsivity), which in later years can lead to conduct disturbance. As these children reach elementary school age, aggressive tendencies with adults and peers continue. Early onset tends to predict a poorer outcome.

Adolescent-onset conduct disorder results in less aggressive behaviors and more normal peer relationships. These individuals are likely to have a better outcome. These pre-adults tend to act out their misconduct with their peer group (e.g., truancy, early-onset sexual behaviors, drinking, substance use, and risk-taking behaviors). Males are more likely to fight, steal, vandalize, and have school discipline problems, whereas girls lie, run away, and engage in prostitution.

Epidemiology

Prevalence rates rise from childhood to adolescence and are higher in males than females. The rate among boys ranges from 6% to 16%. Girls have a rate of about 2% to 9%.

Risk Factors

Conduct disorder is the result of both genetic and environmental risk, because having either a biological or adopted parent or sibling with the disorder increases the risk. Slower resting heart rate and decreased skin conductance-symptoms linked to fearlessness and aggression are present in this population. ODD commonly occurs before childhood-onset conduct disorder. Affect regulation, affect processing, and frontotemporal-limbic connections between the prefrontal cortex and amygdala are different in people with this diagnosis. As with ODD, inconsistent, harsh, and neglectful parenting is associated with conduct disorder.

Treatment

Conduct disorders may require inpatient hospitalization for crisis intervention, evaluation, and treatment planning. These individuals may be subsequently transferred to therapeutic foster care or long-term residential treatment. Multisystemic therapy, an evidence-based model that emphasizes the home environment and the empowerment of families through several hours of treatment each week, has been found to be helpful in treating this population.

To control aggressive behaviors, a wide variety of pharmacological agents have been used, including antipsychotics, mood stabilizers (lithium carbonate and anticonvulsants), antidepressants, and beta-adrenergic blockers. Cognitive–behavioral therapy is used to change the pattern of misconduct by fostering the development of internal controls, both cognitive and emotional. Important components of the treatment program include learning problem-solving techniques, conflict resolution, and empathy.

Assessment Guidelines

Attention-Deficit/Hyperactivity Disorder

1. Assess the child for level of physical activity, attention span, talkativeness, and the ability to follow directions and control impulses.
2. Assess the quality of the relationship between the child and parent or caregiver for evidence of bonding, anxiety, tension, and difficulty of fit between the parents' and child's temperament, which can contribute to the development of disruptive behaviors.
3. Assess the parent's or caregiver's understanding of growth and development, parenting skills, and handling of problematic behaviors, because lack of knowledge contributes to the development of these problems.
4. Assess for difficulty in making friends and performing in school. Academic failures and poor peer relationships

lead to low self-esteem, depression, and further acting out.
5. Assess for enuresis and encopresis.

Oppositional Defiant Disorder

1. Identify issues that lead to power struggles, including when they began and how they are handled.
2. Assess the severity of the defiant behavior and its impact on the child's life at home, at school, and with peers.
3. How does the child respond to limits? Being told "no"? Having to wait, share, or end a favorite activity?

Conduct Disorder

1. Assess the seriousness of the disruptive behavior, when it started, and what has been done to manage it.
2. Assess the child's level of anxiety, aggression, anger, and hostility toward others and the ability to control negative impulses.
3. Assess the child's moral development for the ability to understand the impact of the hurtful behavior on others, empathize with others, and feel remorse.
4. Assess cognitive, psychosocial, and moral development for lags or deficits, because immature developmental competencies result in disruptive behaviors.

Patient Problems

Children and adolescents with ADHD, conduct disorder, and oppositional defiant disorder all display disruptive behaviors that are impulsive, angry or aggressive, and often dangerous. Therefore *potential for violence* is a primary focus. Conflict with authority figures, refusal to comply with requests, and inappropriate ways of getting needs met are addressed with *defensive coping. Impaired social functioning* addresses difficulty making or keeping friends. Interpersonal and academic problems lead to *decreased self-esteem.* Because parents or caregivers participation in therapeutic programs is essential, *parenting problems* applies.

Intervention Guidelines

Disruptive Behavior Disorders

Help the child reach his or her full potential by fostering developmental competencies and coping skills:

1. Protect the child or adolescent from harm and provide for biological and psychosocial needs while acting as a parental surrogate and role model.
2. Provide immediate nonthreatening feedback for unacceptable behaviors.
3. Increase the child's or adolescent's ability to trust and use interpersonal skills to maintain satisfying relationships with adults and peers.
4. Provide immediate positive feedback for acceptable behaviors.
5. Increase the child's or adolescent's ability to control impulses, tolerate frustration, and modulate the expression of affect.
6. Foster the child's or adolescent's identification with positive role models so that positive attitudes and moral values can develop that enable the youth to experience feelings of empathy, remorse, shame, and pride.
7. Use role-play to help the child or adolescent respond in a more acceptable manner when feeling frustrated or aggressive.
8. Foster the development of a realistic self-identity and self-esteem based on achievements and the formation of realistic goals.
9. Provide support, education, and guidance for parents or caregivers.

Nursing Care for Disruptive Behavior Disorders

Potential for Violence

Due to:

- Impaired neurological function
- Impulsivity
- Inability to control temper
- Psychotic symptoms (e.g., hallucinations, delusions, illogical thought processes)
- Emotional dysregulation (e.g., hopelessness, despair, increased anxiety, panic, anger, hostility)

Desired Outcome:
The patient will demonstrate the ability to control aggressive impulses and delay gratification.

Assessment/Interventions (Rationales)

1. Use one-to-one or appropriate level of observation to monitor rising levels of anxiety; determine emotional and situational triggers. (External controls are needed for ego support and to prevent acts of aggression and violence.)
2. Intervene early to calm the patient and defuse a potential incident. (Learning can take place before the patient loses control; new ways to cope can be discussed and role-modeled.)
3. Implement techniques for managing disruptive behaviors (Table 4.1). (Techniques such as signals or warnings, proximity and touch control, humor, and attention are effective in reducing antisocial behavior.)
4. Set clear, consistent limits in a calm, nonjudgmental manner; remind the patient of the consequences of acting out. (A child gains a sense of security with clear limits and calm adults who follow through on a consistent basis.)
5. Avoid power struggles and repeated negotiations about rules and limits. (When limits are realistic and enforceable, manipulation can be minimized.)
6. Use strategic removal if the patient cannot respond to limits (e.g., time out, a quiet room). (Removal allows the patient to express feelings and discuss problems without losing face in front of peers.)
7. Process incidents with the patient to make it a learning experience. (Reality testing, problem solving, and testing new behaviors are necessary to foster cognitive growth.)
8. Use a behavior modification program that rewards the patient for seeking help with handling feelings and controlling impulses to act out. (Rewarding the patient's efforts can increase positive behaviors and foster development of self-esteem.)
9. Redirect expressions of disruptive feelings into nondestructive, age-appropriate behaviors; channel excess energy into physical activities. (Learning how to modulate the expression of feelings and use anger constructively are essential for self-control.)
10. Help the patient see how acting out hurts others; appeal to the child's sense of "fairness" for all. (These children

Table 4.1 **Techniques for Managing Disruptive Behaviors in Children**

Technique	Description
Planned ignoring	Evaluate surface behavior, and intervene when intensity is escalating.
Use of signals or gestures	Use a word, gesture, or eye contact to remind the child or adolescent to use self-control.
Physical distance and touch control	Move closer to the child or adolescent for a calming effect—maybe put an arm around the child or adolescent.
Increased involvement in an activity	Redirect the child's or adolescent's attention to an activity and away from a distracting behavior by asking a question.
Additional affection	Ignore the provocative content of the behavior, and give the child emotional support for the current problem.
Use of humor	Use well-timed kidding as a diversion to help the child or adolescent save face and relieve feelings of guilt or fear.
Direct appeals	Appeal to the child's or adolescent's developing self-control (e.g., "Please, not now.")
Extra assistance	Provide early help to a child or adolescent who "blows up" and is easily frustrated when trying to achieve a goal.
Clarification as intervention	Help the child or adolescent understand the situation and his or her motivation for the behavior.
Restructuring	Change the activity in ways that will lower the stimulation or the frustration (e.g., shorten a story or change to a physical activity).
Regrouping	Use total or partial changes in the group's composition to reduce conflict and contagious behaviors.
Strategic removal	Remove a child or adolescent who is disrupting or using dangerous behaviors.
Setting limits and giving permission	Use firm, clear statements about what behavior is not allowed, and give permission for the behavior that is expected.

Continued

Table 4.1 **Techniques for Managing Disruptive Behaviors in Children—cont'd**

Technique	Description
Promises and rewards	Use carefully and infrequently to prevent situations in which the child or adolescent bargains for a reward.
Threats and punishment	Use threats of punishment and punishment carefully. Brief punishment (e.g., time out or loss of dessert) must happen soon after misbehavior.

are insensitive to the feelings of others. However, they can understand the concept of "fairness" and generalize it to other persons.)

11. Encourage feelings of concern for others and remorse for misdeeds. (Development of empathy is a therapeutic goal with these children.)
12. Use medication if indicated to reduce anxiety and aggression or to modulate moods. (A variety of medications are effective in children who experience a lack of control.)

Defensive Coping

Due to:

- Impaired neurological development or dysfunction
- Low level of self-confidence
- Fear of failure/humiliation
- Disturbance in pattern of tension release (problems in impulse control and frustration tolerance)
- Temperament (highly reactive, difficult to comfort, high motor activity)
- Disturbed relationship with parent or caregiver (lack of trust, abuse, neglect, conflicts, inadequate role models, disorganized family system)
- Deficient support system

Desired Outcome:

The patient will:

- Accept responsibility for behavior.
- Demonstrate an absence of tantrums, rage reactions, or other acting-out behaviors.

Assessment/Interventions (Rationales)

1. Use one-to-one or an appropriate level of observation to monitor rising levels of frustration; determine emotional

and situational triggers. (External controls are needed for emotional support and to prevent tantrums and rage reactions.)

2. Intervene early to calm the patient, problem-solve, and defuse a potential outburst. (Learning can take place before the patient loses control; new solutions and compromises can be proposed.)
3. Avoid power struggles and "no-win" situations. (Therapeutic goals are lost in power struggles.)
4. Use a behavior modification program to reward tolerating frustration, delaying gratification, and responding to requests and behavioral limits. (Rewarding the patient's efforts will increase positive behaviors and help with the development of self-control.)
5. Allow the patient to question the requests or limits within reason; give a simple, understandable rationale for requests or limits. (Discussion allows the patient to maintain some sense of autonomy and power. The rationale is tailored to the developmental age and promotes socialization.)
6. Use medication if indicated to reduce anxiety, rage, and aggression and to modulate moods. (A variety of medications are effective in children who experience behavioral and emotional lack of control.)
7. When feasible, negotiate an agreement on the expected behaviors. Avoid bribes or allowing the patient to manipulate the situation. (An agreement on expected behavior will result in better compliance. However, constant negotiations can result in increased manipulation and testing of limits.)

Impaired Social Functioning

Due to:

- Impaired neurological development or dysfunction
- Lack of appropriate role models
- Poor impulse control, frustration tolerance, or empathy for others
- Disturbed relationship with parents or caregivers
- Identification with aggressive/abusive models
- Loss of friendships due to disruptions in family life and living situation

Desired Outcome:

The patient will interact with others using age-appropriate and acceptable behavior

Assessment/Interventions (Rationales)

1. Use the one-to-one relationship to engage the patient in a working relationship. (The patient needs positive role models for healthy identification.)
2. Monitor for negative behaviors and identify maladaptive interaction patterns. (Negative behaviors are identified and targeted for replacement with age-appropriate social skills.)
3. Intervene early; give feedback and alternative ways to handle the situation. (Children learn from feedback; early intervention prevents rejection by peers and provides immediate ways to cope.)
4. Use therapeutic play to teach social skills such as sharing, cooperation, realistic competition, and manners. (Learning new ways to interact with others through play allows the development of satisfying friendships and self-esteem.)
5. Use role-playing, stories, therapeutic games, and the like to practice skills. (Solidifies new skills in a safe environment.)
6. Help the patient find and develop a special friend; set up one-on-one play situations; be available to problem-solve peer relationship conflicts; role model social skills. (The abilities to reality test, problem solve, and resolve conflicts in peer relationships are important competencies needed for interpersonal skills.)
7. Help the patient develop equal-status peer relationships with honest and appropriate expression of feelings and needs. (When patients can identify personal feelings and needs, they are better prepared to use more direct communication rather than manipulation and/or intimidation.)

Decreased Self-Esteem

Due to:

- Perceived lack of belonging
- Perceived lack of respect from others
- Lack of success in role functioning
- Psychiatric disorder
- Disturbed relationship with parent or caregiver (lack of trust, abuse, neglect, conflicts, inadequate role models, disorganized family system)
- Targeted by peers for rejection or abuse

Desired Outcomes:
The patient will:
- Describe self in positive ways
- Fulfill personally significant roles
- Engage in meaningful interaction with others

Assessment/Interventions (Rationales)
1. Give unconditional positive regard without reinforcing negative behaviors. (The patient often sets up situations in which behaviors cause rejection and further confirms the lack of self-worth.)
2. Reinforce the patient's self-worth with time and attention. (Giving one-to-one time or attention in a group activity supports the patient's self-worth.)
3. Help the patient identify positive qualities and accomplishments. (An accurate appraisal of accomplishments can help dispel unrealistic expectations.)
4. Help the patient identify behaviors needing change and set realistic goals. (To change, the patient needs goals and knowledge of new behaviors.)
5. Use a behavior modification program that rewards the patient for practicing new behaviors and evaluates results. (Rewarding the patient's efforts will increase the positive behaviors and foster the development of increased self-esteem.)

Parenting Problems

Due to:
- Physical illness (impaired neurological development or dysfunction; handicapped condition)
- Attention-deficit/hyperactivity disorder in the child
- Lack of knowledge about parenting/child development or the special needs of the child
- Role strain or overload (multiple stressors)
- Mental or physical illness, in either the parent(s) or child
- History of being abused or history of being abusive
- Lack of parent or caregiver fit with the child

Desired Outcome:
The parent or caregiver will demonstrate effective coping skills in parenting a child with problematic behavior.

Assessment/Interventions (Rationales)
1. Explore the impact of the problematic behavior on the life of the family. (Helps the nurse understand the

parent or caregiver situation. Feeling understood and supported can help foster an alliance.)

2. Assess the parent's or caregiver's knowledge of childhood growth and development and parenting skills. (Problem identification and analysis of learning needs are necessary before intervention begins.)
3. Assess the parent's or caregiver's understanding of the child's diagnosis, treatment, and medications. (Knowledge will increase parent or caregiver participation, motivation, and satisfaction.)
4. Help the parent or caregiver identify the child's biological and psychosocial needs. (Adequate parenting involves being able to identify the child's actual age-appropriate needs.)
5. Involve the parent in identifying a realistic plan for how these needs will be met when the patient is at home. (Parents or caregivers have the opportunity to learn the skills necessary to meet the child's needs.)
6. Work with the parent or caregiver to set behavioral goals; help set realistic goals for when the child is at home. (Mutually setting goals provides continuity and prevents the child from using splitting or manipulation to sabotage treatment.)
7. Teach behavior modification techniques; give the parent or caregiver support in using them and evaluating the effectiveness. (Education and follow-up support are key to a successful treatment program.)
8. Assess the parent or caregiver support system; use referrals to establish additional supports. (Self-help groups and special programs such as respite care can increase the caregiver's ability to cope.)
9. Give information on legal rights and available resources that can assist in advocating for child services. (The parent or caregiver commonly lacks information on how to secure services for the child.)

AUTISM SPECTRUM DISORDERS

Autism spectrum disorders (ASDs) are complex neurobiological and developmental disabilities that typically appear during the first 3 years of life. Autism affects the normal development of social interaction and communication skills. It ranges in severity from mild to moderate to severe.

Symptoms associated with ASDs include deficits in social relatedness. There are deficits in developing and maintaining relationships. Other behaviors include stereotypical repetitive speech, obsessive focus on specific objects, overadherence to routines or rituals, hyperreactivity or hyporeactivity to sensory input, and extreme resistance to change. The symptoms first occur in childhood and cause impairments in everyday functioning.

Epidemiology

The prevalence of ASDs is 1 in 68 children (Christensen et al., 2016). The prevalence is significantly higher in boys (23.6 per 1000) than girls (5.3 per 1000). The rate is significantly higher in non-Hispanic white and black children (15.5 per 1000 and 13.2 per 1000) compared with Hispanic children (10.1 per 1000).

Risk Factors

There is a genetic component to autism. The concordance rate for monozygotic (identical) twins is 70% to 90%, meaning that most of the time if one twin is affected, the other is as well. ASDs are associated with certain conditions such as fragile X syndrome and tuberous sclerosis (Centers for Disease Control and Prevention, 2016). The drugs valproic acid and thalidomide have been linked to a higher incidence of ASDs. Children born to older parents are also more likely to be affected.

Treatment

Children with ASDs are treated in therapeutic nursery schools, day treatment programs, and special education classes in public schools, because their education and treatment is mandated under the Children With Disabilities Act. Treatment plans include teaching parents how to modify the child's behavior and to foster the development of skills when the child is home.

Pharmacological agents target specific symptoms and may be used to improve relatedness and decrease anxiety, compulsive behaviors, or agitation. The second-generation antipsychotics risperidone (Risperdal) and aripiprazole (Abilify) have U.S. Food and Drug Administration (US

FDA, 2017) approval for treating children 5 and 6 years of age and older, respectively. These drugs improve irritability that is associated with severe temper tantrums, aggression, and self-injurious behavior.

Selective serotonin reuptake inhibitors (SSRIs) are the most popular medication used in this population. They improve mood and reduce anxiety, which provides the patient with a higher degree of tolerance for new situations. Stimulant medications may be used to target hyperactivity, impulsivity, or inattention.

Assessment Guidelines

Autism Spectrum Disorder

1. Assess for developmental spurts or lags, uneven development, or loss of previously acquired abilities.
2. Assess the quality of the relationship between the child and parent or caregiver for evidence of bonding, anxiety, or tension; look for antagonism between the parent's and child's temperaments.
3. Be aware that children with behavioral and developmental problems are at risk for abuse.
4. Assess for co-occurring conditions (e.g., intellectual developmental disorder may be present, especially with the lowest functioning individuals).
5. Assess for the child's strengths.

Patient Problems

In ASD the severity of the impairment is demonstrated by the child's lack of responsiveness to or interest in others, a deficiency of empathy or sharing with peers, and little or no cooperative or imaginative play with peers. Therefore *impaired social functioning* is always present. Language delay or absence of language and the unusual stereotyped or repetitive use of language is another area for nursing making *impaired communication* a useful focus. Stereotyped and repetitive motor movements can include behaviors such as head banging, face slapping, and hand biting. The child's apparent indifference to pain can result in serious self-injury, so *potential for injury* can become a priority. Individuals with ASDs often lack an interest in activities outside of self and they frequently disregard bodily needs.

These deficiencies interfere with the development of a personal identity, so *disturbed personal identity* might also be the focus for care.

Nursing Care for Autism Spectrum Disorders

Impaired Social Functioning

Due to:

- Self-concept disturbance (immaturity or developmental deviation)
- Absence of available significant others or peers
- Disturbed thought processes
- Impaired neurological development or dysfunction
- Disturbance in response to external stimuli
- Disturbance in attachment or bonding with the parent or caregiver

Desired Outcomes:

The patient will demonstrate an increase in quantity and quality of social interactions.

Assessment/Interventions (Rationales)

1. Use one-to-one interaction to engage the patient in a therapeutic relationship. (Assigning the same primary nurse, who will be a parental surrogate, can promote attachment.)
2. Monitor for signs of anxiety or distress. Intervene early to provide comfort. (Anticipating the need for help in managing stress will enhance the patient's feelings of security.)
3. Provide emotional support and guidance for ADLs and other activities; use a system of rewards for attempts and successes. (Behavior change occurs through meaningful social interactions involving imitation, modeling, feedback, and reinforcement.)
4. Set up social interactions beginning parallel play and moving toward cooperative play. (Learning to play with peers is sequential.)
5. Help the patient find a special friend. (Having a special friend enhances the learning experience.)
6. Role model social interaction skills (interest, empathy, sharing, waiting, and required language). (Role modeling facilitates the development of necessary social and emotional skills.)

7. Reward attempts to interact and play with peers and the use of appropriate emotional expressions. (Behaviors that are rewarded are repeated.)
8. Role play situations that involve conflicts in social interactions to teach reality testing, cause and effect, and problem solving. (These cognitive skills are needed for successful social and emotional reciprocity.)

Impaired Communication

Due to:

- Physiological conditions and/or emotional conditions
- Impaired neurological development or dysfunction
- Disturbance in attachment or bonding with the parent or caregiver

Desired Outcome:

The patient will communicate basic needs such as hunger, thirst, fatigue, and pain, verbally or through gestures and body language

Assessment/Interventions (Rationales)

1. Use one-to-one interaction to engage the patient in nonverbal play. (The nurse enters the patient's world using a nonthreatening interaction to form a trusting relationship.)
2. Recognize subtle cues indicating the patient is paying attention or attempting to communicate. (Cues are often difficult to recognize [glancing out of the corner of the eye].)
3. Describe to the patient what is happening, and put into words what the patient might be experiencing. (Naming objects and describing actions, thoughts, and feelings help the patient to use symbolic language.)
4. Encourage vocalizations with sound games and songs. (Children learn through play and enjoyable activities.)
5. Identify desired behaviors and reward them (e.g., hugs, treats, tokens, points, or food). (Behaviors that are rewarded will increase in frequency. The desire for food is a powerful incentive in modifying behavior.)
6. Use names frequently, and encourage the use of correct pronouns (e.g., I, me, he). (Problems with self-identification and pronoun reversal are common.)
7. Encourage verbal communication with peers during play activities using role-modeling, feedback, and

reinforcement. (Play is the normal medium for learning in a child's development.)

8. Increase verbal interaction with parents and siblings by teaching them how to facilitate language development. (Education and emotional support help parents and siblings become more therapeutic in their interactions with the patient.)

Potential for Injury

Due to:

- Autism spectrum disorder
- History of self-directed violence (head banging, biting, scratching, hair pulling when frustrated or angry)
- Reduction of tension by self-mutilation
- Impaired neurological development or dysfunction
- Unable to express self verbally
- Lack of impulse control
- Self-injurious behavior in response to change

Desired Outcome:

The patient will be free of self-inflicted injury.

Assessment/Interventions (Rationales)

1. Monitor the patient's behavior for signs of increasing anxiety. (Behavioral cues signal increasing anxiety.)
2. Determine emotional and situational triggers. (Knowledge of triggers is used in planning ways to prevent or manage outbursts.)
3. Intervene early with verbal comments or limits or removal from the situation. (Potential outbursts can be defused through early recognition, verbal interventions, or removal.)
4. Give plenty of notice when having to change routines or rituals or end pleasurable activities. (These children often react to change with catastrophic reactions and need time to adjust.)
5. Provide support for the recognition of feelings, reality testing, and impulse control. (These competencies are often underdeveloped in this population.)
6. Help the patient connect feelings and anxiety to self-injurious behaviors. (Self-control is enhanced through understanding the relationship between feelings and behaviors.)

7. Help the patient develop ways to express feelings and reduce anxiety verbally and through play activities. Use various types of motor and imaginative play (e.g., swinging, tumbling, role playing, drawing, and singing). (Methods for modulating and directing the expression of emotions and anxiety must be learned to control destructive impulses.)

Disturbed Personal Identity

Due to:

- Impaired neurological development or dysfunction
- Failure to develop attachment behaviors
- Biochemical imbalance
- Interrupted or incomplete separation and individuation process

Desired Outcome:
The patient will demonstrate an increase in self-awareness and other-awareness.

Assessment/Interventions (Rationales)

1. Use one-to-one interaction to engage the patient in a safe relationship with the nurse or caregiver. (A consistent caregiver provides for the development of trust needed for a sense of safety and security.)
2. Use names and descriptions of others to reinforce their separateness. (Consistent reinforcement will help break into the patient's world.)
3. Draw the patient's attention to the activities of others and events that are happening in the environment. (Interrupts the patient's self-absorption and stimulates outside interests.)
4. Limit self-stimulating and ritualistic behaviors by providing alternative play activities or by providing comfort when stressed. (Redirecting the patient's attention to favorite or new activities increases interaction and personal identity.)
5. Foster self-concept development; reinforce identity, and body boundaries through drawing, stories, and play activities. (Learning body parts helps to establish self-identity and a differentiation from others.)
6. Help the patient distinguish body sensations and how to meet bodily needs by picking up on cues and using ADLs to teach self-care. (The lack of self-awareness contributes to problems with self-care, especially toileting.)

7. Provide play opportunities for the patient to identify the feelings of others (e.g., stories, puppet play, and peer interactions). (Consistent feedback about the feelings of others helps with self-differentiation and the development of empathy.)

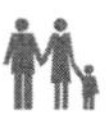

Nurse, Patient, and Family Resources

American Academy of Child and Adolescent Psychiatry
www.aacap.org

American Psychiatric Nurses Association (search child)
www.apna.org

Asperger/Autism Network
www.aane.org

Autism Resources
www.autism-resources.com

Autism Society
www.autism-society.org

Children and Adults With Attention-Deficit/ Hyperactivity Disorder
www.chadd.org

Conduct Disorders Support Site
www.conductdisorders.com

CHAPTER 5

Schizophrenia Spectrum Disorders

Schizophrenia spectrum disorders are disorders that share features with schizophrenia. These disorders are characterized by *psychosis,* which refers to altered cognition, altered perception, or an impaired ability to determine what is or is not real (an ability that is known as *reality testing*).

SCHIZOTYPAL PERSONALITY DISORDER (DELUSIONAL DISORDER)

Schizotypal personality disorder is characterized by delusions (false thoughts) that have lasted 1 month or longer. The delusions tend to have a general theme that includes grandiosity, persecution, and self-reference. These delusions are usually not severe enough to impair occupational or daily functioning. Individuals with this personality disorder do not tend to behave strangely or bizarrely, but they do have severe social anxiety.

BRIEF PSYCHOTIC DISORDER

Brief psychotic disorder is characterized by the sudden onset of at least one of the following: delusions, hallucinations (false sensory perception), disorganized speech, and disorganized or catatonic (severely decreased motor activity) behavior. The symptoms must last longer than 1 day but no longer than 1 month with the expectation of a return to normal functioning.

SCHIZOPHRENIFORM DISORDER

The essential features of schizophreniform disorder are exactly like those of schizophrenia, except that the symptoms last for a much shorter period (at least 1 month, but less than 6 months). Also, impaired social or occupational functioning during some part of the illness is not apparent (although it might occur). It is difficult to know the prognosis of a schizophreniform disorder, because some individuals return to their previous level of functioning, whereas others have more difficulties in moving forward.

SCHIZOAFFECTIVE DISORDER

Schizoaffective disorder is characterized by alterations in mood. Symptoms of this disorder include an uninterrupted period of illness during which there is a major depressive, manic, or mixed episode. At the same time individuals experience delusions, hallucinations, and disorganized speech. The symptoms must not be caused by any substance use or abuse or general medical condition.

SUBSTANCE-INDUCED PSYCHOTIC DISORDER AND PSYCHOTIC DISORDER RELATED TO ANOTHER MEDICAL CONDITION

Substances such as drugs, alcohol, medications, or toxin exposure can induce delusions or hallucinations. Hallucinations or delusions can also be caused by a general medical condition such as delirium, neurological problems, hepatic or renal diseases, and many others. Substance use and medical conditions should always be ruled out before a primary diagnosis of schizophrenia or other psychotic disorder is made.

SCHIZOPHRENIA

Schizophrenia is a potentially devastating brain disorder. It affects more than 1% of adults (3.2 million people in the United States) and can be among the most disruptive and disabling of psychiatric disorders. Schizophrenia targets young people in their teens or early 20s at the beginning of their productive lives (15–25 years of age for men, 25–35 years of age for women).

The presentation of schizophrenia varies considerably from person to person, and it is believed that what has traditionally been called *schizophrenia* is actually a collection of eight or more disorders that, although sharing core features such as impaired reality testing, vary in the type and severity of symptoms, responsiveness to treatment, and prognosis. Some people with schizophrenia can function well with the aid of medications and social supports. Others are more disabled and need a higher level of support in terms of housing, health maintenance, financial aid, and more.

People with schizophrenia compose a large percentage of the homeless population. The longer the individual with psychoses remains untreated, the poorer the prognosis. About 95% of affected individuals experience the disorder throughout their lifetime. People who develop paranoid features usually have a later time of onset. Although schizophrenia is not caused by psychological events, stressful life events can trigger an exacerbation of the illness.

KEY FEATURES OF PSYCHOTIC DISORDERS

Psychotic disorders are characterized by the so-called *positive symptoms,* which include delusions, hallucinations, and disorganized thinking and speech. The *negative symptoms* refer to the absence of human qualities that make life enjoyable.

Positive Symptoms

Hallucinations

Hallucinations refer to perceptual events in the absence of any actual external stimulus. The hallucinations seem so real it is hard for the person to separate what is going on in his or her head from what is going on in the environment. Auditory hallucinations, or hearing voices, are the most common hallucination in the schizophrenia spectrum disorders. The voices may seem like they are coming from inside the person's head or outside. The content of the auditory hallucination may be degrading (e.g., calling the person worthless), persecutory (e.g., telling the person the doctor will kill him), or commanding (e.g., instructing the person to kill herself or hurt others).

Delusions

Delusions are strongly held beliefs that do not change despite evidence of the contrary. There are several types of delusions:

- Grandiose delusions center on feeling special, being exceptionally talented, or being extremely important (e.g., "I have a personal relationship with the U.S. President").
- Persecutory delusions result in feeling singled out for harassment, persecution, or harm (e.g., "People break into my house when I am not home and read my email").
- Somatic delusions are obsessions with the health and functioning of specific bodily organs (e.g., "My heart has mold growing on it").
- Referential delusions are a belief that events going on in the environment or with other people are personally directed (e.g., "The newscaster commented about sunshine because she knows about my golf plans").

Disorganized Thinking and Speech

Disorganized thinking results in disorganized speech. Patients may behave in a trivial and careless manner or they may be agitated. Poverty of thought, poor problem solving, poor decision making, and illogical thinking most profoundly affect the individual's ability to engage in normal social and occupational experiences.

Negative Symptoms

Unlike positive symptoms, qualities that are abnormally present with psychotic disorders, negative symptoms are qualities that should be present but are not. Emotional expression tends to be diminished in facial emotion; eye contact; tone of speech; and the usual movements of the hands, head, and face that normally accompany verbalizations. Lack of motivation (avolition), diminished speech (alogia), an inability to experience joy or pleasure (anhedonia), and lack of interest in interaction (asociality) characterize these disorders.

Phases of Schizophrenia

Schizophrenia is divided into three phases:

Phase I: Onset. This phase (acute phase) includes prodromal symptoms (e.g., acute or chronic anxiety, phobias, obsessions, compulsions, dissociative features) and acute psychotic symptoms (hallucinations, delusions, or disorganized thinking).

Phase II: Years after onset. Patterns that characterize this phase are the ebb and flow of the intensity and disruption caused by symptoms, which might in some cases be followed by complete or relatively complete recovery.

Phase III: Long-term course and outcome. This is the course a severely and persistently mentally ill patient follows when the disease becomes chronic. For some patients, the intensity of the psychosis might diminish with age, but the long-term dysfunctional effects of the disorder are not as amenable to change.

Assessment

Signs and Symptoms

Positive-symptoms of schizophrenia occur suddenly. Positive symptoms are active and include alterations in the following:

- Perceptions (hallucinations and delusions)
- Thinking (disorganized)
- Language (looseness of association, poverty of speech)
- Agitation and emotional dysregulation

Hallucinations and delusions can be very frightening to the patient. They also can be very disconcerting and frightening to nurses and other health care team members, as well as family and friends. Communicating with patients who are delusional, have hallucinations, and exhibit disorganized thinking is a learned skill.

Negative symptoms usually begin in childhood. These children may view these children as odd and withdrawn. Negative symptoms are more insidious and are also very damaging to the patient's quality of life. Alterations are evident in the following:

- Emotions: apathy, anhedonia, depression, feelings of emptiness, avolition
- Social behavior: aggression, bizarre conduct, or extreme withdrawal

Cognitive symptoms are perhaps the most crucial because they interfere with the person's ability to function in all areas of life (e.g., learn, hold a job, have friends). Cognitive symptoms that are altered in schizophrenia include the following:

- Working memory
- Attention and vigilance
- Verbal learning and memory
- Reasoning and problem-solving

- Speed of processing
- Social learning and cognition

Co-occurring depression is a common complication in people with schizophrenia, as are substance use problems and disorders.

Assessment Guidelines

Positive Symptoms

1. Assess for command hallucinations (e.g., voices telling the person to harm self or another). If present, ask the following:
   a. Do you plan to follow the command?
   b. Do you believe the voices are real?
2. Assess for delusions. Determine whether the patient has a fragmented, poorly organized, well-organized, systematized, or extensive system of beliefs that are not supported by reality. If so, follow-up is necessary:
   a. Assess whether delusions have to do with someone trying to harm the patient and whether the patient is planning to retaliate against a person or organization.
   b. Assess whether precautions need to be taken.
   c. Assess for pervasive suspiciousness about everyone and their actions (paranoia)—for example, whether the patient is:
      1) On guard, hyperalert, vigilant
      2) Blaming others for consequences of own behavior
      3) Hostile, argumentative, or threatening in verbalization or behavior

Negative Symptoms

1. Assess for negative symptoms of schizophrenia.
2. Assess whether the patient is on medications, what the medications are, and whether the patient is adherent with medications.
3. Identify how the family responds to the patient's symptoms? Are they overprotective? Hostile? Suspicious?
4. How do family members and the patient relate?
5. Assess the support system. Is the family well informed about the disorder?
6. Does the family understand the need for medication adherence? Is the family familiar with family support groups in the community or where to go for respite and family support?

Cognitive Symptoms

1. Assess the severity of the cognitive symptoms.
2. Assess how the cognitive symptoms interfere with the patient's functioning.
3. Identify the patient's strengths and personal attributes that can be gateways to interventions.

Patient Problems

Relating to people with schizophrenia can be a challenge, especially in the acute phase. The patient problem *impaired communication* addresses this challenge. Again, during the acute phase, relating to others is difficult. Guidelines for interacting and gradually adding social skills are addressed with *impaired social functioning*. Hearing voices that seem to originate either inside or outside of the person is addressed with the patient problem of *auditory hallucinations*. Because of delusions and disorganized thinking, *altered thought processes* is an focus. Due to uncomfortable and often intolerable side effects, coupled with the belief that medication is unnecessary, the patient problem *nonadherence* provides direction for useful interventions. Finally, *altered family processes* addresses the exhaustive needs of families dealing with symptoms of schizophrenia.

Nursing Care for Schizophrenia

Impaired Communication

Due to:

- Biochemical alterations in the brain
- Psychological barriers (psychosis, lack of stimuli)
- Side effects of medication
- Altered perceptions

Desired Outcomes:
The patient will communicate in a manner that can be understood by others.

Assessment/Interventions (Rationales)

1. Assess whether incoherence in speech is chronic or more sudden, as in an exacerbation of symptoms. (Establishing a baseline facilitates the development of realistic goals, the cornerstone for planning effective care.)
2. Identify how long the patient has been on antipsychotic medication (see Chapter 22 for information about

antipsychotics). (Therapeutic levels of an antipsychotic medication can help clear thinking and diminish looseness of association.)

3. Plan short, frequent periods with the patient throughout the day. (Short periods are less stressful, and periodic meetings give the patient a chance to develop familiarity and safety.)
4. Use simple words, and keep directions simple. (The patient might have difficulty processing even simple sentences.)
5. Keep your voice low, and speak slowly. (A high-pitched or loud tone of voice can raise anxiety levels; slow speaking aids understanding.)
6. Look for themes in what is said, even though spoken words appear incoherent (e.g., anxiety, fear, sadness). (Often the patient's choice of words is symbolic of unspoken feelings.)
7. When you do not understand a patient, let him or her know you are having difficulty understanding (e.g., "I want to understand what you are saying, but I am having difficulty.") (Pretending to understand when you do not limits your credibility in the eyes of the patient and decreases the potential for trust.)
8. Use therapeutic techniques to try to understand the patient's concerns (e.g., "Are you saying…?" "You mentioned demons many times. Are you feeling frightened?"). (Even if the words are hard to understand, try getting to the feelings behind them.)
9. Focus on and direct the patient's attention to concrete things in the environment. (Helps draw focus away from delusions and focus on an objective reality.)
10. Keep the environment quiet and as free of stimuli as possible. (Helps to prevent anxiety from escalating and may reduce confusion, hallucinations, and delusions.)
11. Use simple, concrete, and literal explanations. (Minimizes the patient misunderstanding and incorporating those misunderstandings into delusional systems.)
12. Introduce tactics that can lower anxiety and minimize voices and "worrying" thoughts. Take time out, read out loud, seek out another supportive person, listen to music, replace irrational thoughts with rational statements, replace bad thoughts with constructive thoughts, and practice deep breathing. (Help the patient to use tactics to lower anxiety, which can enhance functional speech.)

Impaired Social Functioning

Due to:

- Self-concept disturbance
- Difficulty with communication
- Inappropriate or inadequate emotional responses
- Feeling threatened in social situations
- Exaggerated response to stimuli
- Difficulty with concentration
- Impaired thought processes (hallucinations or delusions)

Desired Outcomes:

The patient will use appropriate skills to initiate and maintain interactions.

Assessment/Interventions (Rationales)

1. Assess whether medication has reached therapeutic levels. (Many of the positive symptoms [paranoia, delusions, and hallucinations] will subside with medications, which will facilitate interactions.)
2. Ensure that the goals set are realistic, whether in the hospital or community. (Attainable goals relieve pressure from the patient and prevents a sense of failure on the part of the nurse and family. This sense of failure can lead to mutual withdrawal.)
3. Keep the patient in an environment as free of stimuli (e.g., loud noises, high traffic areas) as possible. (The patient might respond to noises and crowding with agitation, anxiety, and increased inability to concentrate on outside events.)
4. Avoid touching the patient. (Touch can be misinterpreted as a threatening or sexual gesture. This is particularly true for a patient with paranoia.)
5. If the patient is unable to respond verbally or in a coherent manner, spend frequent, short periods with him or her. (An interested presence can provide a sense of being worthwhile and of safety.)
6. Structure times each day to include brief interactions and activities with the patient on a one-on-one basis. (Helps to develop rapport and helps the patient develop a sense of safety in a nonthreatening environment.)
7. If the patient is delusional or hallucinating or is having trouble concentrating, provide very simple, concrete activities (e.g., looking at a picture book with a nurse, family member, or friend; drawing; painting). (Even

simple activities may shift the patient's attention from delusional thinking to reality in the environment.)

8. Structure activities that work at the patient's pace and ability. (The patient can lose interest in activities that are too ambitious, which can increase a sense of failure.)
9. Try to incorporate the strengths and interests the patient had when less impaired into the activities planned. (Increases the likelihood of the patient's participation and enjoyment.)
10. If the patient is experiencing paranoid thoughts, solitary or one-on-one activities that require concentration are appropriate. (The patient is free to choose the level of interaction; however, the concentration can help minimize distressing paranoid thoughts or voices [e.g., chess].)
11. If the patient is very withdrawn, one-on-one activities with a "safe" person initially should be planned. (Learns to feel safe with one person, then gradually might participate in a structured group activity.)
12. As the patient's recovery progresses, gradually provide activities according to level of tolerance, such as simple games with one person; add a third person slowly to "safe" activities; add simple group activities; and then groups in which patients participate more. (Gradually the patient learns to feel safe and competent with increased social demands.)
13. Eventually engage other patients and significant others in social interaction and activities with the patient (e.g., card games, ping-pong, singing, group outings) at the patient's level. (Patient continues to feel safe and competent in a graduated hierarchy of interactions.)
14. Identify the role that anxiety plays in precipitating paranoia, agitation, and aggressiveness. (Increased anxiety can intensify agitation, aggressiveness, and suspiciousness.)
15. Teach the patient to find a quiet space when feeling agitated and work on anxiety-relief exercises (e.g., deep breathing, thought stopping). (Teaches the patient skills in dealing with anxiety and increases sense of control.)
16. Provide opportunities for the patient to learn adaptive social skills such as good eye contact, maintaining appropriate personal space, and using a moderate voice tone in a nonthreatening environment. (Social

skills training helps the patient adapt and function at a higher level in society and increases patient's quality of life. These simple skills might take time for a patient with schizophrenia but can increase both self-confidence and positive responses from others.)

17. Give acknowledgment and recognition for positive steps the patient takes in increasing social skills and appropriate interactions with others. (Recognition and appreciation go a long way toward sustaining and increasing a specific behavior.)

Auditory Hallucinations

A change in the amount or patterning of incoming stimuli accompanied by a diminished, exaggerated, distorted, or impaired response to such stimuli

Due to:

- Schizophrenia
- Panic level of anxiety
- Environmental stressors
- Neurochemical alterations in the brain

Desired Outcome:

The patient will report a cessation of auditory hallucinations.

or

The patient will manage auditory hallucinations effectively.

Assessment/Interventions (Rationales)

1. If auditory hallucinations are suspected, ask the patient directly if he or she is hearing something. (Since hearing voices is a subjective experience and not measurable, directly asking about hallucinations is necessary.)
2. Assess the nature of the hallucinations: Is the content of the hallucination positive (e.g., providing reassurance or praise) or negative (e.g., degrading, insulting, or angry)? (Gaining an understanding of the patient's internal world will help to address the resulting emotions.)
3. Assess whether the voices are commanding the patient to engage in self-harm or to harm others. (Understanding the impact of hallucinations on the patient's feeling of safety or the safety of others is essential in planning precautions.)

4. Let the patient know that although the voices seem real, that you cannot hear them. (Instilling reasonable doubt as to the reality of the voices is supportive when carefully presented.)
5. Explore methods of distraction to reduce the voices. Methods include singing, listening to music, reading, or a hobby such as gardening. (Distraction is an important part of managing auditory hallucinations.)
6. Teach thought-stopping techniques such as simply using the word "Stop!" until the voice(s) subsides. (Self-help methods such as thought-stopping can give the patient a sense of agency. Using the word "stop" can be a distraction from the hallucination.)
7. Help the patient identify the times that the hallucinations are most prevalent and frightening. Keeping a diary of the voices and exploring the impact of stressors on their frequency may help some patients. (Anxiety has been implicated in provoking auditory hallucinations. Identifying triggers provides points of intervention.)
8. Decrease environmental stimuli when possible. (Reduces the potential for anxiety that might trigger hallucinations.)
9. Encourage the patient to test reality by validating hallucinations with trusted others. (Validation provides reassurance and grounding.)
10. Discuss medication management of this distressing symptom. Identify potential adherence issues and encourage the patient to take on the role of self-advocate in this treatment. (Medication adherence is an essential part of reducing auditory hallucinations. Ownership of the illness, its symptoms, and its treatment is essential for recovery.)
11. Educate family and significant others about ways to deal with a patient who is experiencing hallucinations. (Educating others in the patient's environment provides an additional level of safety and security for the patient.)

Altered Thought Processes

A disruption in mental activities in which a person experiences disturbed thinking, reality orientation, problem solving, and judgment

Due to:

- Schizophrenia
- Neurochemical alterations in the brain

Desired Outcome:

The patient will demonstrate an accurate interpretation of the environment, maintain reality orientation, and communicate clearly with others.

Assessment/Interventions (Rationales)

1. Initiate safety measures to protect the patient and others if the patient feels threated by others. (During the acute phase of psychosis, the patient's delusional thinking might put others at risk for self-protection. External controls may be needed.)
2. Attempt to understand the significance of false beliefs to the patient. (Important clues to underlying fears and issues can be found in the patient's seemingly illogical fantasies.)
3. Be aware that the patient's delusions represent the way that he or she experiences reality. (Identifying the patient's experience allows the nurse to understand the patient's feelings.)
4. Identify feelings related to delusions. (When patients believe that they are understood, anxiety might lessen.)
5. Do not argue with the patient's beliefs or try to correct false beliefs using facts. (Arguing will reinforce false beliefs. This will result in the patient feeling even more isolated and misunderstood.)
6. Do not touch the patient unless necessary for care activities (e.g., blood pressure). (A person with psychosis might misinterpret touch as threatening. Patients with altered thought need increased personal space.)
7. Use distraction to minimize the focus on delusional thoughts. For example, engage the patient in cards, simple board games, and arts and crafts projects. (When thinking is focused on reality-based activities, the patient is free from delusional thinking during that time. This helps focus attention externally.)
8. Encourage healthy habits to optimize functioning, such as maintaining a regular sleep pattern, abstaining from alcohol and drug use, maintaining self-care, and adhering to the medication regimen. (Psychotic illness interferes with sleep, results in self-medication,

reduces the completion of ADLs, and reduces medication adherence.)

9. Teach the patient coping skills that minimize troubling thoughts, including talking to a trusted person, phoning a helpline, going to a gym, and thought-stopping techniques. (Self-care strategies promote recovery.)

Nonadherence (Medication)

Lack of follow-through with an agreed-upon medication regimen

Due to:

- Side effects of medication
- Inability to acquire medication
- Financial limitations
- Biochemical alterations in the brain
- Disagreement with medication regimen

Desired Outcome:

The patient will participate in an acceptable medication regimen

Assessment/Interventions (Rationales)

1. Evaluate the medication response and side effects. (Identify drugs and dosages that have increased therapeutic value and decreased side effects.)
2. Convey empathy and support while educating about how to manage side effects so that they are less disruptive. (Reduces patient distress and resulting resistance caused by side effects, increasing the patient's sense of control.)
3. Guide the patient to see areas where medications help meet goals (e.g., eliminate hallucinations). (Seeing that medication helps the patient to achieve goals will increase the motivation for treatment.)
4. Discuss a possible medication change with the patient's medication prescriber. (Patient advocacy and functioning as part of a team are primary nurse roles.)

Altered Family Processes

Due to:

- Deterioration of the health status of a family member
- Situational crisis or transition

- Family role shift
- Developmental crisis or transition
- Psychiatric disorder of a family member

Desired Outcomes:
Family members and significant others will support the ill family member in maintaining optimum health and receive personal support through community resources.

Assessment/Interventions (Rationales)
1. Assess the family's ability to cope (e.g., experience of loss, caregiver burden, needed supports). (The family's needs must be addressed to stabilize the family unit.)
2. Provide an opportunity for the family to discuss feelings related to the ill family member, and identify their immediate concerns. (Nurses and staff can best intervene when they understand the family's experience and needs.)
3. Assess the family's current level of knowledge about the disease and medications used for treatment. (The family might have misconceptions and misinformation about schizophrenia and treatment, or no knowledge at all. Teach at the patient's and family's level of understanding and readiness to learn.)
4. Provide information on the disease and treatment strategies at the family's level of knowledge. (Meet the family members' needs for information.)
5. Inform the patient and family in clear, simple terms about medication therapy: purpose, dosage, the need to take medications as prescribed, side effects, and toxic effects. Give written information to the patient and family members. (Understanding the disease and its treatment encourages greater family support and patient adherence.)
6. Provide information on patient and family community resources after discharge, such as support groups, organizations, day hospitals, psychoeducational programs, and respite centers. (Schizophrenia is an overwhelming disease for both the patient and family. Agencies, support groups, and psychoeducational centers can help.)
7. Teach the patient and family the warning symptoms of potential relapse. (Rapid recognition of early warning symptoms can help ward off potential relapse when immediate medical attention is sought.)

TREATMENT FOR SCHIZOPHRENIA SPECTRUM DISORDERS

Biological Approaches

Pharmacological Therapy

Prior to the 1950s there were no effective medications for the treatment of the often dramatic symptoms of schizophrenia spectrum disorders. Since then, a variety of drugs have been introduced that address both positive and negative symptoms. A combination of antipsychotic medications along with psychosocial support provide symptom control and allow most people with these disorders to live and be treated in the community. See Chapter 22 for information about antipsychotic medications.

Brain Stimulation Therapy

Several brain stimulation therapies are used in treating the symptoms associated with schizophrenia spectrum disorders. Electroconvulsive therapy is used successfully for treatment-resistant schizophrenia along with clozapine (an antipsychotic) with relatively minor side effects (Kaster et al., 2017). Deep brain stimulation, a surgical procedure involving the implantation of a thin flexible wire into the brain, has been used successfully in treating the negative symptoms of schizophrenia (American Association of Neurological Surgeons, 2017). Repetitive transcranial magnetic stimulation has shown promise in relieving positive and negative symptoms of schizophrenia, particularly auditory hallucinations (Cole et al., 2015). See Chapter 30 for more discussion of brain stimulation therapies.

Psychotherapeutic Approaches

A variety of psychotherapeutic approaches are utilized to address the needs of individuals and families who are affected by a schizophrenia spectrum disorder. A brief overview of these approaches is identified here. Chapter 29 provides more detail about specific therapies.

Individual Therapy

Supportive therapy that includes problem-solving techniques and social skills training helps reduce relapse and enhance social and occupational functioning. It works especially well when combined with medication treatment. Cognitive–behavioral therapy (CBT), cognitive rehabilitation, and social skills training are particularly helpful in people with chronic schizophrenia who have cognitive impairments.

Family Intervention

Families with a member who has schizophrenia endure considerable hardships while coping with the psychotic and residual symptoms of schizophrenia. Often families are the sole caretakers of an individual with schizophrenia and need education, guidance, support, and training to help them manage. Psychoeducational, family, group, and behavioral approaches can help patients increase their social skills, maximize their ability in self-care and independent living, maintain medical adherence, and, most important, increase their quality of life. Patient and family education greatly improves the management of schizophrenia. Families can be helped through several approaches:

- Understanding the disease and the role of medications
- Setting realistic goals for the family member with schizophrenia
- Developing problem-solving skills for handling tensions and misunderstanding within the family environment
- Identifying early signs of relapse
- Having knowledge of where they can go for guidance and support within the community and nationally

Group Therapy

The goals of group therapy are to increase problem-solving ability, enable realistic goal planning, facilitate social interactions, and manage medication side effects. Groups can help patients develop interpersonal skills, work on family problems, and use community supports, as well as increase medication adherence by teaching patients to deal with troubling side effects.

The Recovery Model

The recovery model is based on the principle that recovery has many pathways, and each person is unique; treatment needs to be personalized and holistic. The recovery model includes support by peers and allies as well as through relationships and social networks. Because patients are from different backgrounds and cultural subgroups, recovery needs to be culturally based.

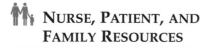

Nurse, Patient, and Family Resources

Brain and Behavior Research Foundation
www.bbrfoundation.org

National Alliance on Mental Illness (NAMI)
www.nami.org

Schizophrenia and Related Disorders Alliance of America (SARDAA)
https:sardaa.org

Schizophrenia.com
www.schizophrenia.com

Schizophrenic.com
www.schizophrenic.com

CHAPTER 6

Bipolar Disorders

Bipolar spectrum disorders are among the most serious of the neurobiological psychiatric disorders. They often result in the loss of partners, families, friendships, employment, and financial security.

Bipolar disorders consist of diagnoses that are characterized by one or more episodes of mania or hypomania and usually one or more depressive episodes.

- Mania is a period of intense mood disturbance with persistent elevation, expansiveness, irritability, and extreme goal-directed activity or energy. These periods last at least 1 week for most of the day, every day. An acute manic phase usually requires hospitalization to protect and stabilize the patient.
- Hypomania refers to a low-level and less dramatic mania. The hypomania of bipolar II disorder tends to be euphoric and often increases functioning. Psychosis is never present in hypomania, and hospitalization is rarely necessary.
- A depressive episode is a sustained (2 weeks or more) depressed mood and/or a loss of interest or pleasure in everyday activities. Concentration and decision-making are usually impaired. People with depression feel empty, hopeless, anxious, worthless, guilty, and/or irritable. The depression in people with a bipolar disorder can be profound and dangerous because of suicidal ideation and the potential for psychotic symptoms.

The bipolar spectrum consists of three main disorders: (1) cyclothymia, (2) bipolar I, and (3) bipolar II. Additional associated disorders are the result of other problems. They are substance- or medication-induced bipolar disorder and bipolar disorder related to another medical condition.

CYCLOTHYMIA

Cyclothymia is a chronic mood disturbance that lasts 2 years or more. Symptoms of hypomania alternate with depression, but these symptoms do not meet the full diagnostic criteria for hypomania or major depressive disorder. People with cyclothymia do not have severe impairment in their social or occupational functioning, nor do they experience psychotic symptoms such as delusions.

BIPOLAR I

Bipolar I consists of one or more periods of clear-cut mania. Prior to or following the manic episode, individuals may experience a hypomanic or major depressive episode. For this diagnosis, the manic episode must last for at least 1 week.

Considerable impairment in social, occupational, and interpersonal functioning exists. Hospitalization is often required to protect the person from the consequences of poor judgment and hyperactivity.

BIPOLAR II

Bipolar II consists of at least one hypomanic episode *and* a major depressive episode. Psychosis is never present in hypomania but may be a feature of the depressed episode. The hypomanic episode must last at least 4 days, while the major depressive episode must last 2 weeks.

PHASES OF BIPOLAR DISORDER

Bipolar I disorder can be grouped into three phases:

1. Acute phase: Hospitalization is usually indicated for patients in the acute manic phase of bipolar disorder. Hospitalization protects patients from harm (e.g., exhaustion, financial loss) and allows time for medication stabilization.
2. Continuation phase (continuation of treatment): Usually lasts for 4 to 9 months, and the goal during this phase is to prevent relapse.
3. Maintenance treatment phase: Aimed at preventing the recurrence of an episode of bipolar illness.

Many of the interventions discussed in this chapter address the patient in the acute phase, because this phase often requires hospitalization and immediate and complex nursing care. For interventions addressing the serious depression associated with the bipolar disorders, see Chapter 7.

ASSESSMENT

Signs and Symptoms

- Periods of hyperactivity (pacing, restlessness, accelerated actions)
- Overconfident, exaggerated view of own abilities
- Decreased need for sleep; no acknowledgment of fatigue
- Increased energy
- Poor social judgment, engaging in reckless and self-destructive activities (risky business ventures, sexual indiscretions spending sprees)
- Rapid speech, pressured speech, loud talking, rhyming or punning
- Brief attention span, easily distractible, flight of ideas, loose associations
- Expansive, irritable, or paranoid behaviors
- Impatient, uncooperative, abusive, obscene, manipulative

Assessment Tools

The Altman Self-Rating Mania Scale (ASRM) (Altman et al., 1997) is a five-item scale to assess the presence or severity of symptoms of mania over the past 7 days. The individual can complete the scale or, if he or she is too impaired to complete the form, a knowledgeable friend, family member, or clinician can do so. See Table 6.1 for the rating scale.

Assessment Guidelines

Manic Phase

1. Assess whether the patient is a danger to self or others (see Table 6.2 for the continuum of mania):
   - Patients with mania can exhaust themselves.
   - The patient might not eat or sleep for days at a time.
   - Poor impulse control might result in harm to others or self.
   - Uncontrolled spending can leave individuals and their families destitute.
2. Patients might give away all of their money or possessions and thus might need controls to protect them from financial ruin.

3. Assess for the need for hospitalization to safeguard and stabilize the patient.
4. Assess the patient's medical status. A thorough medical examination helps determine whether mania is primary or secondary. Mania can be either of the following:
   - Secondary to a general medical condition
   - Substance induced (use of a drug or medication or toxin exposure)
5. Assess the patient's and family's understanding of bipolar disorder and knowledge of medications, support groups, and organizations that provide information on bipolar disorder.

Table 6.1 **Altman Self-Rating Mania Scale**

Choose the one statement in each group that best describes the way you (the individual receiving care) have been feeling for **the past week.**

Points		Score
	Question 1	
1	I do not feel happier or more cheerful than usual.	
2	I occasionally feel happier or more cheerful than usual.	
3	I often feel happier or more cheerful than usual.	
4	I feel happier or more cheerful than usual most of the time.	
5	I feel happier or more cheerful than usual all of the time.	
	Question 2	
1	I do not feel more self-confident than usual.	
2	I occasionally feel more self-confident than usual.	
3	I often feel more self-confident than usual.	
4	I frequently feel more self-confident than usual.	
5	I feel extremely self-confident all of the time.	
	Question 3	
1	I do not need less sleep than usual.	
2	I occasionally need less sleep than usual.	
3	I often need less sleep than usual.	
4	I frequently need less sleep than usual.	
5	I can go all day and all night without any sleep and still not feel tired.	

Table 6.1 **Altman Self-Rating Mania Scale—cont'd**

Points		Score
	Question 4	
1	I do not talk more than usual.	
2	I occasionally talk more than usual.	
3	I often talk more than usual.	
4	I frequently talk more than usual.	
5	I talk constantly and cannot be interrupted.	
	Question 5	
1	I have not been more active (either socially, sexually, at work, home, or school) than usual.	
2	I have occasionally been more active than usual.	
3	I have often been more active than usual.	
4	I have frequently been more active than usual.	
5	I am constantly more active or on the go all the time.	

Reprinted by permission of Elsevier from Altman, E.G., Hedeker, D., Peterson, J.L., & Davis, J.M. (1997). The Altman Self-Rating Mania Scale. *Biological Psychiatry* 42, 948–955, by the Society of Biological Psychiatry.

Table 6.2 **Mania on a Continuum**

Hypomania	Acute Mania
Communication	
1. Talks and jokes incessantly, is life of the party, and gets irritated when not center of attention.	1. Mood is labile—may change suddenly from laughing to anger or sadness.
2. Far more outgoing and sociable as usual	2. Inappropriately demanding of people's attention; intrusive
3. Talk is often sexual, can be obscene, inappropriate propositions to strangers.	3. Speech may contain profanities and crude sexual remarks.
4. Jumps from one topic to the next; marked by pressured speech.	4. Flight of ideas, jumps from topic to topic, complains of racing thoughts.

Continued

Table 6.2 **Mania on a Continuum—cont'd**

Hypomania	Acute Mania
Affect and Thinking	
1. Full of energy and humor, feelings of euphoria and sociability.	1. Humor gives way to irritability and hostility and short-lived periods of rage, especially when not getting his or her way or when limits are set for behaviors. Mood may shift from hostile to calm.
2. Increase in goal-directed activity and planning; may be more creative.	2. Delusional thinking may result in grandiose plans and schemes or paranoid plans for protection.
3. Judgment often poor, but usually not severe enough for hospitalization.	3. Judgment is so poor hospitalization is often necessary.
4. May write large quantities of mail or make calls to famous people regarding schemes.	4. May attempt to contact famous people; severe mania may interfere with planning.
5. Decreased attention span to internal and external cues.	5. Decreased attention span and distractibility are intensified.
Physical Behavior	
1. Overactive, distractible, buoyant, and busily occupied with grandiose plans; goes from one action to the next.	1. Extremely restless and chaotic. May have outbursts such as throwing things. May be dangerous, disoriented, and agitated.
2. Increased sexual appetite; sexually irresponsible and indiscreet. Illegitimate pregnancies in hypomanic women and sexually transmitted disease may occur.	2. No time for sex—too busy. Poor concentration, distractibility, and restlessness are severe.
3. May have voracious appetite, eat on the run, or gobble food during brief periods.	3. No time to eat—too distracted and disorganized.
4. May go without sleeping; feels rested after 3 hours of sleep. However, may be able to take short naps.	4. No time for sleep—psychomotor activity too high.
5. Financially extravagant, goes on spending sprees, gives money and gifts away freely, can easily go into debt.	5. Same as in hypomania, but in the extreme.

Patient Problems

Because of the patient's poor judgment, excessive and constant motor activity, probable dehydration, and difficulty evaluating reality, the patient has a *potential for injury*. Aggression is a common feature in mania; therefore addressing the problem of *potential for violence* is essential.

Because of the patient's grandiose thinking, extremely poor judgment, and hyperactivity, *impulsivity* is usually part of the picture. Distorted thinking and impaired reality testing make *altered thought processes* an essential part of the plan of care. Patients have limited ability to engage in social activities, making *impaired social functioning* an appropriate focus of nursing care. Diminished levels of self-care in hygiene, dressing, feeding, and toileting due to mania is addressed with the patient problem of *impaired activities of daily living*.

Intervention Guidelines

Specific behaviors demonstrated by patients with mania should be addressed separately, as follows in this chapter. Overall guidelines that are effective with bipolar patients during periods of mania include the following:

1. Use a firm and calm approach.
2. Use short, concise explanations or statements.
3. Remain neutral; avoid power struggles.
4. Provide a consistent and structured environment.
5. Firmly redirect energy into appropriate and constructive channels.
6. Decrease environmental stimuli whenever possible.
7. Provide structured solitary activities; tasks that take minimal concentration are best. Avoid groups and stimulating activities until the patient can tolerate that level of activity.
8. Spend one-on-one time with the patient if he or she is psychotic or anxious.
9. Provide frequent rest periods.
10. Provide high-calorie fluids and finger foods frequently throughout the day.
11. Monitor the following:
    - Sleep pattern
    - Food intake
    - Elimination (constipation is a common problem)

12. Teach the patient and family about the illness, and be sure the patient has written information regarding his or her medications.
13. Ascertain that the patient and family have information on supportive services in their community for further information and support.

Nursing Care for Mania

The following sections identify primary patient problems for use with a patient who is experiencing mania, particularly in the acute and severely manic phases of the illness.

Potential for Injury

Due to:
- Biochemical dysfunction
- Cognitive, affective, and psychomotor factors
- Alteration in cognitive functioning
- Alteration in psychomotor functioning
- Compromised nutrition
- Malnutrition
- Alteration in affective orientation

Desired Outcome
The patient will be free from injury.

Assessment/Interventions (Rationales)
1. Maintain a low level of stimuli in the patient's environment (e.g., away from loud noises, bright lights, and people). (Helps decrease the escalation of anxiety.)
2. Provide structured solitary activities with a nurse or aide. (Structure provides security and focus.)
3. Provide frequent high-calorie fluids. (Nutritional status may be compromised due to lack of interest in food and liquids. Regularly offering fluids increases the success of acceptance.)
4. Provide frequent rest periods in a darkened room even if sleep is not possible. (Prevents exhaustion.)
5. Redirect aggressive behavior and encourage exercise. (Physical exercise can decrease tension and provide focus.)
6. Provide prescribed as-needed antipsychotic or antianxiety agents. (Exhaustion, dehydration, lack of sleep, and

increased confusion are the result of constant physical activity. Medication will reduce this activity.)
7. Observe for signs of lithium toxicity. (There is a small margin of safety between therapeutic and toxic doses.)
8. Hold valuables in the hospital safe or send them home. (Protect the patient from giving away money and possessions.)

Potential for Violence

Due to:
- Alteration in cognitive functioning
- Impulsiveness
- Excessive energy and agitation
- Delusional thinking

Desired Outcome
The patient will refrain from assaultive, combative, or destructive behaviors toward others.

Assessment/Interventions (Rationales)
1. Use a calm and firm approach. (Provides structure and control for a patient who is out of control.)
2. Use short and concise explanations or statements. (A short attention span limits comprehension to small bits of information.)
3. Maintain a consistent approach, employ consistent expectations, and provide a structured environment. (Clear and consistent limits and expectations minimize the potential for the patient to manipulate the staff.)
4. Remain neutral: Avoid power struggles and value judgments. (The patient can use inconsistencies and value judgments as justification for arguing which may result in escalating mania.)
5. Decrease environmental stimuli (keep away from loud music and noises, people, and bright lights). (A calm environment decreases the escalation of anxiety and manic symptoms.)
6. Assess the patient's behavior frequently (e.g., every 15 minutes) for signs of increased agitation and hyperactivity. (Early detection and intervention of escalating mania might help prevent harm to the patient or others and decrease the need for seclusion.)

7. Redirect agitation with physical outlets in area of low stimulation (e.g., punching bag, exercise bike). (Relieves agitation and muscle tension.)
8. Alert staff if the potential for restraint or seclusion appears imminent. The usual priority of interventions is (1) setting limits, (2) encouraging time out, (3) offering as-needed medication, and (4) restraint or seclusion. (A team approach to aggression is essential. Always use the least restrictive intervention when intervening with potentially violent behavior.)
9. Document the patient behaviors, interventions, what seemed to escalate agitation, what helped to calm agitation, if and when as-needed medications were given and their effect, and what proved most helpful. (Documentation provides staff with guidelines for future interventions.)

Impulsivity

Due to:
- Alteration in cognitive functioning
- Mania

Desired Outcome

The patient will demonstrate self-restraint of impulsive behaviors.

Assessment/Interventions (Rationales)

1. Administer an antimanic medication and as-needed antianxiety agents or antipsychotics, as ordered, and evaluate for efficacy, side effects, and toxic effects. (Bipolar spectrum disorders are caused by biochemical imbalances in the brain. Medication is effective in stabilizing dysregulated mood.)
2. Observe for destructive behavior toward self or others. Intervene in the early phases of escalation of manic behavior. (Hostile verbal behaviors, poor impulse control, and violent acting out against others or property are seen in acute mania. (Early detection and intervention can prevent harm to the patient or others in the environment.)
3. Have valuables, credit cards, and cash sent home with family or put in the hospital safe until the patient is discharged. (During manic episodes, individuals may give

away valuables and money indiscriminately to strangers, often leaving themselves in debt.)
4. Maintain a firm, calm, and neutral approach at all times. Avoid power struggles and arguing. (Professional behavior by the staff will reduce the chance for conflict and escalation.)
5. Provide hospital legal service when and if a patient is involved in making or signing important legal documents during an acute manic phase. (Judgment and reality testing are both impaired during acute mania. Patients might need legal advice and protection against making important decisions that are not in their best interest.)
6. Assess and recognize early signs of manipulative behavior and intervene appropriately. (Consistently setting limits is important when intervening in manipulative behaviors.)

Altered Thought Processes

Due to:
- Mania
- Disruption in cognitive operations and activities
- Sleep deprivation
- Biochemical alterations

Desired Outcome
The patient will sustain concentration and attention to complete tasks and function independently.

Assessment/Interventions (Rationales)
1. Meet with the patient for short periods each day. (Short, consistent meetings help establish contact and decrease anxiety.)
2. Convey acceptance of the patient's need for a false belief; at the same time, let the patient know that you do not share the belief. (Acceptance will help to develop rapport and support the patient. Expressing reasonable doubt is a good first step in challenging delusions.)
3. Explore the content of hallucinations. (Understanding the content of auditory hallucinations helps to determine whether they are dangerous [e.g., command hallucinations telling the patient to harm someone].)
4. Decrease environmental stimuli if possible. Respond to cues of increased agitation by removing stimuli. A

private room may be helpful. (Disturbed thought processes are challenging enough for the patient. Reducing a stressful environment will help to decrease agitation and confusion.)

5. Reinforce reality by talking about actual events and topics such as unit activities. (Engaging the patient into reality and present issues can increase a here-and-now focus.)

Impaired Social Functioning

Due to:

- Disturbance in thought processes
- Biochemical disturbances in the brain
- Excessive hyperactivity and agitation
- Mania

Desired Outcome

The patient will participate in unit activities without disruption or demonstrating inappropriate behavior.

Assessment/Interventions (Rationales)

1. When possible, provide an environment with minimal stimuli (e.g., quiet, soft music; dim lighting). (Reduction in stimuli lessens distractibility.)
2. Initially, suggest solitary activities that require a short attention span with mild physical exertion (e.g., writing, painting [finger painting, murals], woodworking, or walks with staff). (Solitary activities minimize stimuli; mild physical activities release tension constructively.)
3. When less manic, encourage the patient to join one or two other patients in quiet, nonstimulating activities (e.g., board games, drawing, cards). *Avoid competitive games.* (As mania subsides, involvement in activities that provide focus and social contact becomes more appropriate. Competitive games can stimulate aggression and increase psychomotor activity.)

Impaired Activities of Daily Living

Due to:

- Alteration in cognitive functioning
- Hyperactivity

Desired Outcome

The patient will conduct optimal self-care activities based on personal abilities.

Assessment/Interventions (Rationales)

Insufficient Nutritional Intake

1. Monitor intake and output. (Supports interventions for adequate fluid and caloric intake; minimizes dehydration.)
2. Encourage frequent high-calorie protein drinks and finger foods (e.g., sandwiches, fruit, milkshakes). (Constant fluid and calorie replacement are needed. The patient might be too active to sit at meals. Finger foods allow for "eating on the run.")
3. Frequently remind the patient to eat (e.g., "Tom, finish your milkshake." "Sally, eat this banana."). (The patient is unaware of bodily needs is easily distracted and requires supervision to eat.)

Sleep Pattern Disturbance

4. Encourage frequent rest periods during the day. (Lack of sleep can lead to exhaustion and exacerbate manic symptoms.)
5. Keep the patient in areas of low stimulation. (Promotes relaxation and reduces manic behavior.)
6. At night, encourage warm baths, soothing music, and medication when indicated. Avoid giving the patient caffeine. (Promotes relaxation, rest, and sleep.)

Dressing or Grooming Problems

7. If warranted, supervise the choice of clothes; minimize bizarre dress and sexually suggestive clothing. (Lessens the potential for inappropriate attention, which can increase level of mania, or ridicule, which lowers self-esteem. Assists patient in maintaining dignity.)
8. Give simple step-by-step reminders for hygiene and dress (e.g., "Here is your razor. Shave the left side … now the right side." "Here is your toothbrush. Put the toothpaste on the brush."). (Distractibility and poor concentration are countered by simple, concrete instructions.)

Constipation

9. Monitor bowel habits; offer fluids and foods that are high in fiber. Evaluate the need for a laxative. Encourage

the patient to go to the bathroom. (Promotes regular toileting. Prevents fecal impaction resulting from dehydration and decreased peristalsis.)

TREATMENT FOR BIPOLAR DISORDERS

Biological Approaches

Pharmacological Therapy

Patients with bipolar disorder often resist medication. Many patients want to maintain the higher level of energy, creativity, and confidence. Unfortunately, if left untreated, the high invariably deteriorates into a more disastrous mania or painful depression. Chapter 23 provides an overview of mood stabilizers along with treatment for bipolar depression.

Brain Stimulation Therapy

Electroconvulsive therapy (ECT) is a primary consideration when a patient is unable to wait until a medication starts to become effective, cannot tolerate one of the first-line medications listed earlier, or does not respond to the first-line medications. ECT has been found especially effective with rapid-cycling patients (those who suffer four or more episodes of illness per year), as well as those with paranoid-destructive features that often respond poorly to lithium therapy. ECT should be considered for severe mania and those in highly agitated states. ECT should also be considered for pregnant women. See Chapter 30 for an overview of ECT.

Psychotherapeutic Approaches

The primary goal of all therapies is to reduce the patient's distress, improve the patient's ability to function between episodes, and decrease the frequency of future episodes. Because of the behaviors associated with the disorder, there are usually severe psychosocial consequences from past episodes. Many patients do not fully recover between episodes. Therefore it becomes clear that additional psychotherapeutic treatments are necessary along with medications.

The most successful approach in therapy is one that enforces clear limits. A number of psychotherapeutic approaches can be helpful to some patients. Group and family therapy focuses on acceptance of the disease, the need for long-term medication treatment, and medication teaching. Therapy with medication-stabilized patients includes cognitive–behavioral therapy and psychoeducation.

See Chapter 23 for more information on mood stabilizing medications.

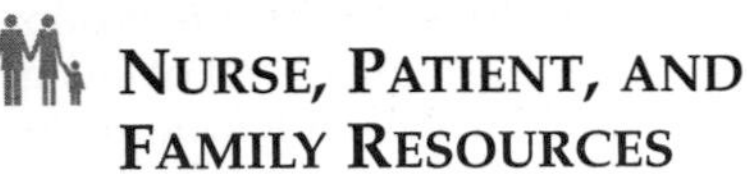

Nurse, Patient, and Family Resources

Bipolar Disorder Guide
www.bipolar.about.com

Bipolar Disorder Page
www.mentalhelp.net (search Bipolar)

Bipolar Support
www.bipolarsupport.org

Depression and Bipolar Support Alliance
www.dbsalliance.org

National Alliance on Mental Illness (NAMI)
www.nami.org

National Institute of Mental Health
www.nimh.nih.gov

CHAPTER 7

Depressive Disorders

Happiness and unhappiness are appropriate responses to life events. When sadness, grief, or elation is extremely intense and the mood prolonged, a depressive disorder may be the cause.

Depressive symptoms often coexist in people with alcohol or substance use problems. Depressive symptoms are common in people who have other psychiatric disorders such as anxiety disorders, eating disorders, personality disorders, and schizophrenia. Depression is highly comorbid in individuals who have been physically or mentally abused. Depression might also be a critical symptom of another medical disorder or condition such as hepatitis, mononucleosis, multiple sclerosis, dementia, cancer, diabetes, or chronic pain.

The two *Diagnostic and Statistical Manual of Mental Disorders,* fifth edition *(DSM-5)* (American Psychiatric Association, 2013) depressive disorders discussed here are major depressive disorder and persistent depressive disorder (dysthymia).

MAJOR DEPRESSIVE DISORDER

In major depressive disorder, a severely depressed mood, usually recurrent, causes clinically significant distress or impairment in social, occupational, or other important areas of the person's life. The depressed mood can be distinguished from the person's usual functioning and might occur suddenly or gradually.

Major depression involves changes in receptor neurotransmitter relationships in the limbic system, prefrontal cortex, hippocampus, and amygdala. The primary neurotransmitters involved with depression are serotonin and norepinephrine, although dopamine is also related to depression. Genetic factors and biochemical and brain scans also reveal anomalies in some individuals suffering from depression.

People with major depression may have other problems, such as the following:

- Anxious distress: Feeling tense, restless, fearful (e.g., something bad might happen, loss of control), worrying, poor concentration
- Psychotic features: delusions or hallucinations
- Catatonia: for example, peculiarities of voluntary movement, motor immobility, purposeless motor activity, echolalia, or echopraxia
- Melancholic features: severe symptoms, loss of feelings of pleasure, exacerbation in morning, early morning awakening, significant weight loss, excessive feelings of guilt
- Peripartum onset: during pregnancy or within 4 weeks of delivery
- Seasonal pattern: most prominent during certain seasons (e.g., winter or summer); more prevalent in climates with longer periods of darkness in a 24-hour cycle

Epidemiology

Major depressive disorder is the leading cause of disability in the United States. In 2014 it affected approximately 16 million adults in the United States, or nearly 7% of the population (Center for Behavioral Health Statistics and Quality, 2015). Nearly 3 million (about 11%) individuals between 13 and 18 years of age experienced depression in 2014. Beginning in early adolescence, females are more likely than males to be affected by depression at a rate of 1:2.

About 1% to 5% of older adults who live in the community have depression. This statistic rises to 11.5% of hospitalized older adults and 13.5% for those requiring home care (National Institute of Mental Health, 2012). A disproportionate number of older adults with depression are likely to die by suicide.

The length of a depressive episode may be 5 to 6 months (McInnis et al., 2014). About 20% of cases become chronic (i.e., lasting more than 2 years). Although depression begins with a single occurrence, most people experience recurrent episodes. People experience a recurrence within the first year about 50% of the time and within a lifetime up to 85% of the time.

The high variability in symptom manifestation, response to treatment, and course of the illness supports the supposition that depression may result from a complex

Box 7.1 Primary Risk Factors for Depression

- Female sex
- Adverse childhood experiences
- Stressful life events
- First-degree family members with major depressive disorder
- Neuroticism (a negative personality trait characterized by anxiety, fear, moodiness, worry, envy, frustration, jealousy, and loneliness)
- Other disorders such as substance use, anxiety, and personality disorders
- Chronic or disabling medical conditions

interaction of causes. For example, genetic predisposition to the illness combined with childhood stress may lead to significant changes in the central nervous system that result in depression. However, there seem to be several common risk factors for depression. These risk factors are listed in Box 7.1.

PERSISTENT DEPRESSIVE DISORDER (DYSTHYMIA)

Persistent depressive disorder (dysthymia) is characterized by less severe, usually chronic depressive symptoms that have been present for a longer period (e.g., 2 years or longer). The symptoms of persistent depressive disorder are very similar to those of major depression, which makes an accurate diagnosis difficult.

Although the symptoms and functional impairment are not as severe with persistent depressive disorder (dysthymia) as they are in major depressive disorder, symptoms can cause significant distress or impairment in major areas of the person's life. Individuals with dysthymia are usually able to function at work and in social situations, but not at optimal levels. There are no psychotic symptoms in people with persistent depressive disorder.

The prevalence of persistent depressive disorder ranges from 0.5% to 1.5%. The problem tends to have an early onset and, as the name suggests, it is a chronic illness.

Assessment

Signs and Symptoms

- Mood of sadness, despair, emptiness
- Diminished interest or pleasure in almost all activities (anhedonia)
- Vegetative signs: alterations in eating, sleeping, activity level (fatigue), and libido
- Agitated symptoms: anger, irritability, rumination (i.e., overthinking things), pacing
- Feelings of worthlessness or guilt
- Difficulty with concentration, memory, and making decisions
- Recurrent thoughts of death or self-harm
- Apathy, low motivation, and social withdrawal
- Excessive emotional sensitivity
- Possibly complaints of pain, such as backache or headache, that does not seem to have a physical cause

Assessment Tools

Many useful tools are available to assess for depression. The PROMIS Emotional Distress–Depression short form is an excellent screening tool (Fig. 7.1). Professionals using this tool use sophisticated scoring methods. For our purposes, higher scores may indicate depression and the need for follow-up.

Assessment Guidelines

1. A thorough physical and neurological examination helps determine whether the depression is primary or secondary to another disorder. Depression is a mood that can be secondary to many medical or other psychiatric disorders, as well as drugs or medications. Essentially, the nurse evaluates whether the following are evident:
   - The patient is experiencing a psychosis
   - The patient has ingested drugs or alcohol
   - Medical conditions are present
2. Always evaluate the patient's risk for harm to self or others. Overt hostility is highly correlated with suicide.

PROMIS Emotional Distress—Depression—Short Form

							Use
In the past SEVEN (7) DAYS....							Item Score
		Never	Rarely	Sometimes	Often	Always	
1.	I felt worthless.	☐ 1	☐ 2	☐ 3	☐ 4	☐ 5	
2.	I felt that I had nothing to look forward to.	☐ 1	☐ 2	☐ 3	☐ 4	☐ 5	
3.	I felt helpless.	☐ 1	☐ 2	☐ 3	☐ 4	☐ 5	
4.	I felt sad.	☐ 1	☐ 2	☐ 3	☐ 4	☐ 5	
5.	I felt like a failure.	☐ 1	☐ 2	☐ 3	☐ 4	☐ 5	
6.	I felt depressed.	☐ 1	☐ 2	☐ 3	☐ 4	☐ 5	
7.	I felt unhappy.	☐ 1	☐ 2	☐ 3	☐ 4	☐ 5	
8.	I felt hopeless.	☐ 1	☐ 2	☐ 3	☐ 4	☐ 5	
						Total Score	

Fig. 7.1 PROMIS Emotional Distress–Depression Short Form.

Patient Problems

Depression can drastically affect many areas of a person's life. Due to the potential for lethal consequences, *potential for suicide* is the first priority for assessment and intervention. Poor concentration, lack of judgment, and difficulties with memory can all affect a person's ability to cope with his or her confused thoughts and profound feelings of despair. Therefore *impaired coping* is almost always present. Feelings of self-worth plummet, resulting in *decreased self-esteem,* and the ability to gain strength from usual religious activities dwindle, resulting in *spiritual distress.*

Feelings of hopelessness are common. Most noticeably, the ability to interact and gain solace from others is markedly reduced making *impaired social functioning* a valuable focus. Depression can lead to physical complications such as lack of sleep, change in eating patterns, and change in elimination. Therefore *impaired activities of daily living* is often used in this population.

Intervention Guidelines

1. Convey caring, empathy, and potential for change by spending time with the patient, even in silence, and anticipating the patient's needs.
2. Note that the instillation of hope is a key tool for recovery.
3. Enhance the patient's sense of self by highlighting past accomplishments and strengths.
4. Whether in the hospital or in the community, the following are important:
   - Assess the patient's needs for self-care, and offer support when appropriate.
   - Monitor and intervene to help the patient maintain adequate nutrition, hydration, and elimination.
   - Monitor and intervene to help provide an adequate balance of rest, sleep, and activity.
   - Monitor and record increases and decreases in symptoms and which nursing interventions are effective.
   - Involve the patient's support system, and find supports for the patient and family members in the community that are appropriate to their needs.
5. The dysfunctional attitude or learned helplessness and hopelessness seen with depressed individuals can be alleviated through cognitive-behavioral techniques.
6. Continually assess for the possibility of suicidal thoughts and ideation throughout the patient's course of recovery.
7. Primary depression is a medical disease. People respond well to psychopharmacology and electroconvulsive therapy (ECT). Be sure patients and those closely involved with them understand the nature of the disease and have written information about the specific medications the patient is taking. Education and a support system are essential.
8. Assess the family's and significant other's needs for teaching, counseling, self-help groups, and knowledge of community resources.

Nursing Care Plans for Major Depressive Disorder

Potential for Suicide

Due to:

- Depressive disorders
- Physical health problems
- Hopelessness
- Helplessness
- Loss
- Suicidal ideation
- Suicide plan
- Lack of personal resources (e.g., coping skills, insight, judgment)
- Lack of social resources (e.g., socially isolated, unresponsive family)
- Conflictual interpersonal relationships

Desired Outcome

The patient will be free from self-harm.

Assessment/Interventions (Rationales)

1. Monitor periodically or continually depending on the level of suicidal ideation. (Patients with active suicidal thoughts, particularly with a plan, should be placed on 1:1 observation.)
2. Determine the level of suicide precautions needed. If high, does the patient need hospitalization? If low, will the patient be safe to go home with supervision from a friend or family member? (A high-risk patient will need constant supervision and a safe environment.)
3. Depending on the medication, determine whether the patient has more than 1 week's supply of medication. (Most commonly prescribed antidepressants, such as the selective serotonin reuptake inhibitors [SSRIs], are rarely fatal in overdose. Some other medications, such as the tricyclics, are more dangerous. Limiting supplies for more lethal medications is essential.)
4. Encourage the patient to talk freely about feelings (anger, disappointments), and help the patient plan alternative ways to handle anger and frustration. (The patient can learn alternative coping methods for dealing with overwhelming emotions and gain a sense of control over his or her life.)

5. Develop a safety plan with the patient for dealing with feelings of intense hopelessness and despair. (Reinforces actions the patient can take when feeling suicidal.)
6. Contact the patient's family and arrange for crisis counseling. Activate links to self-help groups. (Patients need a network of resources to help diminish personal feelings of worthlessness, isolation, and helplessness.)

Impaired Coping

Due to:

- Neurobiological imbalances
- Inability to deal with stressors
- Inadequate resources
- Overwhelming life circumstances
- Prolonged grief reaction
- Pathological fatigue, lack of motivation
- Inadequate social support

Desired Outcome

The patient will:

- Demonstrate adaptive coping strategies
- Report a return to a pre-illness level of functioning

Assessment/Interventions (Rationales)

1. Identify the patient's previous level of cognitive functioning (from the patient, family, friends, and medical records). (Establishing a baseline of ability allows for evaluation of the patient's progress.)
2. Encourage the postponement of important major life decisions. (Requires optimal functioning.)
3. Minimize the patient's responsibilities while he or she is severely depressed. (This will decrease feelings of pressure and anxiety and minimize feelings of guilt.)
4. Use simple, concrete words. (Slowed thinking and difficulty concentrating impair comprehension.)
5. Allow the patient plenty of time to think and frame responses. (Slowed thinking necessitates time to formulate a response.)
6. Help the patient and significant others structure an environment that can help reestablish set schedules and predictable routines during severe depression. (A routine that is fairly repetitive and nondemanding is easier to both follow and remember.)

7. Allow more time than usual for the patient to finish the usual activities of daily living, such as dressing and eating. (The usual tasks might take a long time; demanding that the patient hurry only increases anxiety and slows the patient's ability to think clearly.)
8. Teach the patient to recognize negative thinking and thoughts. Teach the patient to reframe or refute negative thoughts. (Negative ruminations add to feelings of hopelessness and are part of a depressed person's faulty thought processes. Intervening in this process aids in a healthier and more useful outlook.)

Decreased Self-Esteem

Due to:

Major depressive disorder

- Past failures
- Negative reinforcement from others
- Lack of social support
- Lack of family support
- Negative self-appraisal
- Unrealistic expectations of self

Desired Outcome

The patient will report a positive self-appraisal and optimism for the future.

Assessment/Interventions (Rationales)

1. Work with the patient to identify cognitive distortions that encourage negative self-appraisal. For example, overgeneralizations, self-blame, mind reading, and discounting positive attributes (Cognitive distortions reinforce a negative, inaccurate perception of the self and the world by taking one fact or event and making a general rule of it ["He always"; "I never"], assuming others "do not like me," without any real evidence that assumptions are correct, or focusing on negative qualities.)
2. Teach visualization techniques that help the patient replace negative self-images with more positive thoughts and images. (Promotes a healthier and more realistic self-image by helping the patient choose more positive actions and thoughts.)
3. Work with the patient on areas that he or she would like to improve using problem-solving skills. Evaluate the need for more teaching in this area. (Feelings of low

self-esteem can interfere with the usual problem-solving abilities.)
4. Evaluate the need for assertiveness training to pursue things he or she wants or needs in life. Arrange for training through resources such as community-based programs, personal counseling, and literature. (People with low self-esteem often feel unworthy and have difficulty asking appropriately for what they need and want.)
5. Encourage participation in a support or therapy group where others are experiencing similar thoughts, feelings, and situations. (Participation in such a group can decrease feelings of isolation and provide an atmosphere where positive feedback and a more realistic appraisal of self are available.)

Spiritual Distress

Due to:
- Isolation
- Death or dying of self or others
- Chronic illness of self or others
- Life changes
- Pain
- Lack of purpose and meaning in life
- Questions belief in God or higher power

Desired Outcome

The patient will express deriving comfort and meaning from personal belief system.

Assessment/Interventions (Rationales)
1. Assess what spiritual practices have offered comfort and meaning to the patient's life when not ill. (This assessment will evaluate neglected areas in patient's life that, if reactivated, might add comfort and meaning during a painful depression.)
2. Discuss what has given meaning and comfort to the patient in the past. (When depressed, patients often struggle for meaning in life and reasons to go on when feeling hopeless and despondent.)
3. Encourage the patient to write in a journal every day, expressing daily thoughts and reflections. (Journal writing can help the patient to identify significant personal issues and thoughts and feelings surrounding

spiritual issues. Journal writing is an excellent way to explore deeper meanings of life.)
4. If the patient is unable to write, encourage the use of a tape recorder. (Speaking aloud often helps the patient clarify thinking and explore issues.)
5. Provide information on referrals, when needed, for religious or spiritual information (e.g., readings, programs, tapes, community resources). (When a patient is hospitalized, spiritual tapes and readings can be useful; when the patient is in the community, he or she might express other needs.)
6. Suggest that the spiritual advisor affiliated with the facility contact the patient. (Spiritual advisors in an institution or community [priests, clergy, rabbis, the spiritual advisors congruent with the individual's lifestyle] are familiar with spiritual distress and might offer comfort to the patient.)

Impaired Social Functioning

Due to:
- Negative view of self
- Absence of significant others or peers
- Disturbed thought processes
- Feelings of worthlessness
- Self-concept disturbance
- Fear of rejection
- Anergia (lack of energy) and avolition (lack of motivation)

Desired Outcome

The patient will state and demonstrate progress in the resumption of sustaining relationships with friends and family members

Assessment/Interventions (Rationales)
1. During the most severely depression, involve the patient in one-to-one activity. (One-to-one activities can maximize the potential for interactions while minimizing anxiety levels.)
2. Engage the patient in gross-motor activities that call for limited concentration (e.g., walking). (Physical activities can help relieve tension and might help to elevate mood.)

3. Initially, provide activities that require little concentration (e.g., playing simple card games, looking through a magazine, or drawing). (Concentration and memory are poor in people with depression. Activities that have no "right or wrong" or "winners or losers" minimize opportunities for self-diminishment.)
4. Eventually increase the patient's contacts with others (e.g., first one other, then two others). (Contact with others distracts the patient from self-preoccupation.)
5. Eventually involve the patient in group activities (e.g., dance therapy, art therapy, group discussions). (Socialization decreases feelings of isolation. Genuine regard for others can increase self-worth.)
6. Refer both the patient and family to self-help groups and/or psychoeducational groups within the community. (Both the patient and family can gain tremendous support and insight from people through sharing their experiences and learning more about the disease.)

Impaired Activities of Daily Living

Due to:

- Perceptual or cognitive impairment
- Decreased or lack of motivation (anergia)
- Fatigue
- Severe preoccupation
- Severe anxiety

Desired Outcome

The patient will conduct optimal self-care activities based on personal abilities.

Assessment/Interventions (Rationales)

Insufficient Nutritional Intake

1. Encourage small, high-calorie, high-protein snacks and fluids frequently throughout the day and evening if weight loss exists. (Minimizes weight loss, dehydration, and constipation.)
2. Encourage eating with others. (For many people, eating is a social event. Eating with others increases socialization; decreases the focus on food.)
3. Help the patient to select foods or drinks. (Patients are more likely to eat foods they like.)

4. Weigh the patient weekly, and observe the patient's eating patterns. (Weighing provides the information needed for revising the intervention.)

Sleep Pattern Disturbance

5. Encourage rest periods after activities. (Fatigue can intensify feelings of depression.)
6. Encourage the patient to get up and dress and to stay out of bed during the day. (Minimizing sleep during the day increases the likelihood of sleep at night.)
7. Encourage relaxation measures in the evening (e.g., back massage, warm bath, or warm milk). (These measures induce relaxation and sleep.)
8. Reduce environmental and physical stimulants in the evening; provide decaffeinated coffee, soft lights, soft music, and quiet activities. (Decreasing caffeine and epinephrine levels increases the possibility of sleep.)
9. Teach relaxation exercises. (Besides deeply relaxing the body, relaxation exercises often lead to sleep.)

Bathing or Hygiene Problems

10. Encourage the use of a toothbrush, washcloth, soap, makeup, shaving equipment, and other grooming items. (Being clean and well groomed can temporarily raise self-esteem.)
11. Give step-by-step reminders, such as "Wash the right side of your face, now the left." (Slowed thinking and difficulty concentrating make organizing simple tasks difficult.)

Constipation

12. Monitor intake and output, especially bowel movements. (Many depressed patients are constipated. If this condition is not addressed, fecal impaction can occur.)
13. Offer foods that are high in fiber, and provide periods of exercise. (Intake of fiber and regular exercise stimulate peristalsis and help evacuation of fecal material.)
14. Encourage the intake of nonalcoholic/noncaffeinated fluids (6–8 glasses per day). (Fluids help prevent constipation.)
15. Evaluate the need for laxatives and enemas. (These prevent the occurrence of fecal impaction.)

TREATMENT FOR MAJOR DEPRESSIVE DISORDERS

Biological Approaches

Pharmacological Therapy

Depression is a recurring disorder. More than one half of people with primary depression have multiple episodes. However, the discovery of effective antidepressants has resulted in depression being one of the most treatable disorders. The following has been noted about depression:

- Most patients with depression respond to antidepressant treatment.
- Approximately one fourth to one third of patients with major depression fail to respond meaningfully to currently available treatment.
- Waiting too long to start treatment can lead to the following:
  - Greater morbidity
  - Greater disability
  - Greater expense
  - Greater resistance to treatment and increased potential for relapse

Antidepressant drugs can improve poor self-concept, degree of withdrawal, vegetative signs of depression, and activity level. Refer to Chapter 24 for pharmacology used in the treatment of major depressive disorder.

Brain Stimulation Therapy

Electroconvulsive therapy (ECT) is considered the best treatment for severe (psychotic) depression and for treatment-resistant depression. ECT is useful in treating patients with major depressive and bipolar depressive disorders, especially when psychotic symptoms are present (e.g., delusions of guilt, somatic delusions, or delusions of infidelity). ECT is also indicated in individuals who present with catatonic stupor, severe suicidality, extreme mania, or self-starvation. After a course of ECT, maintenance ECT (once a week to once a month) helps prevent relapse when used in conjunction with an antidepressant.

The following list describes when ECT may be indicated:

- There is a need for a rapid, definitive response when a patient is suicidal or homicidal.

- The patient is in extreme agitation or stupor.
- The patient's life is threatened because of refusal of foods and fluids.
- The patient has a history of poor drug response, a history of good ECT response, or both.
- Standard medical treatment has no effect.

ECT may be contraindicated in patients with various medical conditions. Patients with cardiovascular disease, increased intracranial pressure, or cerebrovascular fragility would be poor candidates and would require a careful pretreatment medical workup.

Vagus nerve stimulation (VNS) is used to treat intractable epilepsy and was approved in 2009 by the U.S. Food and Drug Administration (FDA) as an adjunctive, long-term treatment for patients with treatment-resistant depression. *Treatment-resistant depression* refers to depression in those with chronic or recurrent major depressive disorder who have failed a minimum of four antidepressant medication trials, ECT, or both. See Chapter 30 for a description of VNS.

Rapid transcranial magnetic stimulation (rTMS) applies the principles of electromagnetism to deliver an electrical field to the cerebral cortices. Unlike ECT, the waves do not result in generalized seizure activity. An electrical magnetic coil is placed on the scalp, not implanted. Pulsed high-intensity current passes through the coil, creating powerful magnetic fields that change the way brain cells function. Chapter 30 provides more information related to rTMS.

Complementary and Integrated Therapy

Light therapy is the first-line treatment for seasonal affective disorder (SAD) with or without medication. Full-spectrum wavelength light is the specific type of light used. People with SAD often live in climates with marked seasonal differences in the amount of daylight. Seasonal variations in mood disorders in the Southern Hemisphere are the reverse of those in the Northern Hemisphere. Light therapy also may be useful as an adjunct to medications in treating chronic major depressive disorder or dysthymia with seasonal exacerbations.

St. John's wort *(Hypericum perforatum)* is a whole plant product with antidepressant properties that is not regulated by the FDA. The herb is not to be taken by certain patient populations, such as those who have major depressive disorder or are pregnant. To date, any efficacy is found for people who have mild depression. St. John's wort poses potentially harmful drug interactions that can result in significant toxic effects on the liver. Some drugs that need to be avoided when taking St. John's wort are amphetamines or other stimulants, other antidepressants (monoamine oxidase inhibitors, selective serotonin reuptake inhibitors), warfarin, theophylline, digoxin, and other prescription and over-the-counter drugs.

S-adenosylmethionine (SAMe) is a synthetic form of a chemical produced naturally in the body and is sold as an over-the-counter dietary supplement. SAMe is well tolerated, safe, and effective as an adjunctive treatment in patients with major depressive disorder who are nonresponsive to medications. SAMe should be used with caution in persons with bipolar disorder, because it may induce mania. It should not be taken with any other serotonin-enhancing drugs, because it may increase the risk of serotonin syndrome. Visit http://consumerlab.com for reputable brands of herbal and dietary supplements.

Psychotherapeutic Approaches

Cognitive–behavioral therapy (CBT), interpersonal therapy (IPT), and behavioral therapy have been proven effective in the treatment of depression. However, only CBT and IPT demonstrate superiority in the maintenance phase. CBT helps people change their negative styles of thinking and behaving, whereas IPT focuses on working through personal relationships that may contribute to depression. Outcome research has consistently found that CBT and medication are largely comparable. CBT helps guard against relapse, because people learn skills on how to reshape their thinking and behaviors. See Chapter 29 for more information about models of therapy.

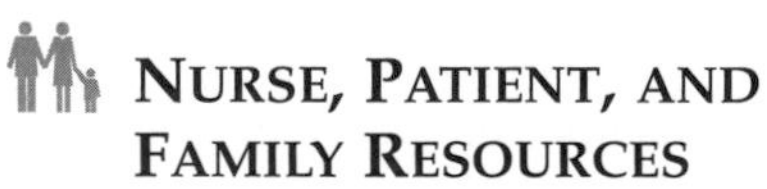

Nurse, Patient, and Family Resources

Depressed Anonymous: Recovery From Depression
www.depressedanon.com

Depression and Bipolar Support Alliance
www.dbsalliance.org

Depression Central
www.psycom.net/depression.central

Internet Mental Health
www.mentalhealth.com

National Alliance on Mental Illness (NAMI)
www.nami.org

National Foundation for Depressive Illness
www.depression.org

National Institute of Mental Health (NIMH): Depression
www.nimh.nih.gov/publicat/depression.cfm

CHAPTER 8

Anxiety and Obsessive–Compulsive Disorders

The negative feelings of anxiety are related to the negative emotion of fear. However, anxiety affects us at a deeper and more profound level. Anxiety is a feeling of apprehension, uneasiness, uncertainty, or dread about future events and the ability to predict or deal with the events. The negative emotion of anxiety results from a threat whose actual source is unknown or unrecognized. Fear, on the other hand, is the emotional response to a clear and current danger.

Anxiety is a normal response to threatening situations. Anxiety is experienced at four levels: mild, moderate, severe, and panic (Peplau, 1968). The boundaries between these levels are not distinct, and the behaviors and characteristics of individuals experiencing anxiety can and often do overlap. Identification of the specific level of anxiety is essential, because interventions are based on the *degree* of the patient's anxiety.

MILD ANXIETY

Mild anxiety occurs in everyday living and allows an individual to perceive reality in sharp focus. In mild anxiety a person sees, hears, and grasps more information, and problem solving becomes more effective. Physical symptoms may include slight discomfort, restlessness, irritability, or mild tension-relieving behaviors (e.g., nail biting, foot or finger tapping, fidgeting).

MODERATE ANXIETY

As anxiety increases, the perceptual field narrows, and details may be excluded from attention. The person sees, hears, and grasps less information and may demonstrate selective inattention. The ability to think clearly is hampered, but learning and problem solving can still take place. Sympathetic nervous system responses result in tension, pounding heart, increased pulse and respiratory rate, perspiration, and mild somatic symptoms (e.g., gastric discomfort, headache, urinary urgency). Voice tremors and shaking may be noticed.

SEVERE ANXIETY

In severe anxiety the perceptual field is greatly reduced. A person may focus on one particular detail or on scattered details. Learning and problem solving are not possible, and the person may be dazed and confused. Behavior is aimed at reducing or relieving anxiety. Symptoms (e.g., headache, nausea, dizziness, insomnia) often increase. Trembling and a pounding heart are common, and the person may hyperventilate or feel doom or dread.

PANIC

Panic results in markedly disturbed behavior. In this state the person is unable to process what is going on in the environment and may lose touch with reality. Behaviors include pacing, running, shouting, screaming, or withdrawal. Hallucinations, or false sensory perceptions (e.g., hearing voices), may be experienced. Physical behavior may become erratic, uncoordinated, and impulsive. Acute panic may lead to exhaustion.

ANXIETY DISORDERS

Anxiety disorders are among the most common of all psychiatric disorders. Individuals with anxiety disorders use rigid, repetitive, and ineffective behaviors to try to control anxiety. The degree of anxiety is so high that it interferes with work, social, and family functions. Anxiety disorders tend to be chronic, persistent, and are often disabling.

People may suffer from more than one anxiety disorder, and anxiety and depression often occur together. Anxiety disorders can be painful for those who experience them. These individuals might self-medicate with alcohol or drugs, and they might be at risk for suicide.

Nurses need to be aware that anxiety can be a symptom of a physical disease, a medical problem, or substance use. Medical causes and drug-induced anxiety must be ruled out before a diagnosis of anxiety disorder can be made. People who have anxiety disorders are usually treated in the community setting. Rarely is hospitalization necessary unless the patient is suicidal or the symptoms are severely out of control, such as self-mutilation.

Anxiety disorders that will be discussed here are:

- Separation anxiety disorder
- Specific phobia
- Social anxiety disorder
- Panic disorder
- Generalized anxiety disorder

An additional group of problems with prominent anxiety features is also addressed in this chapter, the obsessive–compulsive disorders. These disorders are characterized by obsessions, which are recurrent and persistent thoughts, and compulsions, which are repetitive behaviors or mental acts in response to the obsession. They include the following:

- Obsessive–compulsive disorder
- Body dysmorphic disorder
- Hoarding disorder
- Trichotillomania (hair-pulling) disorder
- Excoriation (skin-picking) disorder

SEPARATION ANXIETY DISORDER

Developmentally inappropriate levels of concern about being apart from a significant other characterize separation anxiety disorder. This problem is typically diagnosed before the age of 18 years after about a month of symptoms. An adult form of this disorder may begin either in childhood or in adulthood. The subject of the attachment—a parent, a spouse, a child, or a friend—may resent the constant neediness and clinginess. In fact, adults with this disorder often have extreme difficulties in romantic relationships and are more likely to be unmarried.

The 12-month prevalence rate of separation anxiety disorder in adults, adolescents, and children is 0.9% to 1.9%, 1.6%, and 4%, respectively. It is the most common anxiety disorder in children. Females are more likely to be affected.

Identifying and acknowledging specific fears is the first step in managing separation anxiety. Desensitization is useful. For example, if a child is afraid to sleep in his own bed, he may be gradually moved from his parents' room to his own. Selective serotonin reuptake inhibitors (SSRIs) and benzodiazepines such as lorazepam (Ativan) may help during the early stages of treatment.

SPECIFIC PHOBIA

A phobia is a persistent, irrational fear of a specific object, activity, or situation. This fear leads to a desire for avoidance, or actual avoidance, of the object, activity, or situation, even though the individual recognizes that dreading these objects or situations is irrational. Phobias may focus on dogs, spiders, heights, storms, water, blood, closed spaces, tunnels, and bridges. Specific phobias are common and usually do not cause much difficulty, because people can find ways to avoid the feared object.

The 12-month prevalence rates for specific phobias in children, adolescents, and adults are 5%, 16%, and 8%, respectively. Females are affected twice as often as males. Parental overprotection, abuse, and loss are associated with this disorder. First-degree relatives of someone with a specific phobia are significantly more likely to have the same problem.

Few people are seen in health care settings for treatment of phobias. In general, they seek help for comorbid conditions including major depression, anxiety, and substance use. Systematic desensitization is the most common treatment method. In this therapy, patients are gradually exposed to anxiety-provoking stimuli along with antianxiety medication, hypnosis, and relaxation methods.

SOCIAL ANXIETY DISORDER

Social anxiety disorder is characterized by severe anxiety or fear provoked by exposure to a social situation or a performance situation (e.g., fear of saying something that sounds foolish in public, fear of being unable to answer questions in a classroom, fear of eating in the presence of others, fear of performing on stage).

Social anxiety disorders are common, and the 12-month prevalence is about 7% (American Psychiatric Association [APA], 2013). Females are affected more often than males. This disorder seems to run in families and is associated with traits of behavioral inhibition. Some evidence suggests a dopaminergic dysfunction in this population.

Treatment consists of both psychotherapy and pharmacology. Medications with US Food and Drug Administration (FDA) approval for this disorder include the SSRIs paroxetine (Paxil) and sertraline (Zoloft) and a serotonin norepinephrine reuptake inhibitor (SNRI) venlafaxine (Effexor). Buspirone (BuSpar), a non-immediate acting antianxiety agent, may be used in conjunction with the antidepressants. Beta-adrenergic receptor antagonists such as atenolol (Tenormin) and propranolol are useful in performance situations to reduce autonomic arousal.

PANIC DISORDER

A panic attack is the key feature of panic disorders. A panic attack is the sudden onset of extreme apprehension or fear, usually associated with feelings of impending doom, "I am going to die." The feelings of terror during a panic attack are so severe that normal functioning is suspended, the perceptual field is severely limited, and misinterpretation of reality may occur. Physical symptoms include palpitations, chest pain, diaphoresis, muscle tension, urinary frequency, hyperventilation, breathing difficulties, nausea, and a choking sensation. Panic attacks typically occur suddenly, last 1 or 2 minutes, and then subside.

The 12-month prevalence rate for panic disorder is fairly low—about 2% to 3% of adults and adolescents (APA, 2013). People who tend to experience negative emotions and people who believe that anxiety is harmful are prone to this disorder. It is probably genetically transmitted.

Panic disorder responds well to treatment. Cognitive–behavioral therapy (CBT) helps patients to recognize false beliefs about panic attacks, especially beliefs that they are life threatening.

Four antidepressants have FDA approval for treating panic disorder. They are the SSRIs fluoxetine (Prozac), paroxetine (Paxil), and setraline (Zoloft), and an SNRI venlafaxine (Effexor). Two antianxiety agent benzodiazepines are also FDA approved for panic—alprazolam (Xanax) and clonazepam (Klonopin).

GENERALIZED ANXIETY DISORDER

Persistent anxiety and excessive worrying are the cardinal symptoms of generalized anxiety disorder. Other symptoms include restlessness, fatigue, poor concentration, irritability, muscle tension, difficulty concentrating (mind goes blank), and sleep disturbance. The individual's worry is out of proportion to the actual situation. Sleep disturbance is common because of rumination (overthinking) of concerns during the hours of sleep. Decision-making is difficult because of poor concentration and dread of making a mistake.

Generalized anxiety disorder prevalence is about 1% for adolescents and nearly 3% for adults (APA, 2013). Women are twice as likely to receive this diagnosis. About one third of the risk for developing this problem is inherited. The temperamental traits of neuroticism and harm avoidance are associated with generalized anxiety disorder.

Treatment for this disorder includes CBT, supportive therapy, and insight-oriented approaches. Pharmacological first-line therapy are antidepressants. The FDA approved SSRI antidepressants are escitalopram (Lexapro) and paroxetine (Paxil), and SNRI antidepressants are venlafaxine (Effexor) and duloxetine (Cymbalta). Buspirone (BuSpar), a non-addicting antianxiety agent, is also approved for this disorder. Benzodiazepines may be used on a short-term basis. Some tricyclic antidepressants, antihistamines, and B-adrenergic antagonists are also used.

OBSESSIVE–COMPULSIVE DISORDER

Obsessive–compulsive disorder results in severe emotional suffering. Obsessions are persistent and recurring thoughts, impulses, or images that cannot be dismissed. Common obsessions include fears of hurting a loved one, contamination, violence, sex, or religion. Compulsions are ritualistic behaviors based on the obsession that an individual feels driven to perform in an attempt to relieve anxiety. Common compulsions are repetitive hand washing, chewing one's food 100 times, jumping through doorways, and checking a door multiple times to make sure it is locked. Patients recognize these behaviors as unreasonable.

Fortunately, this disorder is fairly rare, affecting about 1.2% in a 12-month time period (APA, 2013). It is more common in males during childhood and more common in females during adulthood. Internalizing symptoms, negative emotions, and childhood shyness and abuse are risk factors. Infectious agents are associated with sudden onset in children. Obsessive–compulsive disorder is genetically mediated, with a concordance rate in identical twins of 0.57.

Although behavioral therapy may be helpful, due to the biological nature of this illness, most treatment is pharmacological. SSRIs are extremely helpful and are FDA approved for obsessive–compulsive disorder. Another drug with FDA approval is clomipramine (Anafranil).

BODY DYSMORPHIC DISORDER

Patients with body dysmorphic disorder are commonly seen in community, psychiatric, cosmetic surgery, and dermatological settings. Although patients tend to have a normal appearance, their preoccupation with an imagined defective body part results in obsessional thinking and compulsive behavior, such as mirror checking and camouflaging. People may be either well aware that their thoughts are distorted, or they may be completely sure of the existence of the defect.

The prevalence of body dysmorphic disorder is slightly higher in females (2.5%) than males (2.2%). The rate of this problem is higher among cosmetic surgery patients, dermatology patients, adult orthodontia patients, and oral and maxillofacial surgery patients. Individuals with the disorder often come from homes with abuse and neglect. Body dysmorphic disorder seems to be related to obsessive–compulsive disorder because first-degree relatives often share those conditions.

Treatment with SSRIs and the tricyclic antidepressant clomipramine (Anafranil) reduces symptoms in about 50% of patients (Sadock et al., 2015).

HOARDING DISORDER

Excessive collecting and the failure to discard characterize compulsive hoarding syndrome. Symptoms result in the accumulation of a large number of possessions (often worthless trash) that collect and clutter active living areas at home or the workplace to the extent that their intended use is no longer possible; clutter is so severe it necessitates interventions of third parties (e.g., family members, cleaners, authorities). Hoarding causes distress or interference in social, occupational, or other areas of functioning. Depression often co-occurs in people with hoarding disorder.

Exact prevalence is difficult to determine. Some surveys suggest the prevalence is between 2% and 6% (APA, 2013). The character trait of indecisiveness, stress, and trauma are risk factors. About 50% of people who hoard have family members who have the same behavior.

Hoarding disorder is difficult to treat because of poor insight, low motivation, and resistance to treatment. CBT with training in decision-making and categorizing, cognitive restructuring, and behavioral exposure and habituation to discarding has proven to be helpful (Sadock et al., 2015). Medication may be used for anxiety and depression.

TRICHOTILLOMANIA DISORDER AND EXCORIATION DISORDER

Trichotillomania (hair pulling) disorder and excoriation (skin picking) disorder are distressing problems that result in varying degrees of disability, social stigma, and altered appearance. Both activities are irresistible to the individual, who typically tries to hide the activity. These disorders have been linked to symptoms of obsessive–compulsive disorder.

The disorder seems to run in families. Individuals with relatives who have obsessive–compulsive disorder tend to have higher rates of trichotillomania.

The SSRIs are the most commonly used treatment method. In the case of skin-picking disorder, a joint treatment with a psychiatric professional and a dermatologist may be the best approach.

Assessment

Signs and Symptoms

- Narrowing of perceptions, difficulty concentrating, inefficient problem solving
- Increased vital signs (blood pressure, pulse, respirations), increased muscle tension, activated sweat glands, dilated pupils
- Palpitations, urinary urgency or frequency, nausea, tightening of the throat, unsteady voice
- Complaints of fatigue, difficulty sleeping, irritability, disorganization
- Panic attacks, obsessions, compulsions, phobias, compulsive hoarding, free-floating anxiety interfering with the ability to function at optimal levels

- A sense of impending doom or feeling as though he or she is going to die

Assessment Tools

A number of tools can help the health care worker assess for anxiety symptoms. One common measure is the PROMIS Emotional Distress tool in Fig. 8.1. While professionally trained clinicians use an advanced scoring method, for the purpose of nursing students it is helpful to see the questions and understand their relevance to anxiety.

Assessment Guidelines

A thorough physical and neurological examination helps determine whether the anxiety is primary or secondary to another psychiatric disorder, a medical condition, or substance abuse.

- Assess for a history of childhood abuse.
- Assess for potential for self-harm. Severe anxiety disorder is associated with suicide attempts or completion, as well as certain overuse of medications or illicit drugs.
- Assess the patient's community for appropriate clinics, groups, and counselors who offer anxiety-reduction techniques.
- Be aware that differences in culture can affect how anxiety is manifested.

Patient Problems

Not surprisingly, the patient problem *anxiety* is most often used to address these disorders. When focusing on *anxiety,* the nurse needs to clarify the level of anxiety, because different levels of anxiety call for different intervention strategies. *Impaired coping* is another common problem, because high levels of anxiety lead to interference in ability to work, disruptions in relationships, and changes in ability to interact satisfactorily with others.

The patient problem *need for health teaching* indicates that there is an absence or deficiency of cognitive information for individuals to obtain resources to learn new coping skills, use anxiety-reduction techniques, or receive therapy. People with anxiety often have difficulty falling

PROMIS Emotional Distress—Anxiety—Short Form

							Use
In the past SEVEN (7) DAYS....							Item Score
		Never	Rarely	Sometimes	Often	Always	
1.	I felt fearful.	❑ 1	❑ 2	❑ 3	❑ 4	❑ 5	
2.	I felt anxious.	❑ 1	❑ 2	❑ 3	❑ 4	❑ 5	
3.	I felt worried.	❑ 1	❑ 2	❑ 3	❑ 4	❑ 5	
4.	I found it hard to focus on anything other than my anxiety.	❑ 1	❑ 2	❑ 3	❑ 4	❑ 5	
5.	I felt nervous.	❑ 1	❑ 2	❑ 3	❑ 4	❑ 5	
6.	I felt uneasy.	❑ 1	❑ 2	❑ 3	❑ 4	❑ 5	
7.	I felt tense.	❑ 1	❑ 2	❑ 3	❑ 4	❑ 5	
						Total Score	

Fig. 8.1 PROMIS Emotional Distress–Anxiety–Short Form. (PROMIS Health)

asleep, difficulty maintaining sleep, and early-morning awakening, These sleep disruptions can lead to impaired functioning at work, at school, and in social situations. Therefore, the problem of *insomnia* is essential when caring for this population.

Intervention Guidelines

- Identify community resources that can help the patient to develop new skills.
- Identify community support groups for people with specific anxiety disorders.
- Assess the need for interventions with families and significant others (support groups, family therapy), and help with issues that might lead to relationship stress and turmoil.

When medications are used in conjunction with therapy, patients and their significant others will need thorough teaching. Give written information and instructions to the patient, family, or partner.

Nursing Care for Anxiety and Obsessive-Compulsive Disorders

Anxiety

A feeling of apprehension, uneasiness, uncertainty, or dread resulting from a real or perceived threat (Halter, 2018, p. 271)

Due to:
- External stressors (e.g., economic, job loss, housing problems)
- Internal stressors (e.g., illness, altered self-concept)
- Deficient resources
- Substance use
- Crisis (situational, maturational adventitious)
- Exposure to phobic object or situation
- Ritualistic behavior
- Fear of panic attack
- Intrusive, unwanted thoughts

Desired Outcomes
The patient will experience the elimination of maladaptive anxiety.

Assessment/Interventions (Rationales)
1. Provide a safe, calm environment by decreasing environmental stimuli. (Stimulating environments increase anxiety.)
2. Listen to and reassure the patient that he or she can feel more in control. (When people feel fearful and vulnerable, a sense of connectedness with someone can reduce anxiety.)
3. Encourage the patient to talk about feelings and concerns. (When concerns are stated out loud, problems can be discussed and feelings of isolation decreased.)
4. Reframe the problem in a way that is solvable. Provide a new perspective, and correct distorted perceptions. (Correcting distortions increases the possibility of finding workable solutions to a realistically defined problem.)
5. Identify thoughts or feelings before the onset of anxiety: "What were you doing/thinking right before you started to feel anxious?" (Identifies triggers for escalating anxiety and a chance to understand why these triggers are so frightening to the patient.)

6. Teach relaxation techniques (e.g., deep breathing exercises, meditation, progressive muscle relaxation). (When patients learn to lower their levels of anxiety, their ability to assess a situation and use their own problem-solving skills are improved.)
7. Identify negative self-talk or messages (e.g., "I'll never be able to do this right." "This means I'll never succeed in anything."). (Cognitive skills can be used to help the patient to reframe his or her thinking so that problems can be solved.)
8. Refer the patient and significant others to support groups, self-help programs, or advocacy groups when appropriate. (Patients with specific problems are known to greatly benefit from being around others who are grappling with similar issues. This provides the patient with information and support and decreases feelings of isolation in stressful and difficult situations.)
9. Administer medications, or obtain an order for medications when appropriate. (Use the least restrictive interventions to decrease anxiety.)

Impaired Coping

Due to:

- Severe to panic levels of anxiety—panic attack, generalized anxiety disorder
- Excessive negative beliefs about self
- Presence of obsessions and compulsions
- Avoidance behavior
- Compulsive hoarding

Desired Outcome

The patient will verbally demonstrate the ability to cope effectively with anxiety.

Assessment/Interventions (Rationales)

1. Monitor and reinforce the patient's use of positive coping skills and healthy defense mechanisms. (Identifies what does and does not work for the patient. The nurse uses the patient's strengths to build upon.)
2. Teach new coping skills to substitute for ineffective ones. (Provides more adaptive options.)
3. At the patient's level of understanding, explain the fight-or-flight response and the relaxation response of

the autonomic nervous system. Address how breathing can be used to elicit the relaxation response. (Understanding the physiological aspects of anxiety and that people have some degree of control over their physiological responses gives patients hope and a sense of control in their lives. Such knowledge aids them in mastering relaxation techniques.)

4. When the patient's level of anxiety is mild to moderate, teach the patient proper breathing techniques, and breathe with the patient. (Breathing techniques can prevent anxiety from escalating. Doing exercises with the patient helps foster adherence.)
5. When the patient's level of anxiety is mild to moderate, teach the patient relaxation techniques (such as imaging or visualization). (Help the patient gain some control over switching the autonomic nervous system from the fight-or-flight response to the relaxation response.)
6. Identify therapies that are effective with individuals who have the same disorder (cognitive, behavioral). (Not only do cognitive and behavioral approaches work to decrease the patient's anxiety and improve quality of life, they also foster chemical changes in the brain that decrease the brain's response to anxiety.)
7. Use a cognitive approach. (Helps the patient recognize that thoughts and beliefs can cause anxiety.)
8. Teach the patient proven behavioral techniques. The patient can become desensitized to a feared object or situation over time. (Behavioral techniques are extremely effective interventions for treating anxiety disorders. Once they are learned, patients can draw upon these skills for the rest of their lives.)
9. Keep focus on manageable problems; define them simply and concretely. (Concrete, well-defined problems lend themselves to intervention.)
10. Provide behavioral rehearsals (role play) for anticipated stressful situations. (Determination of previous effective or new coping strategies, along with practice, increases potential for success.)
11. Some patients respond well to biofeedback and feel more comfortable with physiological manipulations than one-on-one therapy. (Biofeedback is extremely useful for decreasing anxiety levels. Some patients might feel less shame in getting help.)

12. Provide education including the medication's purpose, length of time until benefits are apparent, side effects, and adverse responses. This information should always be given to patients in writing after the nurse verbally explains it. (Anxiety disorders respond to medications along with therapy and medication education is essential.)

Need for Health Teaching

Due to:

- Exaggerated behaviors (fears of objects or situations, panic attack)
- Inappropriate behaviors (compulsive behaviors [repetitive nonfunctional actions]), hoarding
- Distractibility
- Intrusive thoughts, obsessive thinking, feelings of helplessness or hopelessness to change behaviors, feelings, and thoughts
- Lack of control to change behaviors, feelings, and thoughts

Desired Outcomes

The patient will recognize escalating anxiety and demonstrate techniques to reduce the anxiety.

Assessment/Interventions (Rationales)

1. Explore the thoughts that lead to the patient's anxious feelings and relief behaviors. (Recognition of precipitating thoughts or feelings leading to anxiety behaviors might give clues about how to arrest escalating anxiety.)
2. Link the patient's relief behaviors to thoughts and feelings. (The patient becomes aware of how anxiety can be the result of thoughts and realizes that with practice, people can have some control over their thoughts and therefore their anxiety levels.)
3. Teach cognitive principles. Anxiety is the result of dysfunctional appraisal of a situation, and anxiety is the result of automatic thinking. (Again, introduces the concept to patients that they can have some control over their thoughts and feelings; instills hope and stimulates trying new ways of thinking.)
4. Teach some brief cognitive techniques that the patient can try out right away. (Increases self-awareness while

distancing the patient from his or her own anxiety. In a sense, it helps distract the patient from feelings of anxiety and allows him or her to be more of an observer.)

5. Teach the patient behavioral techniques that can interrupt intrusive, unwanted thoughts. (Can help distract the patient and interrupt escalating anxiety. During this time, alternative coping skills can be used.)
6. Role play and rehearse with the patient alternative coping strategies that can be used in threatening or anxiety-provoking situations. (Gives the patient a chance to be proactive, giving the patient a choice of alternatives instead of the patient using the usual unsatisfactory automatic reactions.)
7. Encourage the patient to keep a daily journal of thoughts and situations that seem to precede anxiety and the coping strategies used. (Allows the patient to monitor "triggers" and evaluate useful coping strategies over time.)
8. Teach the patient to rate his or her anxiety levels on a scale from 1 to 10, where 1 is the least and 10 the highest. Encourage the patient to record situations and anxiety levels in a journal. (Allows the patient to evaluate the effectiveness of coping strategies and monitor the decrease in anxiety levels over time.)
9. Review the journal with the patient, and identify which strategies worked and which did not work. (Helps the patient to see what seems to be working and what does not, and encourages adherence when going through phases of feeling discouraged.)
10. Review with the patient progress made, and give credit for the patient's hard work. (Positive feedback helps to reinforce learning.)
11. Refer the patient to support groups in the community in which people are dealing with similar issues. (Groups can foster a sense of belonging and diminish feelings of isolation and alienation. Positive feedback from others helps foster adherence and enhances self-esteem.)
12. Review stress-reduction techniques with the patient, family, and significant others during family and patient teaching. Encourage the patient and family members to practice relaxation techniques; give handouts and references. (Anxiety is communicated interpersonally. Sometimes simple steps make big differences in people's lives.)

13. Refer family members and significant others to resources in the community such as family therapy, couples counseling, financial counseling, support groups, or relaxation classes. (Family and others close to the patient might need support and may benefit from learning new coping strategies.)

Insomnia

Due to:

- Anxiety disorder
- Fear
- Anxiety
- Inadequate sleep hygiene
- Biochemical agents
- Obsessional thoughts
- Fears (dark, intrusion, death)
- Panic attacks

Desired Outcome

The patient will report satisfaction with falling asleep, maintaining sleep, and time upon awakening.

Assessment/Interventions (Rationales)

1. Assess the patient's usual sleep patterns, changes that have occurred, and what was happening at the time the sleep problem began. Identify whether there was a precipitating event around the onset of the sleep problem or whether it is chronic. (Understanding the baseline sleep pattern provides direction for eliminating the sleep disruption.)
2. Identify the patient's usual sleep patterns, including bedtime rituals, time of rising, time of retiring, use of alcohol or caffeine before sleep, and use of sleep aids (prescribed or over-the-counter medications). (Establishing a baseline helps to determine useful interventions.)
3. Develop a sleep relaxation program with the patient (e.g., self-hypnosis, progressive muscle relaxation, imagery). (Using both physical and mental relaxation can help minimize anxiety and promote sleep.)
4. Demonstrate and rehearse these techniques with the patient until he or she feels relaxed and is able to practice them at bedtime. (Have the patient practice the

chosen relaxation method with a nurse. Allow time for the patient to begin to feel the results of the relaxation.)

5. Suggest the use of relaxation recordings. (If the patient has racing thoughts or is troubled by a problem, relaxation recordings can help the patient focus on relaxation.)
6. Encourage the patient to use decaffeinated beverages until the sleep pattern improves; limit fluid intake 3 to 5 hours before retiring; increase physical activity during the day, even if fatigued; avoid daytime naps; establish regular times of retiring and waking. (These measures are known sleep aids.)
7. Establish with the patient a sleep program that incorporates the elements of good sleep hygiene and relaxation tools. (The patient is more likely to follow the plan if he or she is involved with the incorporation of known effective techniques.)
8. Suggest that if the patient does not feel drowsy after 20 minutes, he or she should get up and engage in a quiet activity that is "boring"—*not* stimulating. (Waiting for sleep that will not come can increase anxiety and frustration. Doing something monotonous at bedtime might help the patient become drowsy.)
9. Encourage patient to practice the agreed-upon bedtime routine for 2 weeks, even if there does not seem to be a benefit. (It might take 2 weeks or longer for habits to settle in.)
10. Encourage the patient to simultaneously identify issues that might be adversely affecting sleep (e.g., anxiety disorders, social or personal problems, job-related issues, interpersonal difficulties). Offer referrals when appropriate. (Disturbances in sleep are often secondary to other issues, either emotional or physical. If such issues are present, they need to be addressed.)

TREATMENT FOR ANXIETY AND OBSESSIVE–COMPULSIVE DISORDERS

Biological Approaches

Pharmacological Therapy

There are a variety of antianxiety medications available for treating these anxiety-related disorders. Some of them were discussed previously in this chapter along with an overview of the specific disorders. Antidepressants are typically a first-line of defense when treating anxiety as well as depression. See Chapter 24 for a discussion of this drug classification. Chapter 25 introduces the antianxiety agents.

Psychotherapeutic Approaches

Many psychotherapeutic techniques have proven useful in treating individuals with anxiety-related disorders. Some include:

- Cognitive restructuring
- Relaxation training
- Modeling techniques
- Systematic desensitization or graduated exposure
- Flooding (implosion therapy)
- Behavior therapy

See Chapter 29 for more discussion on psychotherapeutic models.

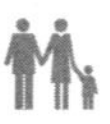

Nurse, Patient, and Family Resources

Anxiety and Depression Association of America
www.adaa.org

International OCD Foundation
www.iocdf.org

Mental Help Net
www.mentalhelp.net

Panic Disorder
www.nlm.nih.gov/medlineplus/panicdisorder.html

Panic/Anxiety Disorders Guide
www.panicdisorder.about.com

CHAPTER 9

Trauma-Related Disorders

Traumatic life events can result in a wide range of psychiatric disorders and other medical disorders. Trauma responses can be the result of tragic, yet day-to-day experiences, such as prolonged and severe child abuse. Traumatic responses can also be the result from out of the ordinary horrific events such as war or disasters.

Understanding trauma is essential in order to provide the most effective interventions. Integrating trauma-informed care into all healthcare settings can reduce or prevent the damaging psychological and physical consequences of trauma. Figure 9.1) illustrates the harm that is caused by long-term stress responses.

TRAUMA RELATED DISORDERS

Two specific stress disorders identified in the *Diagnostic and Statistical Manual of Mental Disorders,* fifth edition *(DSM-5)* (American Psychiatric Association, 2013) are posttraumatic stress disorder (PTSD) and acute stress disorder. Both disorders follow exposure to an extremely traumatic event, usually outside the range of normal experience. These events include natural disasters, crime-related events, acts of terrorism, bombings, car or train wrecks, torture or kidnap, military combat, sexual assault, witnessing a violent death or mutilation, or diagnosis of a life-threatening disease. Patients feel not only fear, but also a sense of hopelessness and horror. The common element in all of these experiences is the individual's extraordinary helplessness or powerlessness in the face of such stressors.

The main difference between PTSD and acute stress disorder is timing. Acute stress disorder symptoms must be evident within 1 month of the traumatic event and resolve within that month. If symptoms last longer than 1

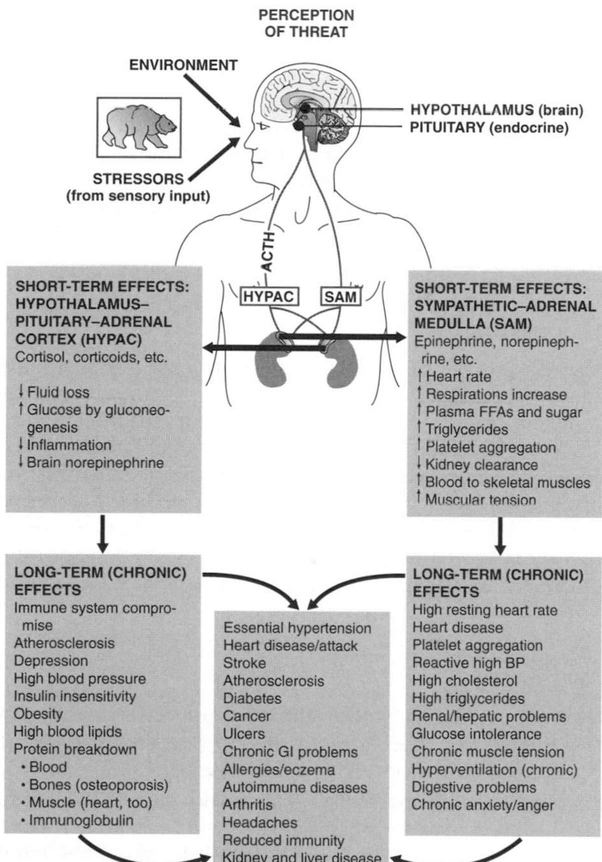

Fig. 9.1 "The Stress Response, Figure p. 72" by Dierdre Davis Brigham, from IMAGERY FOR GETTING WELL: CLINICAL APPLICATIONS FOR BEHAVIORAL MEDICINE by Deirdre Davis Brigham. Copyright © 1994 by Deirdre Davis Brigham. Used by permission of W. W. Norton & Company, Inc.

month, the diagnosis is changed from acute stress disorder to PTSD. Other stress disorders are listed in the *DSM-5*. They are:

- Reactive attachment disorder: Children whose trauma leaves them unable to respond emotionally to caregivers.
- Disinhibited social engagement disorder: Children whose trauma leads them to superficially and indiscriminately bond to unfamiliar adults.
- Adjustment disorder: Emotional or behavioral symptoms in response to stress that are out of proportion to the stress.

Epidemiology

Most (55%–90%) people experience at least one traumatic event in their lifetimes, with an average of five traumatic events reported per person (Centers for Disease Control and Prevention, 2010). After a traumatic event, nearly 8% of people will develop PTSD (Kessler et al., 1995), with some populations particularly vulnerable. The lifetime prevalence for PTSD is 3.5% of the adult population (National Institute of Mental Health, 2015). Women are more than twice as likely as men (10% versus 4%) to develop PTSD.

Assessment

Obtaining a history about the time of onset, frequency, course, severity, level of distress, and degree of functional impairment is important. Further assessment for suicidal or violent ideation, family and social supports, insomnia, social withdrawal, functional impairment, current life stressors, medication, past medical and psychiatric history, and a mental status examination are indicated. The diagnosis of acute stress disorder or PTSD involves a comprehensive clinical assessment of all symptoms collectively.

There are a variety of screening tools available to quantify symptoms related to trauma. The Severity of Posttraumatic Stress Scale by Kilpatrick et al. (2013) is provided in Fig. 9.2. When experienced clinicians use this scale, the scoring system is more advanced. Students can use this scale to get an idea of target questions for trauma and the severity of symptoms that may be experienced.

Severity of Posttraumatic Stress Symptoms—Adult*

***National Stressful Events Survey PTSD Short Scale (NSESSS)**

Instructions: People sometimes have problems after extremely stressful events or experiences. How much have you been bothered during the PAST SEVEN (7) DAYS by each of the following problems that occurred or became worse after an extremely stressful event/experience? **Please respond to each item by marking (✓ or x) one box per row.**

							Clinician Use
		Not at all	A little bit	Moderately	Quite a bit	Extremely	Item score
1.	Having "flashbacks," that is, you suddenly acted or felt as if a stressful experience from the past was happening all over again (for example, you reexperienced parts of a stressful experience by seeing, hearing, smelling, or physically feeling parts of the experience)?	❑ 0	❑ 1	❑ 2	❑ 3	❑ 4	
2.	Feeling very emotionally upset when something reminded you of a stressful experience?	❑ 0	❑ 1	❑ 2	❑ 3	❑ 4	
3.	Trying to avoid thoughts, feelings, or physical sensations that reminded you of a stressful experience?	❑ 0	❑ 1	❑ 2	❑ 3	❑ 4	
4.	Thinking that a stressful event happened because you or someone else (who didn't directly harm you) did something wrong or didn't do everything possible to prevent it, or because of something about you?	❑ 0	❑ 1	❑ 2	❑ 3	❑ 4	
5.	Having a very negative emotional state (for example, you were experiencing lots of fear, anger, guilt, shame, or horror) after a stressful experience?	❑ 0	❑ 1	❑ 2	❑ 3	❑ 4	
6.	Losing interest in activities you used to enjoy before having a stressful experience?	❑ 0	❑ 1	❑ 2	❑ 3	❑ 4	
7.	Being "super alert," on guard, or constantly on the lookout for danger?	❑ 0	❑ 1	❑ 2	❑ 3	❑ 4	
8.	Feeling jumpy or easily startled when you hear an unexpected noise?	❑ 0	❑ 1	❑ 2	❑ 3	❑ 4	
9.	Being extremely irritable or angry to the point where you yelled at other people, got into fights, or destroyed things?	❑ 0	❑ 1	❑ 2	❑ 3	❑ 4	
						Total Score	

Fig. 9.2 Severity of Posttraumatic Stress Scale.

Nursing Care for Trauma Related Disorders

Posttrauma Syndrome

Due to:

- War
- Sexual assault or violence
- Terrorism
- Torture
- Disasters
- Military combat
- Physical and psychological abuse
- Serious accidents
- Witnessing violet death or mutilations
- Motor vehicle and industrial accidents
- Being a prisoner of war

- Natural and man-made disasters
- Hospitalization in an intensive care unit

Desired Outcome
The patient will report a return to the pre-trauma level of functioning.

Assessment/Interventions (Rationales)

1. Assess for suicidal or homicidal thoughts and feelings. (The priority concern and nursing measures are for the patient's and others' safety.)
2. Assess the patient's anxiety level. (Identify what level of intervention might be needed to minimize escalation of anxiety.)
3. Assess for alcohol or drug use. If the patient is misusing alcohol or drugs, assess readiness for substance abuse therapies (e.g., support groups, counseling). Offer referrals if the patient is ready. (Patients cannot effectively participate in learning coping skills, reliving traumatic memories, and making positive changes while impaired.)
4. Identify the patient's symptoms and clarify that they are anxiety related and not the product of a physiological condition (e.g., chest tightness, headaches, dizziness, numbness). (Physical causes of symptoms must be ruled out before assumptions of psychological causes are made [e.g., a patient might have PTSD along with a cardiac problem].)
5. Identify and document psychological responses the patient is experiencing (e.g., shock, anger, withdrawal, panic, confusion, psychosis, emotional instability, nightmares, flashbacks). (The psychological symptoms are often many, and different ones might require different intervention strategies. When the symptoms begin to diminish, you know that goals are being reached.)
6. Identify whether the patient is in or has been in support groups with others who deal with similar traumatic issues. If not, offer referrals to groups in the patient's community. (Support groups of people with similar experiences are pivotal to healing. They allow for expressing similar feelings in a safe environment.)
7. Spend time with the patient, allowing him or her to set the pace when describing present or past traumatic events. (Often feelings and memories of trauma are buried. It often takes time and trust for a person to

open up to a stranger or discuss a topic he or she might not have shared with anyone.)

8. Monitor your own feelings in response to the individual's experience. (Many of the stories patients tell are horrifying and difficult to listen to.)
9. Avoid interrupting or minimizing the horror or over-identifying with the events. (Venting with other staff or a supervisor helps the nurse process feelings and discharge tensions.)
10. Remain nonjudgmental in your interactions. (Avoid reinforcing blame, shame, and guilt.)
11. Listen attentively to the patient's description of the event. (Although it might be difficult to listen to the trauma, sharing the pain with others can be the beginning of healing.)
12. Encourage expression of feelings through talking, writing, crying, role playing, or other ways in which the patient is comfortable. (The description of the events and the expression of feelings associated with the event are paramount to the healing process.)
13. Teach the patient adaptive cognitive and behavioral strategies to manage symptoms of emotional and physical reactivity: deep breathing, relaxation exercises, cognitive techniques, desensitization, assertive behavior, thought-stopping techniques, and stress-reduction techniques. (Once repressed areas are addressed, accompanying, often unbearable, feelings will emerge.)
14. Assess the family and social support system. Is there a need for family interventions or counseling? (Often family and friends become confused, afraid, hurt, angry, or feel hopeless and depressed over time.)
15. Instruct the patient and family on signs and symptoms of PTSD. (Often when actions and behaviors that seemed totally chaotic and unrelated are viewed in terms of an identifiable syndrome, relief is experienced, especially when treatment is available.)

TREATMENT FOR TRAUMA-RELATED DISORDERS

Biological Approaches

Pharmacological Therapy

The U.S. Food and Drug Administration (FDA) approved two medications for treating PTSD. They are the selective serotonin reuptake inhibitors (SSRIs) sertraline (Zoloft) and paroxetine (Paxil). Other drugs used off-label include phenelzine (Nardil), a monoamine oxidase inhibitor that has been used with some success in PTSD. A serotonin norepinephrine reuptake inhibitor (SNRI) such as venlafaxine (Effexor) may be used to decrease anxiety and depressive symptoms. Tricyclic antidepressants (TCAs) or mirtazapine (Remeron) may be prescribed. See Chapter 24 for more information on antidepressants.

Clonidine (Catapres) is a centrally acting alpha-2 receptor agonist used to address hyperarousal and intrusive symptoms. Prazosin (Minipress) is an alpha-receptor antagonist used for nightmares and sleep disturbances. Propranolol (Inderal), a beta-blocker, is used for hyperarousal and panic. The most difficult-to-tolerate side effect of these medications is hypotension.

Psychotherapeutic Approaches

Psychoeducation

Initial education should include reassurance that reactions to trauma are common and that these reactions do not indicate personal failure or weakness. Strategies to improve coping, enhance self-care, and facilitate recognition of problems are essential. Patients experiencing such severe stress will benefit from relaxation techniques and from the avoidance of caffeine and alcohol.

Psychotherapy

Advanced practice psychiatric professionals commonly use two therapies with this population: cognitive–behavioral therapy (CBT) and eye movement desensitization and reprocessing (EMDR) therapy. CBT works to help patients recognize faulty thinking patterns and to increase positive responses such as "at least I am alive." EMDR therapy helps people process traumatic memories though a specific protocol involving talking about the traumatic event while attending to other activities such as eye movements or tapping one's foot. See Chapter 29 for a more detailed description of these therapies.

Nurse, Patient, and Family Resources

International Society for Traumatic Stress Studies
www.istss.org

National Alliance on Mental Illness [PTSD]
www.nami.org

National Center for PTSD
www.ptsd.va.gov

David Baldwin's Trauma Information Pages
www.trauma-pages.com

Trauma Survivors Network
www.trauasurvivorsnetwork.org

CHAPTER 10

Eating Disorders

People with eating disorders experience a severe disruption in their normal eating patterns and their perception of body shape and weight. Eating disorders can be severe and disabling, and successful treatment requires long-term care and follow-up. Unlike most psychiatric conditions, these disorders can cause substantial physiological damage.

The focus of this chapter is anorexia nervosa, bulimia nervosa, and binge-eating disorder. Three additional feeding problems—pica, rumination disorder, and avoidant/restrictive food intake disorder—are described briefly.

PICA

Pica is the persistent ingestion of substances that have no nutritional value such as dirt or paint. Eating nonfood items may interfere with eating nutritional items, and can also be dangerous. For example, paint may contain lead that can lead to brain damage. Objects such as stones may cause intestinal blockage. Sharp objects such as paperclips may result in intestinal damage or laceration. Bacteria from dirt or other soiled objects may be the source of serious infection. Pica usually begins in early childhood and lasts for a few months. It is associated with intellectual disability and development disorders such as autism.

Monitoring the child's eating behavior is obviously an essential aspect of treating this problem. Behavioral interventions such as rewarding appropriate eating are helpful.

RUMINATION DISORDER

In rumination disorder undigested food is regurgitated and then rechewed, reswallowed, or spit out. Rumination symptoms can occur at any age. The onset in infants is between 3 and 12 months. The symptoms commonly remit spontaneously but may become habitual and result in esophageal erosion, severe malnutrition, and even death. Intellectual disability is associated with rumination, as is neglect.

Interventions include repositioning infants and small children during feeding. Improving the interaction between the caregiver and child and making mealtimes a pleasant experience often reduce rumination. Distracting the child when rumination begins is also helpful. Behavior therapy may be used for individuals with intellectual disability. Family therapy may provide additional support.

AVOIDANT/RESTRICTIVE FOOD INTAKE DISORDER

A lack of interest in food and an aversion to the sensory experience of eating are symptoms of avoidant/restrictive food intake disorder. This disorder goes way beyond picky eating since it results in nutritional deficiencies, weight loss, growth retardation, and interference with emotional and social functioning. It most commonly begins in infancy or early childhood and may continue into adulthood. Anxiety and family anxiety are risk factors. A history of gastrointestinal problems such as reflux is associated with this feeding disorder.

Behavior modification is useful in increasing regular food consumption. Families caring for a child with a feeding disorder often need support and education in specific behavioral techniques. Cognitive-behavioral therapy is also recommended. Treating anxiety and depressive symptoms may be helpful in some cases.

ANOREXIA NERVOSA

Individuals with anorexia nervosa fail to maintain a minimally normal weight for height and express intense fear of gaining weight. The term anorexia, meaning "loss of appetite" is inaccurate, because loss of appetite is rare. Some people with anorexia nervosa exclusively restrict their intake of food, whereas others engage in binge eating and purging.

Anorexia nervosa may start as early as between the ages of 7 and 12 years. Anorexia nervosa is a chronic illness that waxes and wanes. The 1-year relapse rate approaches 50%, and long-term studies show that up to 40% of patients continue to meet some criteria for anorexia nervosa after 4 years (Harrington et al., 2015). Factors that influence recovery include percentage of ideal body weight that has been achieved, the extent to which self-worth is defined by shape and weight, and the amount of disruption existing in the patient's personal life.

Epidemiology

For women, the lifetime incidence of anorexia nervosa is 0.9%; the lifetime incidence for men is 0.24% (Rosenvinge & Petterson, 2015). It is extremely difficult to determine the specific number of people afflicted with eating disorders, because most people do not seek health care for this illness.

Risk Factors

Altered brain serotonin function contributes to dysregulation of appetite, mood, and impulse control in eating disorders. Patients consistently exhibit personality traits of perfectionism, obsessive–compulsiveness, and dysphoric mood, all of which correlate with serotonin pathways in the brain. There may be a difference in the neural reward and executive function area.

From a cognitive–behavioral perspective, anorexia nervosa is rooted in learned behavior with positive reinforcement. For example, a mildly overweight 14-year-old has the flu and loses a little weight. She returns to school, and her friends say, "Wow, you look great." Now she purposefully strives to lose weight. When people say, "You look really skinny," she hears, "Wow, you look great."

Family theorists maintain that eating disorders are a problem of the whole family. In addition, the Western cultural ideal that equates feminine beauty to tall, thin models has received much attention as a factor in anorexia nervosa.

Treatment

A patient with anorexia nervosa will require long-term treatment that might include periodic brief hospital stays and outpatient psychotherapy. The combination of individual, group, couples, and family therapy (especially for younger patients) provides the patient with the greatest chance for a successful outcome.

There are no drugs approved by the U.S. Food and Drug Administration (FDA) for the treatment of anorexia nervosa. The selective serotonin reuptake inhibitor (SSRI) fluoxetine (Prozac), however, has proven useful in reducing obsessive–compulsive behavior *after* the patient has reached a maintenance weight.

Assessment

Signs and Symptoms

Psychological

- Extreme fear of gaining weight
- Poor social adjustment
- Odd food habits (hoarding, hiding food)
- Focuses on exercising
- Mood and/or sleep disturbances
- Obsessive–compulsive food behaviors
- Views self as fat
- Perfectionist
- Introverted
- Intimacy avoidant
- Sexually inactive
- Denies sadness or anger
- Pleasant affect

Physiological

- <85% of ideal body weight
- Blood pressure <90/60
- Heart rate <40 bpm
- Orthostatic hypotension
- Glucose <60 mg/dL
- Temperature <97° F
- Potassium <3 mEq/L
- Electrolyte imbalance
- Dehydration
- Edema
- Cachexia (muscle and weight loss)
- Dry, yellowish skin
- Amenorrhea (loss of menstruation)
- Hair loss
- Lanugo (downy hair on shoulders)
- Decreased metabolic rate
- Constipation
- Fatigue and lack of energy
- Insomnia
- Loss of bone mass, osteoporosis
- Loss of tooth enamel from vomiting

- Scars on knuckles (Russell's sign) from self-induced vomiting
- Parotid gland enlargement

Assessment Guidelines

1. Other medical conditions should be ruled out by a thorough physical examination along with appropriate blood work.
2. Determine whether the patient has medical or psychiatric symptoms severe enough to require hospitalization or if the patient is a candidate for outpatient treatment such as partial hospitalization.
3. Assess the patient's willingness for treatment.
4. Identify the level of family's knowledge about the disorder.
5. Determine the patient's and family's need further teaching or information regarding the treatment plan (e.g., pharmacological interventions, behavioral therapy, cognitive-behavioral therapy, family therapy).
6. Assess the patient's and family's interest desire in a support group and need for referrals.

Patient Problems

Table 10.1 identifies signs and symptoms along with potential patient problems for individuals with anorexia nervosa.

Intervention Guidelines

1. Acknowledge the patient's desire for thinness and control.
2. Do a self-assessment and be aware of reactions that might limit your ability to help the patient. Some nurses might experience the following:
   - Feeling shock or disgust for the patient's behavior or appearance
   - Resenting the patient, believing that the disorder is self-inflicted
   - Feeling helpless to change the patient's behavior, leading to anger and frustration.
   - Becoming overwhelmed by the patient's problems, leading to feelings of hopelessness.

Table 10.1 **Signs and Symptoms and Patient Problems for Anorexia Nervosa**

Signs and Symptoms	Patient Problems
Emaciation, dehydration, arrhythmias, inadequate intake, dry skin, decreased blood pressure, decreased urine output, increased urine concentration, weakness	*Insufficient nutritional intake* *Dehydration* *Potential for cardiac arrhythmia* *Potential for heart failure*
Excessive self-monitoring, describes self as fat despite emaciation	*Body image alteration*
Destructive behavior toward self, poor concentration, inability to meet role expectations, inadequate problem solving	*Impaired coping*
Indecisive behavior, lack of eye contact, passiveness, reports feelings of shame, rejects positive feedback about self	*Decreased self-esteem*

- Engaging in power struggles with the patient, which result in angry feelings in the nurse toward the patient..

3. Limit discussions of food.
4. Monitor laboratory values and report abnormal values to the primary clinician.

Nursing Care for Anorexia Nervosa

Insufficient Nutritional Intake

Due to:

- Psychological factors
- Restricting caloric intake or refusing to eat
- Excessive fear of weight gain
- Excessive physical exertion
- Self-induced vomiting
- Laxative, diuretic, or enema use

Desired Outcome:
By discharge (inpatient) or after two weeks (outpatient) the patient's weight will be maintained within a medically safe range and the patient will consume calories and fluids within normal limits.

Assessment/Interventions (Rationales)

Severely Malnourished Patients: Nutritional Rehabilitation

1. When severely malnourished and refusing nourishment, the patient may require tube feedings, either alone or in conjunction with oral or parenteral nutrition. (Tube feedings may be the only means available to maintain the patient's life. The patient may not tolerate solid foods at first. The use of nasogastric tube feedings decreases the chance of vomiting.)
2. Tube feedings or parenteral nutrition are often given at night. (Nighttime administration helps diminish drawing attention or sympathy from other patients and allows the patient to participate more fully in daytime activities.)
3. After completion of nasogastric tube feeding, supervise the patient for 90 minutes initially, and gradually reduce the time to 30 minutes. (Helps minimize the patient's chance of vomiting or siphoning off feedings.)
4. Assess vital signs at least three times daily until stable, and then daily. Repeat electrocardiogram (EKG) and laboratory tests (electrolytes, acid–base balance, liver enzymes, albumin, and others) until stable. (As the patient's weight begins to increase, cardiovascular status improves to within normal range, and less frequent monitoring is needed.)
5. Administer tube feedings in a matter-of-fact, nonpunishing manner. Tube feedings are not to be used as threats, nor are they to be bargained about. (Tube feedings are medical treatments, not a punishment or bargaining chip. Being consistent and enforcing limits lowers the chance of manipulation and chance of power struggles.)
6. Give the patient the opportunity to take foods or liquid supplements orally, and supplement insufficient intake through tube feedings. (Allows the patient some control over whether he or she needs tube feedings.)
7. Weigh the patient weekly or biweekly at the same time of day each week. Use the following guidelines:
   - Before the morning meal
   - After the patient has voided
   - In a hospital gown and undergarment only

   (Patients are terrified about gaining weight. Staff members should guard against patients trying to manipulate their weight by drinking excess water, having a full bladder, or putting heavy objects in their pockets or on their person before being weighed.)

8. Remain neutral, neither approving nor disapproving. (Keep issues of approval and disapproval separate from issues of health. Weight gain and loss is a health matter, not an area that has to do with the staff's pleasure or disapproval.)

Less Severely Malnourished Patients: Nutritional Maintenance

1. When possible, set up a contract with the patient regarding treatment goals and outcome criteria. (When the patient agrees to take part in establishing goals, he or she is in a position to have some control over his or her care.)
2. Provide a pleasant, calm atmosphere at mealtimes. Mealtimes should be structured. The patient should be told the specific time and duration of a meal (e.g., 30 minutes). (Mealtimes become episodes of high anxiety, and knowledge of regulations decreases tension in the milieu, particularly when the patient has given up so much control by entering treatment.)
3. Observe the patient during meals to prevent hiding or throwing away food. Accompany the patient to the bathroom if purging is suspected. Observe the patient for at least 1 hour after meals and snacks to prevent purging. (These behaviors are difficult for the patient to stop. External control will help until the patient develops more internal resources.)
4. Observe the patient closely for the use of physical activity to control weight. (Patients are often discouraged from engaging in planned exercise programs until their weight reaches 85% of ideal body weight.)
5. Closely monitor and record the following:
   - Fluid and food intake
   - Vital signs
   - Elimination pattern (discourage the use of laxatives, enemas, or suppositories)

   (Fluid and electrolyte balance is crucial to the patient's well being and safety. Abnormal data should alert staff to potential physical crises.)
6. Continue to weigh the patient as described previously. (Objectively monitors progress.)
7. As the patient approaches the target weight, gradually encourage personal choices for menu selection. (Fosters a sense of control and independence.)

8. Privileges are based on weight gain (or loss) when setting limits. When weight loss occurs, decrease privileges. Use this time to focus on circumstances surrounding the weight loss and the feelings of the patient. (By not focusing on eating, physical activity, calorie counts, and the like, there is more emphasis on the patient's feelings and perceptions.)
9. When weight gain occurs, increase privileges. (The patient receives positive reinforcement for healthy outcomes and behaviors.)

Nutritionally Stabilized Patients: Maintenance of Recovery

1. Continue to provide a supportive and empathetic approach as the patient continues to meet target weight. (For patients with anorexia, eating regularly, even within the framework of restoring health, is extremely difficult.)
2. The weight maintenance phase of treatment challenges the patient. This is the ideal time to address more of the issues underlying the patient's attitude toward weight and shape. (At a healthier weight, the patient is cognitively better prepared to examine emotional conflicts and themes.)
3. Use a cognitive–behavioral approach to the patient's expressed fears regarding weight gain. Identify dysfunctional thoughts such as, "If I gain weight, I am a failure." (Confronting dysfunctional thoughts and beliefs is crucial to changing eating behaviors.)
4. Emphasize the social nature of eating. Encourage conversation that does not have the theme of food during mealtimes. (Eating is a social activity, and participating in conversation serves both as a distraction from obsessional preoccupation and as a pleasurable event.)
5. Focus on the patient's strengths, including his or her progress in normalizing weight and eating habits. (The patient has achieved a major accomplishment and should be proud. Explore activities unrelated to eating as sources of gratification.)
6. Encourage the patient to apply all the knowledge, skills, and gains made from the various individual, family, and group therapy sessions. (The patient should have been receiving intensive therapy (cognitive–behavioral) and education that have provided tools and techniques useful for maintaining healthy eating and living behaviors.)

7. Teach and role model assertiveness. (The patient learns to get his or her needs met appropriately, which helps reduce anxiety and acting-out behaviors.)

Stabilized Patients: Follow-Up Care

1. Involve the patient's family and significant others with teaching, treatment, and discharge and follow-up plans. Teaching includes nutrition, medication, and the dynamics of the illness. (Family involvement is a key factor to patient success. Family dynamics are often a significant factor in the patient's illness and distress.)
2. Make arrangements for follow-up therapy for both the patient and family. (Follow-up therapy for both the patient and family is key to relapse prevention.)
3. Offer referrals to the patient and family to local support groups or national groups. (See the list at the end of the chapter for suggestions.) (Support groups offer emotional support, resources, and important information; help minimize feelings of isolation; and encourage healthier coping strategies.)

Body Image Alteration

Due to:

- Cognitive and perceptual factors
- Psychosocial factors
- Chemical/biological imbalances
- Negative perception of body
- Morbid fear of obesity
- Low self-esteem

Desired Outcome:

By discharge (inpatient) or within two weeks (outpatient) the patient will verbalize a realistic perception of body size and shape and refer to body in a more positive way.

Assessment/Interventions (Rationales)

1. Establish a therapeutic alliance with the patient. (Patients with anorexia are highly resistant to giving up unhealthy eating behaviors. A trusting relationship with a nurse is the first step toward recovery.)
2. Give the patient feedback about the low weight and resultant impaired health. Do not argue or challenge the patient's perceptions. (Focuses on health and the benefits of increased energy. Arguments or power struggles will increase the patient's need to control.)

3. Recognize that the patient's distorted image is real to him or her. Avoid minimizing the patient's perceptions while challenging distortions (e.g., "I understand you see yourself as fat. I do not see you that way.") (This recognition acknowledges the patient's perceptions, and he or she feels understood even though your perception is different. This kind of feedback is easier to hear than negation of the patient's beliefs.)
4. Encourage expression of feelings regarding how the patient thinks and feels about self and body. (Promotes a clear understanding of the patient's perceptions and lays the groundwork for future interventions.)
5. Assist the patient to distinguish between thoughts and feelings. Statements such as "I feel fat" should be challenged and reframed. (It is important for the patient to distinguish between feelings and facts. The patient often speaks of feelings as though they are reality.)
6. Use a cognitive–behavioral approach to encourage the patient to keep a journal of thoughts and feelings and teach how to identify and challenge irrational beliefs. (Cognitive–behavioral approaches can be effective in helping the patient challenge irrational beliefs about self and body image. Journaling allows the patient to reflect on thoughts, feelings, and behaviors and facilitates sharing with the nurse.)
7. Encourage the patient to identify positive personal traits of his or her personal appearance. (Helps the patient refocus on strengths and actual physical and other attributes. Disrupts negative rumination.)
8. Educate the family regarding the patient's illness and encourage attendance at family sessions. (The reactions of family members may be triggers of emotional responses and distorted perceptions.)
9. Encourage family therapy for family and significant others. (Families and significant others need assistance in learning how to communicate with and relate to a patient who has anorexia.)

BULIMIA NERVOSA

Individuals with bulimia nervosa engage in repeated episodes of binge eating followed by inappropriate compensatory behaviors such as self-induced vomiting; misuse of laxatives, diuretics, or other medications; fasting; or excessive exercise. This disorder is characterized by a significant disturbance in the perception of body shape and weight. A sense of being out of control accompanies the consumption of large amounts of food, sometimes more than 5000 calories at a time. Bingeing is usually done alone and in secret. After a binge, individuals experience tremendous guilt, depression, or disgust with themselves.

Individuals with bulimia are more socially skilled and sexually active than patients with anorexia nervosa. Poor impulse control can manifest itself in other impulsive behaviors such as shoplifting and promiscuity. Alcohol and substance use is more common with this population.

Epidemiology

The 12-month prevalence of bulimia nervosa among young women is 1% to 1.5%. The lifetime incidence of bulimia nervosa for women is 2.3 and the lifetime incidence for men is 0.5% (Rosenvinge & Petterson, 2015). Bulimia commonly begins in later adolescence, when the prevalence peaks, up to young adulthood. Onset of bulimia nervosa is rare in children younger than 12 years and adults older than 40 years.

Risk Factors

Increased frequency of bulimia nervosa is found in first-degree relatives of people with this disorder. Gene variations that are responsible for serotonin have been implicated in bulimia. Even in recovery from this disorder serotonin levels remain abnormal. Vomiting may increase plasma endorphin levels and resultant feelings of well-being.

Affected individuals have increased gray matter in the medial orbitofrontal cortex, an area of the brain associated with reward responses. Inattention, impulsivity, and poor emotional regulation may result from altered activity in attentional areas of the brain. Accordingly, attention-deficit/hyperactivity disorder is associated with bulimia nervosa.

Temperamental qualities including impulsivity and sensation seeking are associated with this disorder. Triggers for bingeing may include stress, poor body self-image, food, restrictive dieting, or boredom.

Internalization of a thin body ideal increases the risk for weight worries, which in turn increase the risk for bulimia nervosa. There is also some connection between the disorder and childhood sexual or physical abuse. In some cases traumatic events and environmental stress may be contributing factors.

Treatment

Patients who are medically compromised may be referred to an inpatient eating disorder unit for comprehensive treatment of the illness. The cognitive–behavioral principles of treatment, which challenge irrational beliefs and self-defeating thoughts, are highly effective and typically serve as the cornerstone of the therapeutic approach.

Inpatient units designed to treat eating disorders are specially structured to interrupt the cycle of binge eating and purging and to normalize eating habits. The patient is encouraged examine the underlying conflicts and body dissatisfaction that accompany the illness. Evaluation for comorbid disorders, such as major depressive disorder and substance use, is also initiated. In most cases, substance use should be addressed prior to treating the eating disorder.

Antidepressants combined with cognitive–behavioral therapy is the best approach. Fluoxetine (Prozac), an SSRI antidepressant, has FDA approval for acute and maintenance treatment of bulimia nervosa in adult patients. When fluoxetine is used for bulimia, it is typically at a higher dose than is used for depression. Although no other drugs have FDA approval for this disorder, medications such as topiramate (Topamax) have been studied for binge suppression. Tricyclic antidepressants help reduce binge eating and vomiting.

Assessment

Signs and Symptoms

Psychological

- Feels out of control during binges
- Evaluates self based on body shape and weight
- Dissatisfied with body
- Feelings of dissociation during binges
- Ashamed of eating habits and attempts to conceal the behavior
- Binges are preceded by negative feelings and negative self-evaluation

Physiological

- Enlarged parotid glands
- Dental erosion, caries
- Loss of tooth enamel from vomiting
- Scars on knuckles (Russell's sign) from inducing vomiting
- Chronic hoarseness, chronic sore throat
- Cardiac arrhythmias
- Hypotension
- Gastrointestinal problems (e.g., constipation, diarrhea, reflux, and esophagitis)
- Fluid retention or dehydration
- Alkalosis (loss of stomach acid)
- Electrolyte imbalance (e.g., hypokalemia, hypochloremia, hyponatremia)

Assessment Guidelines

1. Medical stabilization is the first priority. Problems resulting from purging include disruptions in electrolyte and fluid balance and cardiac function; a thorough medical examination is vital.
2. Medical evaluation usually includes a thorough physical, as well as interpretation of pertinent laboratory values:
   - Electrolytes
   - Glucose
   - Thyroid function tests
   - Neuroimaging of the pituitary gland
   - Complete blood count
   - EKG
3. A psychiatric evaluation assesses for psychiatric comorbidity.

Patient Problems

Table 10.2 identifies signs and symptoms along with potential patient problems for individuals with bulimia nervosa.

Intervention Guidelines

1. Coexisting disorders (depression, substance use, personality disorders) often complicate the clinical picture,

Table 10.2 **Signs and Symptoms and Patient Problems for Bulimia Nervosa**

Signs and Symptoms	Patient Problems
Electrolyte imbalances, esophageal tears, cardiac problems, excessive vomiting, self-destructive behaviors	*Potential for injury* *Potential for cardiac arrhythmia* *Potential for electrolyte abnormalities*
Obsession with body, denial of problems, dissatisfaction with appearance	*Body image alteration*
Obsession with food, substance use, impulsive responses to problems; inappropriate use of laxatives, diuretics, enemas, fasting; inadequate problem solving	*Impaired coping*
Loss of control with the binge–purge cycle, feelings of shame and guilt, views self as unable to deal with events, excessive seeking of reassurance	*Decreased self-esteem*
Absence of supportive significant other(s), hides eating behaviors from others, reports feeling alone	*Isolation*

and these might require additional treatment and interventions.

2. Cognitive–behavioral techniques have been shown to be useful.
3. Group therapy with other individuals who have bulimia is often part of successful therapy.
4. Because anxiety and feelings of stress often precede bingeing, alternative ways of dealing with anxiety and alternative coping strategies to lessen anxiety are useful tools.
5. Family therapy is helpful and encouraged.

Nursing Care for Bulimia Nervosa

Potential for Injury

Due to:

- Chemical exposure (poisons, overuse of laxatives, diet pills, or diuretics)

- Malnutrition
- Biochemical dysfunction
- Nutritional deficiencies
- Uncontrollable binge–purge cycles
- Inadequate coping mechanisms to deal with anxiety and stress
- Poor impulse control
- Medical complications
    - Electrolyte imbalances
    - Esophageal tears
    - Cardiac problems
    - Altered thyroid and cortisol function

Desired Outcome:
By discharge (inpatient) or within two weeks (outpatient) the patient will break the binge-purge cycle and improve self-evaluation.

Assessment/Interventions (Rationales)

1. Assess for suicidal thoughts and other self-destructive behaviors. (Maintaining physical safety is the priority nursing intervention.)
2. Educate the patient regarding the negative effects of self-induced vomiting (i.e., dental erosion, low potassium level, cardiac problems). (Health teaching is crucial for the patient to know the insidious and unseen effects of purging behavior.)
3. Educate the patient about the binge–purge cycle and its self-perpetuating nature. (The compulsive nature of the binge–purge cycle is maintained by repeated restricting, hunger, bingeing, and then purging accompanied by feelings of guilt.)
4. Identify triggers that produce compulsive eating and purging behaviors. (Being aware of triggers helps the patient to substitute healthier coping when triggers occur.)
5. Explore dysfunctional thoughts that precede the binge–purge cycle. Teach the patient to challenge these thoughts and reframe them in healthier ways. (Cognitive-behavioral techniques can balance and combat distorted thinking. More rational thinking can lead to healthier behaviors, improved self-esteem, body image, and self-worth.)
6. Encourage the patient to record thoughts, feelings, and behaviors in a journal and share it with the nurse.

(Journaling helps to clarify thoughts and feelings and leads to increased self-awareness, problem-solving, and healing. Sharing journal content provides the patient with a sounding board for feedback.)

7. Work with the patient to identify problems and mutually establish short- and long-term goals. (The patient needs to develop tools for dealing with personal problems rather than turning to automatic binge–purge behaviors. Goals support hope and provide direction.)
8. Assess and teach problem-solving skills. (Alternative methods of relieving stress and getting needs met are vital in helping individuals to substitute healthy behaviors for binge eating behaviors.)
9. Arrange for the patient to learn ways to increase interpersonal communication, socialization, and assertiveness skills. (Patients with bulimia are often isolated from close relationships and lack appropriate skills for getting their needs met.)
10. Encourage attendance at support groups, recovery groups, or therapy groups with other individuals with bulimia. Provide information for family members as well. (Eating disorders are chronic diseases, and long-term follow-up therapy and support are critical for success.)

Powerlessness

Due to:

- Unsatisfying interpersonal interactions
- Lifestyle of helplessness
- Inability to control binge eating
- Distortion of body image
- Feelings of low self-worth
- Impulsivity
- Insufficient coping skills

Desired Outcome:

By discharge (inpatient) or within two weeks (outpatient) the patient will verbalize increased feelings of security and autonomy and demonstrate the ability to refrain from binge and purge behaviors.

Interventions (Rationales)

1. Explore the patient's experience of out-of-control eating behavior. (Listening in an empathetic, nonjudgmental

manner helps the patient feel that someone understands his or her experience.)

2. Encourage the patient to keep a journal of thoughts and feelings associated with binge–purge behaviors. (Automatic thoughts and beliefs maintain the binge–purge cycle. A journal is an excellent way to identify these dysfunctional thoughts and underlying assumptions.)
3. Teach the patient how to challenge negative and self-defeating thoughts and beliefs in a systematic manner. (These automatic dysfunctional thoughts must be examined and challenged if a change in patient thinking and behavior is to occur.)
4. Explore the kinds of cognitive distortions that affect feelings, beliefs, and behaviors. (Cognitive distortions reinforce unrealistic views of the self in terms of strengths and future potential. Realistic self-views promote healing and growth.)
5. Encourage the patient's participation in decisions and responsibility in his or her care and future. (Self-advocacy helps the patient gain a sense of control over his or her life and recognizing options for making important changes.)
6. Teach the patient alternative stress-reduction techniques and visualization skills to improve self-confidence and feelings of self-worth. (Visualizing a positive self-image and positive outcomes for life goals stimulates problem-solving toward desired goals.)
7. Encourage the patient to role play new skills in counseling sessions and in group therapy to practice communications with others, particularly family. (Role play allows an opportunity for the patient to become comfortable with new and different ways of relating and responding to others in a safe environment.)
8. Teach the patient that one lapse is not a relapse. One slip of control does not eliminate all positive accomplishments. (At the time of the lapse, it is helpful to examine what led to the lapse, knowing that one lapse does not eliminate all positive accomplishments.)

BINGE-EATING DISORDER

Individuals with binge-eating disorder engage in repeated episodes of out-of-control binge eating, after which they experience significant distress. They eat rapidly, eat until they feel uncomfortable, and eat when they are not hungry. Solitary and hidden binge eating of food is common to conceal the behavior. Inevitably, people feel self-disgust and guilt after the binge. Individuals with binge-eating disorder do not regularly use the compensatory behaviors (e.g., vomiting and laxatives) that are common with bulimia nervosa. Although people who start binge eating have a normal weight, repeated binge eating eventually results in obesity.

Epidemiology

Binge eating is the most common eating disorder. The 12-month prevalence for adults is 1.6% in females and 0.8% in males. For women, the lifetime incidence of binge-eating disorder is 3.6% and the lifetime incidence for men is 2.1% (Rosenvinge & Petterson, 2015). This eating disorder is more prevalent in overweight populations (3%) than in the general population (2%). All racial and ethnic groups seem to be represented fairly equally.

Risk Factors

Binge-eating disorder tends to run in families, which may be the result of addictive genetic influences. Biological abnormalities, such as hormonal irregularities, may be associated with compulsive eating and food addition. Low self-esteem and body dissatisfaction can contribute to binge-eating disorder. Reduced levels of coping ability are also associated with this disorder. Adverse childhood events such as sexual abuse can increase the risk of binge eating. Social pressures to be thin can trigger emotional eating.

Treatment

Several psychotherapeutic models are used in treating this population. Cognitive–behavioral therapy, behavior therapy, dialectical behavior therapy, and interpersonal therapy have all been associated with reduced binge frequency. See Chapter 29 for a description of these models.

Because of their efficacy with bulimia nervosa, SSRIs are used at or near the high end of the dosage range to treat binge-eating disorder. Although they seem to help in the short term, patients regain significant weight after stopping this medication.

Lisdexamfetamine dimesylate (Vyvanse), a central nervous system stimulant used for attention-deficit/

hyperactivity disorder, is the only FDA- approved drug for treating binge-eating disorder. This drug is a stimulant and can be habit-forming and misused. Common side effects include dry mouth and insomnia, but more serious side effects including strokes and heart attacks can occur. Antidepressants are probably a better first option due to more tolerable adverse effects and the lack of misuse risk.

Non-FDA approved drugs are used to treat overweight and individuals with obesity. Antidepressants help by improving mood, thereby reducing compulsive behavior, and also through the side effect of appetite suppression. SSRIs, tricyclic antidepressants, and bupropion (Wellbutrin) are used for reducing binge eating. Anti-seizure drugs such as topiramate (Topamax) are also used to break the binge eating cycle.

Assessment

Signs and Symptoms

Psychological

- Lack of control
- Distress
- Depression
- Grief
- Anxiety
- Shame
- Self-disgust
- Isolation

Physiological

- May be normal weight, overweight, or obese
- Obesity may result in:
  - Type II diabetes
  - High blood pressure
  - High cholesterol
  - Gallbladder disease/gallstones
  - Cardiac disease
  - Joint pain
  - Sleep apnea
  - Cancer (e.g., gallbladder, esophagus)

Patient Problems

Because binge-eating disorder is similar to bulimia nervosa (without the purging behaviors), many of the same patient

Table 10.3 **Signs and Symptoms and Patient Problems for Binge-Eating Disorder**

Signs and Symptoms	Patient Problems
Dysfunctional eating pattern, eating in response to internal cues, sedentary lifestyle, lack of control, intake exceeds metabolic need	*Excessive caloric intake*
Eats as a coping method, absence of other more effective coping methods, eats even when full	*Impaired coping*
Loss of control of eating, feelings of shame and guilt, views self as unable to deal with events	*Decreased self-esteem* *Powerlessness*
Absence of supportive significant other(s), eats normally in the presence of others, hides eating behaviors, reports feeling alone	*Isolation*

problems are applicable. Table 10.3 identifies signs and symptoms and potential patient problems for binge-eating disorder.

Nursing Care for Binge-Eating Disorder

Excessive Caloric Intake

Due to:

- Binge eating
- Lack of control over eating
- Eating rapidly
- Eating until uncomfortably full
- Eating when not hungry

Desire Outcome:

The patient will eliminate maladaptive eating behaviors by recognizing triggers for binge-eating, challenging automatic thoughts that lead to binge-eating, and utilize informal and formal supports.

Assessment/Interventions (Rationales)

1. Encourage the patient to keep a journal recording urges to binge eat, feelings or events immediately before, and responses to urges. (Understanding a pattern of binge eating will help to identify more adaptive responses to the urges.)

2. Identify ways to challenge irrational thoughts that may occur before binge eating. (Correcting faulty thinking is an evidence-based approach to managing this disorder.)
3. Encourage the exploration of alternate and healthy coping strategies. (Patients have been using food to regulate their mood and need new strategies.)
4. Help the patient to develop goals for adopting healthy eating patterns and exercise. (Self-care is promoted through the development of goals within the context of the nurse–patient relationship.)
5. Identify social support through friends and community (locally or online). (Social support makes one feel less alone and stronger, and more likely to achieve goals.)
6. Identify support groups for eating disorders in general or binge-eating disorder specifically. Groups can be local in physical facilities or online forums. (Support groups are a powerful tool for reducing isolation, getting feedback, sharing, helping, and practicing relational skills.)

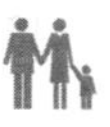

Nurse, Patient, and Family Resources

Anorexia Nervosa and Related Eating Disorders
www.anred.com

Binge Eating Disorder Association
www.bedaonline.com

Families Empowered and Supporting Treatment of Eating Disorders
www.feast-ed.org

KidsHealth (Search for Eating Disorders)
www.kidshealth.org

Mirror Mirror Eating Disorder Help
www.mirror-mirror.org

National Association of Anorexia Nervosa and Associated Disorders (ANAD)
www.anad.org

National Eating Disorders Association
www.nationaleatingdisorders.org

CHAPTER 11

Sleep Disorders

For many people, sleep is an expendable commodity. In a fast-paced society, sleep is often forfeited, and people subject themselves to schedules that disrupt normal sleep patterns. Sleep is given up to meet other social and vocational demands. The amount of time spent working, engaging in academic activities, and traveling to and from work and school are the strongest determinants of total sleep time. The more time devoted to work-related activities, the less time spent sleeping.

Sleep requirements vary from individual to individual and to some degree are probably genetically mediated. Although most adults require 7 to 8 hours of sleep for optimal functioning, a small percentage of individuals are referred to as long sleepers (requiring 10 or more hours per night) or short sleepers (requiring less than 5 hours per night). The amount of sleep necessary to feel fully awake and able to sustain normal levels of performance is known as the basal sleep requirement.

Nurses routinely work with patients who are sleep deprived. Pain, noise, unfamiliar environments, and anxiety disrupt sleep patterns in hospitalized patients. Virtually all psychiatric disorders are associated with sleep disturbance. Sleep disruption itself may be a precipitating factor in triggering psychiatric disorders and increasing the risk for relapse. Depressed patients with sleep disturbances demonstrate greater degrees of suicidal ideation. Long-standing insomnia is common in alcohol use disorder recovery. One of the strongest indications of recovery from any mental illness is a return to normal sleep patterns.

This chapter first examines common sleep disorders. This overview is followed by basic nursing care plans to address these common problems.

INSOMNIA DISORDER

Insomnia is characterized by dissatisfaction with the quantity or quality of sleep (American Psychiatric Association [APA], 2013). People with insomnia may have difficulty initiating sleep. Other people with insomnia may fall asleep easily but have difficulty maintaining sleep. They may wake frequently and then have trouble going back to sleep. Early morning awakening and being unable to go back to sleep is another problem associated with insomnia.

According to Spielman and Glovinsky (2004), three types of factors contribute to insomnia:

1. Predisposing factors create a vulnerability to insomnia. They include a history of poor-quality sleep, depression and anxiety, or a state of hyperarousal.
2. Precipitating factors are external events that trigger insomnia. Personal and work difficulties, medical and psychiatric disorders, grief, and changes in identity (as seen with retirement) are examples.
3. Perpetuating factors are sleep practices and attributes that maintain the sleep complaint, such as excessive caffeine or alcohol use, spending excessive amounts of time in bed or napping, and worrying about the consequences of insomnia.

Epidemiology

Insomnia is the most common sleep disorder and may affect up to 45% of adults (Sadock et al., 2015). Females are more commonly affected, as are older adults.

CIRCADIAN RHYTHM SLEEP DISORDERS

Circadian rhythm sleep disorders occur when there is a misalignment between the timing of the individual's normal circadian rhythm and external factors that affect the timing or duration of sleep. Examples include the following:

- Delayed sleep phase type: A delay of more than 2 hours between the desired time of sleep and actual sleep, which results in delayed waking. Rare in the general population, this type is more common in adolescents (about 7%).

- Advanced sleep phase type: Sleep begins several hours earlier and ends several hours earlier than desired. This problem becomes more common with age.
- Irregular sleep–wake type: Sleep is sporadic and fragmented. The longest sleep period lasts about 4 hours. It is associated with brain disorders such as Alzheimer disease and disruptive environments such as hospitals.
- Non-24-hour sleep–wake type: Sleep tends to occur later and later, eventually resulting in daytime sleeping. This is a significant problem for up to 70% of blind individuals. Medication specifically approved for this problem—tasimelteon (Hetlioz)—works by increasing melatonin.
- Shift work type: Working outside of the normal work hours (late evening and night) results in excessive sleepiness at work and impaired sleep at home.

EPIDEMIOLOGY

The prevalence of delayed sleep problems is about 7% in adolescents, compared with 0.17% of the general population. The prevalence of the other types of circadian rhythm sleep–wake disorders are dependent on environment, comorbid disorders, and work hours.

ASSESSMENT

Signs and Symptoms

- Looks fatigued
- Poor concentration
- Irritability, agitation
- Listlessness
- Complains of drowsiness
- Expresses dissatisfaction with sleep

Assessment Guidelines

The following questions are useful in determining the extent of the sleep problem:

- When did you begin having trouble with sleep?
- What activities do you normally engage in before sleep?
- Are there things in your sleep environment that are hampering your sleep (e.g., noise, light, temperature, or comfort)?

- Do you use your bedroom for things other than sleep or sexual activity?
- What time do you go to bed? How long does it take to fall asleep?
- Once asleep, do you wake? If so, what wakes you up? Are you able to return to sleep?
- If you are unable to sleep, what do you do?
- What time do you wake up?
- How much time do you actually think you sleep?
- Do you sleep longer on weekends or days off?
- Do you nap? If so, for how long? Do you feel refreshed?
- Has any stress or problem contributed to your sleep difficulties?
- What are your daily habits, diet, exercise, and medications?

Patient Problems

Table 11.1 offers signs and symptoms along with potential patient problems for individuals with sleep disorders.

Table 11.1 **Signs and Symptoms and Patient Problems for Sleep Disorders**

Signs and Symptoms	Patient Problems
Appears tired; experiences changes in affect and energy; reports changes in mood, quality of life, concentration, and sleep; reports lack of energy, sleep disturbances, early wakening	*Insomnia*
Confusion, agitation, anxiety, apathy, fatigue, poor concentration, slowed reaction, irritability, lethargy, malaise, perceptual problems, delusions, hallucinations	*Inadequate sleep*
Changes in normal sleep pattern, decreased ability to function, dissatisfaction with sleep, awakening, no difficulty falling asleep, not feeling well rested	*Sleep pattern disturbance*

Intervention Guidelines

Patients should be instructed to do the following:

- Go to bed only when sleepy.
- Use the bed or bedroom only for sleep and intimacy (no television, reading, or other activities in the bedroom).
- Get out of bed if unable to sleep and engage in a quiet activity such as reading or crossword puzzles.
- Avoid lighted activities, which stimulate the retina in the hour before bed (no television or computer).
- Maintain a regular sleep–wake schedule, with getting up at the same time each day being the most important factor.
- Avoid daytime napping. If napping is necessary to prevent an accident or injury, it should be limited to 20 to 30 minutes maximum, and a timer should be set.

Nursing Care for Insomnia

Insomnia

Due to:

- Anxiety
- Pain
- Grieving
- Daytime napping
- Inadequate physical activity
- Psychiatric disorder (e.g., major depressive disorder, schizophrenia)
- Poor sleep hygiene
- Medication
- Caffeine
- Alcohol
- Unsuitable environment

Desired Outcome:

By discharge (inpatient) or within one week (outpatient) patient will obtain 6 to 8 hours of uninterrupted sleep and express feelings of refreshment after sleeping.

Assessment/Interventions (Rationales)

1. Assess the patient's activity pattern and sleep pattern. (Baseline information sets the stage for successful interventions.)

2. Monitor the effects of hypnotic or other medications on the patient's sleep pattern. (If medication is effective, it can be slowly withdrawn as more permanent methods [e.g., antidepressants] take effect.)
3. Teach sleep hygiene measures such as limiting daytime naps, avoiding caffeine and nicotine close to bedtime, increasing daytime exercise, establishing a relaxing bedtime routine, and avoiding light-producing electronics 1 hour before sleep. (Obtaining healthy sleep is important for both physical and mental health.)
4. Provide for a comfortable, cool, quiet, disturbance-free, and dark environment. (Heat, noise, people, and light impair an individual's ability to sleep.)
5. Encourage the use of blackout curtains, eye shades, ear plugs, "white noise" machines or cell phone apps, humidifiers, fans and other devices that can make the bedroom more relaxing. (Nonpharmacological sleep aids are often extremely successful in promoting sleep.)
6. Teach relaxation methods to promote sleep such as slow, deep breathing; guided imagery; and progressive muscle relaxation. (Relaxation methods reduce anxiety and muscle tension that interfere with sleep.)
7. Monitor the patient's sleep for physical problems such as sleep apnea, urinary frequency, or discomfort. (Many physical problems that interfere with sleep can be successfully treated.)
8. Encourage the patient to keep a sleep diary or use an exercise-tracking device. (Understanding and evaluating sleep practices promote self-care. Sometimes perceptions of sleep are inaccurate and tracking sleep can improve self-perception.)

Inadequate Sleep

Due to:

- Physical or psychological pain
- Age-related sleep pattern changes
- Circadian asynchrony
- Restless legs syndrome
- Sleep apnea
- Psychiatric disorder (e.g., bipolar mania, schizophrenia, dementia)
- Poor sleep hygiene
- Nightmares, sleep walking, sleep terrors
- Caffeine
- Sleep interruption for treatments

- Unsuitable environment
- Life demands (caregiving responsibilities, parental duties, night shift work)

Desired Outcome:
By discharge (inpatient) or one week (outpatient) patient will establish a regular sleep and wake time and report feeling refreshed after sleep.

Assessment/Interventions (Rationales)
1. Assess sleep patterns and document findings. (Accurate baseline data will inform interventions and provide a record for improvement or lack of improvement.)
2. Provide sedatives or hypnotics, antipsychotics, or other medications prescribed for sleep. (Medication can prevent sustained sleep loss, which could result in psychosis [i.e., disturbed thinking, delusions, hallucinations].)
3. If sleep deprivation is severe, provide sleep-inducing medication through an intramuscular route. (Psychosis may impair the patient's ability to recognize a need for medication. Inducing sleep is a medical and nursing priority.)
4. Minimize sleep disruption whenever possible by medicating before bed and in the morning, keeping lights dim and voices quiet if medications or treatments must be accomplished at night. (Hospitals are notoriously noisy, and treatments can be intrusive at night. Minimizing sleep disturbances is essential to facilitate recovery.)
5. Promote a regular bedtime and wake time. (Reestablishing a normal period of sleep will improve functioning.)
6. As sleep normalizes, discourage sleep during the day. (Initially, patients may be so sleep deprived that short daytime naps are essential to restoring brain function and body homeostasis. After the crisis period, daytime naps will interfere with sleeping at night.)
7. Limit caffeine-containing drinks and food such as coffee, tea, colas, and chocolate. (Caffeine is a central nervous system stimulant and will interfere with sleep.)

TREATMENT FOR SLEEP DISORDERS

Biological Approaches

Pharmacological Therapy

Many people use sedative or hypnotic medications to address their sleep problems. Nurses can provide education about the benefits of a particular drug, the side effects, and adverse effects. Nurses should explain that medications are usually prescribed for no more than 2 weeks, because tolerance and withdrawal may result. In many settings, the nurse also monitors the effectiveness of the medication. Chapter 26 provides a list of US Food and Drug Administration (FDA) approved drugs for the treatment of insomnia.

Over-the-counter sleeping aids have limited effectiveness. Melatonin, a naturally occurring hormone, is a popular over-the-counter product. To date, there is little data to support its use in the management of insomnia disorder, but new research into prolonged-release forms of melatonin are demonstrating some promise.

Non-FDA approved drugs used for insomnia include antidepressants, anticonvulsants, and antihistamines are also used off-label. Second-generation antipsychotics improve sleep in people using them as indicated for other problems such as schizophrenia. See Chapter 26 for specific sleep-promoting medications.

Psychotherapeutic Approaches

Successful treatment of insomnia involves the integration of basic principles of sleep hygiene (conditions and practices that promote continuous and effective sleep). Modifying poor sleep habits and establishing a regular sleep–wake schedule can be facilitated by using sleep diaries (Fig. 11.1). A period of 2 weeks is helpful in establishing overall sleep patterns and determining overall sleep efficiency ([time in bed divided by total sleep time] × 100). After reviewing sleep diaries, patients are sometimes surprised to discover that their sleep problems are not as bad as previously believed.

Sleep restriction, or limiting the total sleep time, creates a temporary mild state of sleep deprivation and strengthens the sleep homeostatic drive. This helps decrease sleep latency and improves sleep continuity and quality. If, for example, a patient is in bed for 8 hours but sleeping only 6 hours, sleep is restricted to 6 hours, and the bedtime and wake time are adjusted accordingly. Once sleep efficiency is improved, total sleep time is gradually increased by 10- to 20-minute increments.

A specific type of cognitive–behavioral therapy (CBT) is used for insomnia (CBT-I). Patients are encouraged to

Two-week sleep diary

INSTRUCTIONS:

1 Write the date, day of the week, and type of day: Work, School, Day off, or Vacation.
2 Put the letter "C" in the box when you have coffee, cola or tea. Put "M" when you take any medicine. Put "A" when you drink alcohol. Put "E" when you exercise.
3 Put a line (I) to show when you go to bed. Shade in the box that shows when you think you fell asleep.
4 Shade in all the boxes that show when you are asleep at night or when you take a nap during the day.
5 Leave boxes unshaded to show when you wake up at night and when you are awake during the day.

SAMPLE ENTRY BELOW: On a Monday when I worked, I jogged on my lunch break at 1 PM, had a glass of wine with dinner at 6 PM, fell asleep watching TV from 7 to 8 PM, went to bed at 10:30 PM, fell asleep around midnight, woke up and couldn't get back to sleep at about 4 AM, went back to sleep from 5 to 7 AM, and had coffee and medicine at 7:00 in the morning.

Today's Date	Day of the week	Type of Day Work, School, Off, Vacation	Noon	1 PM	2	3	4	5	6 PM	7	8	9	10	11 PM	Midnight	1 AM	2	3	4	5	6 AM	7	8	9	10	11
sample	Mon.	Work		E					A				I									C M				

Week 1

Week 2

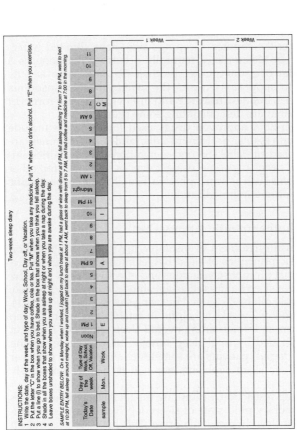

Fig. 11.1 Two Week Sleep Diary Figure 7.2. (Printed with permission from the American Academy of Sleep Medicine. Available from: http://sleepeducation.org/.)

identify misperceptions about sleep (e.g., I need 9 hours). The focus is aimed at the quality of sleep rather than the number of hours slept. Other objectives of CBT-I are directed at identifying and correcting maladaptive attitudes and beliefs about sleep. For example, patients may rationalize maladaptive coping behaviors such as excessive time in bed to catch up on lost sleep and may exhibit unrealistic expectations about sleep.

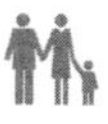

NURSE, PATIENT, AND FAMILY RESOURCES

American Academy of Sleep Medicine
www.aasmnet.org

American Sleep Apnea Association
www.sleepapnea.org

American Sleep Medicine
www.americansleepmedicine.com

Centers for Disease Control and Prevention: Sleep and Sleep Disorders
www.cdc.gov/sleep/resources.html

Narcolepsy Network
www.narcolepsynetwork.org

National Sleep Foundation
www.sleepfoundation.org

Restless Legs Syndrome Foundation
www.rls.org

CHAPTER 12

Substance Use Disorders

Substance use disorders are not disorders of choice. They are complex diseases of the brain characterized by craving, seeking, and using regardless of consequences. Continuous substance use results in actual changes in the brain structure and brain function. Substance use disorders are chronic and relapsing. They result in compromised executive function circuits that mediate self-control and decision making.

More than 21 million individuals, or nearly 9% of the population of the United States, are estimated to have substance use disorders (Substance Abuse and Mental Health Services Administration [SAMHSA], 2015). A substance use disorder is a pathological use of a substance that leads to a disorder of use. Symptoms fall into four major groupings:

- Impaired control
- Social damage
- Risky use
- Physical effects (i.e., intoxication, tolerance, and withdrawal)

Substance use disorders encompass a broad range of products that human beings take into their bodies through various means (e.g., swallowing, inhaling, injecting). They range from fairly innocuous and innocent-seeming substances such as caffeine to absolutely illegal mind-altering drugs such as LSD. No matter the substance, use disorders share many commonalities, intoxication characteristics, and withdrawal attributes.

The American Psychiatric Association's (APA) *Diagnostic and Statistical Manual of Mental Disorders, fifth edition* (*DSM-5;* 2013) provides diagnostic criteria for the following psychoactive substances:

Alcohol
Caffeine
Cannabis
Hallucinogen

Inhalant
Opioid
Sedative, hypnotic, and antianxiety medication
Stimulant
Tobacco

In addition to substances, behaviors can be addictive. In these process addictions, there are no substances being used. Although the physical signs of drug addiction do not accompany these types of addictions, compulsive actions activate the reward or pleasure pathways in the brain similarly to substances (SAMHSA, 2014). The first process addiction, gambling disorder, was added to the *DSM-5* in 2013. Other compulsive behaviors including internet gaming, using social media, shopping, and sexual activity may be added as official disorders in future editions of the *DSM*.

CONCEPTS CENTRAL TO SUBSTANCE USE DISORDERS

Addiction

Addiction is a primary, chronic disease of brain reward, motivation, memory, and related circuitry. It is a disease of dysregulation in the hedonic (pleasure-seeking) or reward pathway of the brain. Individuals with addictions are unable to abstain from the substance or activity or recognize how disturbed their functioning, interpersonal relationships, and emotional responses are. Like other chronic diseases, there are cycles of relapse and remission. Ultimately, without treatment, addiction is progressive and often results in disability or premature death.

Intoxication

When people are using a substance to excess, they are experiencing intoxication. Intoxication varies depending on the substance being used. Terminology varies depending on the substance and the population who is using: alcohol causes intoxication, but cocaine makes you high.

Tolerance

Tolerance occurs when a person no longer responds to the drug in the way that person initially responded. It takes a higher dose of the drug to achieve the same level of early response.

Withdrawal

Withdrawal is a set of physiological symptoms that occur when a person stops using a substance. Withdrawal is specific to the substance being used, and each substance will have its own characteristic syndrome, which may be mild or life threatening. The more intense symptoms a person has, the more likely the person is to start using the substance again to avoid the symptoms.

This chapter focuses on substance use disorders. An overview of each major category is provided. The subject of nursing care for this population is then addressed.

CLINICAL PICTURE

Caffeine

Caffeine is the most widely used psychoactive substance in the world. Excessive caffeine use is not an official use disorder. However, caffeine can result in intoxication and withdrawal. The half-life of caffeine in the human body is 3 to 10 hours, and the peak concentration for most people is 30 to 60 minutes (Sadock et al., 2015).

Caffeine Intoxication

Symptoms of caffeine intoxication include nervousness, excitement, agitation, rambling speech, and inexhaustibility. Patients may have a flushed face, diuresis, gastrointestinal disturbance, muscle twitching, tachycardia, or cardiac arrhythmia. These symptoms are distressing to the individual and result in impairment of normal areas of functioning. Individuals with tolerance may not experience these symptoms. Extremely high doses may result in grand mal seizures, and respiratory failure may cause death.

Caffeine Withdrawal

Removal of caffeine from the daily routine results in headache, drowsiness, irritability, and poor concentration. Some people experience nausea, vomiting, and muscle aches. Symptoms occur within 12 to 24 hours after the last ingestion, peak in 24 to 48 hours, and resolve within 1 week.

Cannabis Use Disorder

Cannabis, or marijuana, comes from the dried leaves, flowers, stems, and seeds from the cannabis plant. The chemical compound tetrahydrocannabinol (THC) is responsible for its mind-altering effects. The 12-month prevalence of cannabis use disorder in adolescents is about 3.5% and in adults is about 1.5% (APA, 2013). Males are more likely to have this disorder, which tends to progress slowly. Users experience craving, tolerance, and withdrawal. The use of this substance results in problems with work, home life, education, and social and physical well-being.

Cannabis Intoxication

Cannabis intoxication heightens users' sensations. They experience brighter colors, they see new details in common stimuli, and time seems to go more slowly. In higher doses, they experience depersonalization and derealization. Motor skills are impacted for 8 to 12 hours, and driving and the use of machinery may be hazardous. Physical symptoms of intoxication include conjunctival injection (red eyes from vessel dilation), increased appetite, dry mouth, and tachycardia.

Cannabis Withdrawal

Withdrawal occurs within 1 week of cessation. Symptoms include irritability, anger, aggression, anxiety, restlessness, and depressed mood. Because marijuana causes sleepiness, insomnia and disturbing dreams may occur without it. A decreased appetite may lead to weight loss. Physical symptoms of withdrawal include abdominal pain, shakiness, sweating, fever, chills, and headache.

Cannabis Treatment

Abstinence and support are the main principles of treatment for cannabis use disorder. Hospitalization or outpatient care may be required. Individual, family, and group therapies can provide support. Antianxiety medication may be useful for short-term relief of withdrawal symptoms. Patients with underlying anxiety and depression may respond to antidepressant therapy.

Hallucinogen Use Disorder

Hallucinogens cause a profound disturbance in reality. Hallucinogens are associated with flashbacks, panic attacks, psychosis, delirium, and mood and anxiety disorders. They are both natural and synthetic substances. Hallucinogens have no medical use. They are found in some plants and mushrooms, or they can be human-made. Classic hallucinogens (e.g., LSD) and dissociative hallucinogens (e.g., phencyclidine [PCP] and ketamine) exist. A use disorder causes significant impairment or distress and includes craving, difficulty with role obligations, impairment, and tolerance.

Hallucinogen Intoxication

Intoxication is characterized by paranoia, impaired judgment, intensified perceptions, depersonalization, and derealization. Illusions, hallucinations, and synesthesias (e.g., hearing colors or seeing sounds) are prominent. Other symptoms include pupillary dilation, tachycardia, sweating, palpitations, blurred vision, tremors, and incoordination.

Hallucinogen Intoxication Treatment

Treatment for hallucinogen intoxication includes talking the patient down. That means reassuring the patient that the symptoms are caused by the drug and that they will subside. In severe cases (Sadock et al., 2015), an antipsychotic such as haloperidol (Haldol) or a benzodiazepine such as diazepam (Valium) can be used in the short term.

Phencyclidine Intoxication

PCP intoxication is a medical emergency. Behavioral symptoms include belligerence, assaultiveness, impulsiveness, and unpredictability. Physical symptoms include nystagmus (involuntary eye movements), hypertension, tachycardia, reduced response to pain, ataxia (loss of voluntary muscle control), dysarthria (unclear speech), muscle rigidity, seizures, coma, and hyperacusis (sensitivity to sound). Hyperthermia and seizure activity may also occur.

Phencyclidine Intoxication Treatment

Patients who have ingested PCP cannot be talked down and may require restraint and a calming medication such as a benzodiazepine. Mechanical cooling may be necessary for severe hyperthermia.

Hallucinogen Withdrawal

There is no official withdrawal syndrome. However, hallucinogen persisting perception disorder may be experienced by about 4% of users, particularly with LSD. The hallmark of this problem is the reexperiencing of perceptual symptoms that were experienced while intoxicated. These symptoms are distressing and impair the individual from normal functioning for weeks, months, or even years.

Inhalant Use Disorder

Inhalants are toxic gases inhaled through the nose or mouth that enter the bloodstream. Misused household products include solvents for glues and adhesives; aerosol propellant paint sprays, hair sprays, and shaving cream; thinners such as paint products and correction fluids; and fuels such as gasoline and propane. Use of inhalants result in increasing use, craving, and tolerance. Inhalants result in impaired life roles and problems in relationships. This disorder occurs primarily between the ages of 12 and 17 years with a 12-month prevalence rate of about 0.4% (APA, 2013).

Inhalant Intoxication

Small doses result in disinhibition and euphoria. High doses can cause fearfulness, illusions, auditory and visual hallucinations, and a distorted body image. Apathy, diminished social and occupational functioning, impaired judgment, and impulsivity and aggression accompany intoxication. Physical responses include nausea, anorexia, nystagmus, depressed reflexes, and diplopia. High doses can lead to stupor, unconsciousness, and amnesia. Delirium, dementia, and psychosis are also possible.

Inhalant Treatment

Although intoxication usually does not usually require treatment, serious responses such as coma, cardiac arrhythmias, or bronchospasm do happen. A psychotic state may be induced by inhalant intoxication. This self-limiting (a few hours to a few weeks) problem may require an antipsychotic such as haloperidol (Haldol) to manage severe agitation.

Opioid Use Disorder

Opioid misuse, particularly with heroin and prescription drugs, is a chronic relapsing disorder. Cravings and tolerance are significant. The misuse of this substance results in significant impairment in life roles and causes interpersonal conflict. The disinhibition from the drug often puts people in physically hazardous situations.

In 2014 about 435,000 people age 12 years or older were current heroin users (SAMHSA, 2015). Opioid use problems usually begin in the late teens or early 20s. With increasing age, fewer people are affected, probably due to factors such as early mortality and a cessation of use after age 40 years.

Opioid Intoxication

Opioid intoxication results in psychomotor retardation, drowsiness, slurred speech, altered mood, and impaired memory and attention. Intoxicated individuals also exhibit pupillary constriction. Intense drowsiness can progress to a comatose state.

Opioid Withdrawal

Withdrawal symptoms occur after a cessation or reduction in use, or after an opioid antagonist has been administered. Symptoms include mood dysphoria, nausea, vomiting, diarrhea, muscle aches, fever, and insomnia. Other classic symptoms of withdrawal are lacrimation (watery eyes), rhinorrhea (runny nose), pupillary dilation, piloerection (bristling of hairs), and yawning. Males may experience sweating and spontaneous ejaculations.

Morphine, heroin, and methadone withdrawal begins at 6 to 8 hours. It intensifies on the second or third day and then subsides during the next week. Meperidine (Demerol) withdrawal begins within 8 to 12 hours from abstinence and lasts about 5 days.

Opioid Overdose

Death usually results from respiratory depression. Symptoms include unresponsiveness, slow respiration, coma, hypothermia, hypotension, and bradycardia. Three symptoms—coma, pinpoint pupils, and respiratory depression—are strongly suggestive of overdose.

Overdose treatment begins with aspirating secretions and inserting an airway. Mechanical ventilation should be used until naloxone, a specific opioid antagonist, can be given. Narcan nasal spray is sprayed into one nostril while patients lie on their back. Evzio is a prefilled auto-injection device that is used to inject naloxone quickly into the outer thigh. Increased respirations and pupillary dilation happen quickly. Too much naloxone may produce withdrawal symptoms. The duration of action for naloxone is short compared with many opioids and repeated administration may be required.

Opioid Treatment

Individual therapy, behavioral therapy, cognitive–behavioral therapy, family therapy, and social skills training are used to manage opioid use disorder. Support groups such as Narcotics Anonymous (NA), a 12-step program, are effective.

A summary of medications used for this disorder follows:

- Methadone (Dolophine, Methadose) is used to decrease symptoms of withdrawal. It reduces the attractiveness of opioids by blocking their euphoric effects.
- Buprenorphine is used to help reduce or quit opioids.
- Naltrexone (Vivitrol) is used to prevent of relapse after detoxification by blocking the euphoric and sedative effects of opioids.

See Chapter 27 for more information on pharmacological treatment for opioid addiction.

Sedative, Hypnotic, and Antianxiety Medication Use Disorder

Sedative, hypnotic, and antianxiety mediation use disorder is applied to the misuse of all prescription sleeping medications and almost all prescription antianxiety drugs: benzodiazepines, benzodiazepine-like drugs (e.g., zolpidem, zaleplon), carbamates, barbiturates (e.g., secobarbital), and barbiturate-like hypnotics (e.g., methaqualone). Use of these depressants negatively affects role performance and relationships. Craving, tolerance, and withdrawal can develop even when taken for their intended indication. However, a psychiatric diagnosis is only given in the presence of clinically significant maladaptive behavior or psychological changes.

The 12-month prevalence of this problem is about 0.2% in adults. It occurs in males slightly more often than in females. These disorders are highest among 18- to 29-year-olds (0.5%) and lowest among individuals 65 and older (0.04%).

Sedative, Hypnotic, and Antianxiety Medication Intoxication

Because they are depressants, intoxication from these drugs results in slurred speech, incoordination, unsteady gait, nystagmus, and impaired thinking. A coma is possible. Inappropriate aggression and sexual behavior, mood fluctuation, and impaired judgment may also be side effects.

Sedative, Hypnotic, and Antianxiety Medication Overdose

Overdose treatment includes gastric lavage, activated charcoal, and vital sign monitoring. If awake after overdosing, patients should be kept awake to prevent a loss of consciousness. If the patient is unconscious, an intravenous fluid line should be started. An endotracheal tube may be required to provide a patent airway, and mechanical ventilation may be necessary. Flumazenil (Romazicon), a benzodiazepine receptor antagonist, is FDA approved for the management of benzodiazepine overdose.

Sedative, Hypnotic, and Antianxiety Medication Withdrawal

Repeated dampening of the central nervous system, along with the body's attempts to return to homeostasis, results in rebound hyperactivity with the removal of the depressant. Hence, autonomic hyperactivity, tremor, insomnia, psychomotor agitation, anxiety, and grand mal seizures occur. The drug's half-life is an important predictor of withdrawal time.

Gradual reduction of benzodiazepines will prevent seizures and other withdrawal symptoms. Barbiturate withdrawal can be aided by using a long-acting barbiturate such as phenobarbital.

Stimulant Use Disorder

Amphetamine-type, cocaine, or other stimulant drugs are second only to cannabis as the most widely used illicit substances in the United States. They typically produce a euphoric feeling and high energy. Long-distance truckers, students studying for examinations, soldiers in wartime, and athletes in competition use these drugs. As with all use disorders, increased use, craving, and tolerance are accompanied by reduced ability to function in major roles. Stimulants represent a significant problem, because a use disorder pattern can occur in as little as 1 week.

The estimated 12-month prevalence for amphetamine-type stimulants is about 0.2% in adults. Both genders are affected equally. Intravenous stimulant use is greater in males, at a rate of around 4:1. Cocaine use disorder is higher, 0.3%, with more male users.

Stimulant Intoxication

Stimulants make people feel elated, euphoric, and sociable. They also make people hypervigilant, sensitive, anxious, tense, and angry. Physical symptoms include chest pain, cardiac arrhythmias, high or low blood pressure, tachycardia or bradycardia, respiratory depression, dilated pupils, perspiration, chills, nausea or vomiting, weight loss, psychomotor agitation or retardation, weakness, confusion, seizures, and coma.

Stimulant Withdrawal

Withdrawal symptoms begin within a few hours to several days. Symptoms include tiredness, vivid nightmares, increased appetite, insomnia or hypersomnia, and psychomotor retardation or agitation. Functionality is impaired during withdrawal. Depression and suicidal thoughts are the most serious side effects of stimulant withdrawal.

Withdrawal Treatment

For amphetamines, an inpatient setting is usually necessary. Depending on the amphetamine used, specific drugs may be used short-term. Antipsychotics may be prescribed for a few days. If there is no psychosis, diazepam (Valium) is useful in treating agitation and hyperactivity.

For cocaine, the 1- to 2-week withdrawal period has no physiological disturbances that require inpatient care. Some patients experience fatigue, mood changes, disturbed sleep, craving, and depression. There are no drugs that reliably reduce the intensity of these symptoms. Hospitalization may be helpful to remove the affected individual from the usual social settings and drug sources.

Tobacco Use Disorder

Craving, persistent use, and tolerance are all symptoms of tobacco use disorder. Dependence happens quickly. The 12-month prevalence of tobacco use disorder is about 13% in adults. Rates are slightly higher in males compared with females. Most people who use tobacco begin before the age of 18 years.

Tobacco Withdrawal

Tobacco withdrawal is distressing and results in irritability, anxiety, depression, difficulty concentrating, restlessness, and insomnia. Within days of smoking cessation, heart rates decrease by 5 to 12 beats per minute. Within the first year of smoking cessation, people gain an average of 4 to 7 pounds.

Withdrawal Treatment

Behavioral therapy helps patients to recognize cravings and respond to them. Hypnosis is used to treat tobacco withdrawal. Nicotine replacement therapies in the form of gum, lozenges, nasal sprays, and patches are successful treatments. The antidepressant bupropion (Zyban) reduces cravings for nicotine. Clonidine (Catapres) decreases sympathetic activity and reduces withdrawal symptoms. Varenicline (Chantix) partially activates nicotinic acetylcholine receptors providing mild nicotine-like effects. It also blocks the effects of nicotine from cigarettes if smoking is resumed.

Gambling Disorder

Gambling is a compulsive activity that causes economic problems and significant disturbances in personal, social, or occupational functioning. Individuals are preoccupied with the behavior, experience an increasing desire to engage in the behavior, and lie to conceal the extent of the problem. They may try to control the behavior, cut back, or stop gambling. Otherwise honest people may commit illegal acts to finance their addiction. They may rely on others to help pay off debts and gamble to recoup losses.

The 1 year prevalence rate in females is about 0.2% and in males is about 0.6%. The lifetime prevalence of gambling disorder is about 0.4% to 1%. Early gambling problems are more common in males, although the progression is more rapid for females. Gambling may be regular or episodic. Heavy gambling may be interspersed with abstinence. Stress and depression may increase this behavior.

Treatment

Legal problems, pressure from family, and other psychiatric problems may bring the person who gambles excessively into treatment. Gamblers Anonymous (GA) is a 12-step program modeled on Alcoholics Anonymous (AA). It involves public confession, peer pressure, and peer counselors who are reformed gamblers. Hospitalization may help by removing patients from gambling environments. Individual, group, and family therapy are useful in supporting the patient.

Medications such as selective serotonin reuptake inhibitors, bupropion (Wellbutrin), mood stabilizers (lithium), and anticonvulsants such as topiramate (Topamax) may be helpful. Second-generation antipsychotics are used. Naltrexone, an opioid antagonist, may be given to individuals with the most severe symptoms of gambling disorder.

ALCOHOL USE DISORDER

Although alcohol is a sedative, it creates an initial feeling of euphoria. This is probably related to decreased inhibitions. A cluster of behavioral and physical symptoms characterizes alcohol use disorder.

Table 12.1 **Maximum Safe Number of Drinks**

	Men	Women	Pregnant	Adolescent	Older Adults
Day	4	3	0	0	3
Week	14	7	0	0	7

US Department of Health and Human Services. (2015). 2015–2020 Dietary guidelines for Americans (8th ed.). Retrieved from http://health.gov/dietaryguidelines/2015/guidelines/.

Types of Problematic Drinking

The amounts of alcohol that is considered safe varies depending on individual factors. Table 12.1 identifies the numbers of drinks that are considered acceptable depending on the gender, age, and pregnancy status.

Excessive drinking is described with two different terms. Binge drinking is a pattern of drinking that brings blood alcohol concentration (BAC) levels to 0.08 g/dL. This level usually happens after 4 drinks for women and 5 drinks for men in about 2 hours (US Department of Health and Human Services, 2015). Heavy drinking is characterized by drinking too much, too often. Consuming eight or more drinks in a week constitutes heavy drinking in women. Men who drink more than 15 drinks in a week are considered heavy drinkers.

Alcohol Intoxication

In the United States a standard drink contains about 14 grams of pure alcohol. This amount is found in 12 ounces of beer with 5% alcohol content, 5 ounces of wine with 12% alcohol content, and 1.5 ounces of distilled spirits with 40% alcohol content.

The legal definition of intoxication in most states requires a blood concentration of 0.08 to 0.10 g/dL. Blood alcohol levels, numbers of drinks, and symptoms of alcohol intoxication are listed in Table 12.2.

Excessive amounts of alcohol may result in blackouts in which new memories cannot be consolidated. During blackouts a person actively engages in behaviors, can perform complicated tasks, and may appear normal.

Alcohol Withdrawal

Alcohol withdrawal occurs after reducing or quitting alcohol after heavy and prolonged use. A summary of

Table 12.2 **Blood Alcohol, Drinks, and Symptoms**

Blood Alcohol	Drinks	Symptoms
0.02 g/dL	2	Slower motor performance, decreased thinking ability, altered mood, and reduced ability to multitask
0.05 g/dL	3	Impaired judgment, exaggerated behavior, euphoria, and lower alertness
0.08 g/dL	4	Poor muscle coordination, altered speech and hearing, difficulty detecting danger, impaired judgment, poor self-control, and decreased reasoning
0.10 g/dL	5	Slurred speech, poor coordination, and slowed thinking
0.15 g/dL	6	Vomiting (unless high tolerance) and major loss of balance
0.20 g/dL	8–10	Memory blackouts, nausea, and vomiting
0.30 g/dL	10+	Reduction of body temperature, blood pressure, respiratory rate, sleepiness, and amnesia
0.40 mg/dL	—	Impaired vital signs and possible death

symptoms is provided below. See Chapter 27 for a more thorough discussion of alcohol withdrawal and treatment.

- Mild symptoms begin 6 to 24 hours after alcohol cessation. These symptoms include agitation, lack of appetite, nausea, vomiting, insomnia, impaired cognition, and mild perceptual changes.
- Moderate symptoms begin 24 to 72 hours after the last drink. Autonomic symptoms are experienced as increased systolic blood pressure, rapid respirations, tachycardia, and mild hyperthermia. More severe symptoms of psychosis and perceptual symptoms may begin.
- Patients undergoing withdrawal to the point of psychosis should be treated promptly because of the risks of unconsciousness, seizures, and delirium.
- Withdrawal seizures may occur within 12 to 24 hours after alcohol cessation. These seizures are generalized and tonic-clonic.
- Alcohol withdrawal delirium, or delirium tremens (DTs) may happen anytime in the first 72 hours. It is a medical

emergency that may kill 20% of untreated patients, usually as a result of pneumonia, renal disease, hepatic insufficiency, or heart failure (Sadock et al., 2015). Autonomic hyperactivity is accompanied by delusions and visual and tactile hallucinations.

Alcohol-Induced Persisting Amnestic Disorder

Wernicke-Korsakoff Syndrome. Heavy alcohol use may result in a memory-reducing problem called Wernicke (alcoholic) encephalopathy, an acute and reversible condition. It is characterized by altered gait, vestibular dysfunction, confusion, and several ocular motility abnormalities. Sluggish reaction to light and anisocoria (unequal pupil size) are also symptoms. Wernicke encephalopathy responds rapidly to large doses of intravenous thiamine two to three times daily for 1 to 2 weeks.

Untreated Wernicke's encephalopathy may progress into Korsakoff's syndrome, the more severe and chronic version of this problem. Treatment of Korsakoff syndrome is also thiamine for 3 to 12 months. Most patients with Korsakoff's syndrome never fully recover, although cognitive improvement may occur with thiamine and nutritional support.

Fetal Alcohol Syndrome

Fetal alcohol syndrome is the leading cause of intellectual disability in the United States (Sadock et al., 2015). Alcohol during pregnancy inhibits intrauterine growth and postnatal development resulting in microcephaly, craniofacial malformations, and limb and heart defects. As adults, affected individuals tend to have a short stature. Pregnant women with alcohol-related disorders have a 35% risk of having a child with defects.

Systemic Effects

Alcohol overuse results in damage to just about every system in the body. Conditions associated with alcohol use disorder include the following:

- Peripheral neuropathy
- Alcoholic myopathy
- Alcoholic cardiomyopathy
- Esophagitis
- Gastritis

- Cirrhosis of the liver
- Leukopenia
- Thrombocytopenia
- Cancer
- Pancreatitis
- Alcoholic hepatitis

TREATMENT FOR ALCOHOL USE DISORDER

Biological Approaches

Pharmacological Therapy

A summary of treatments for alcohol use disorder is provided in Chapter 27.

Psychotherapeutic Approaches

Recovery

Recovery is a lifelong process, and it comes about in steps. Because each patient has different strengths, backgrounds, and supports, the goals of treatment should be tailored to the individual's immediate needs and abilities. The Recovery Model emphasizes hope, social connections, empowerment, coping strategies, and meaning in life. It is a social model of hope rather than a medical model of disability. This model focuses on managing symptoms, reducing psychological disability, and improving role performance.

Support Groups

A 12-step program based on AA is the most effective treatment modality for all addictions. The 12 steps ("working the steps") are designed to help a person refrain from addictive behaviors and to foster individual change and growth. Other substance-based support groups include Narcotics Anonymous (NA), Pills Anonymous (PA), Cocaine Anonymous (CA), and others. These groups help break down denial in an atmosphere of support and acceptance. Other group members who are further along in recovery sponsor new individuals. The more the patient feels socially involved with peers, the greater the likelihood of successful treatment outcome, continuation of treatment, and lower relapse rates.

Family and significant others are dramatically affected by individuals with addictive disorders. They may engage in enabling behaviors such as making excuses for a spouse's hangover or lending money to a drug user so he or she won't be forced to steal. Support groups provide information and methods for identifying and avoiding enabling behaviors. Al-Anon is for friends and family members of individuals with alcohol use disorder. Adult Children of Alcoholics (ACOA) addresses issues common to growing up in alcohol-disordered homes. Narc-Anon is for friends and family members of individuals with opioid use disorder.

ASSESSMENT

Current alcohol or other substance problems can be detected by asking two questions that are easily integrated into a clinical interview:

- In the past year, have you ever gotten drunk or used drugs more than you intended?
- Have you ever felt you wanted or needed to cut down on your drinking or drug use in the past year?

The APA (2013) recommends asking the following questions:

1. How much have you been bothered by drinking at least four drinks of alcohol in a single day?
2. How much have you been bothered by smoking cigarettes, a cigar, or pipe, or using snuff or chewing tobacco?
3. How much have you been bothered by using any of the following medicines on your own, or without a prescription, in greater amounts or longer than prescribed (e.g., painkillers [like Vicodin]; stimulants [like Ritalin or Adderall]; sedatives or tranquilizers [like sleeping pills or Valium]; or drugs like marijuana, cocaine or crack, club drugs [like ecstasy], hallucinogens [like LSD], heroin, inhalants or solvents [like glue], or methamphetamine [like speed])?

Assessment Tool

A simple, crosscutting measure for most misused substances is provided in Table 12.3. This tool helps to identify risky substance use in patients by quantifying the behaviors.

Table 12.3 **National Institute on Drug Abuse Modified ASSIST**

In the past year, how often have you used the following?					
Alcohol[a]	Never	Once or twice	Monthly	Weekly	Daily or almost daily
Tobacco	Never	Once or twice	Monthly	Weekly	Daily or almost daily
Prescription drugs[b]	Never	Once or twice	Monthly	Weekly	Daily or almost daily
Illegal drugs	Never	Once or twice	Monthly	Weekly	Daily or almost daily

[a]Men, 5+ drinks a day; women, 4+ drinks a day
[b]Nonmedical reasons
National Institute on Drug Abuse. NIDA drug screening tool. Retrieved from https://www.drugabuse.gov/nmassist/

Assessment Guidelines

- Is immediate medical attention necessary for a severe or major withdrawal syndrome? For example, alcohol and sedative use can be life threatening during a major withdrawal.
- Is the patient experiencing an overdose to a substance that requires immediate medical attention? For example, opioids or depressants can cause respiratory depression, coma, and death.
- Does the patient have physical complications related to substance use (e.g., AIDS, abscess, tachycardia, hepatitis)?
- Does the patient have suicidal thoughts or indicate, through verbal or nonverbal cues, a potential for self-destructive behaviors?
- Does the patient seem interested in doing something about the substance use problem?

Patient Problems

Nurses care for patients with substance use disorders in a variety of settings and situations. Some conditions call for medical interventions and skilled nursing care, whereas others call for effective use of communication and counseling skills. The following pages offer the nurse guidelines for treatment. Table 12.4 identifies identifies signs and symptoms along with potential patient problems for people who have substance use disorders.

Table 12.4 **Signs and Symptoms and Patient Problems for Substance Use Disorders**

Signs and Symptoms	Patient Problems
Impulsiveness, loss of relationships and occupation because of focus on substances or gambling, legal problems, social isolation	*Potential for suicide*
Impairment from substances; overdose; withdrawal from substances; hallucinations; elevated temperature, pulse, respirations; agitation	*Potential for injury*
Reports not feeling well rested, decreased ability to function, reports awakening multiple times	*Sleep pattern disturbance*
Substitutes substances for healthy foods, lack of appetite, aversion to food	*Insufficient nutritional intake*
Increased appetite from cannabis use, dysfunctional eating pattern, weight 20% over ideal for height and frame, excessive intake in relation to metabolic need	*Excessive nutritional intake* -
Inadequate environmental hygiene, inadequate personal hygiene, nonadherence to health activity	*Inadequate health behaviors*
Substance use or gambling, decreased use of social support, destructive behavior toward self and others, difficulty organizing information, inadequate problem-solving, poor concentration, reports inability to cope	*Impaired coping*
Does not perceive danger of substance use or gambling, minimizes symptoms, refuses health care attention, unable to admit effects of disease on life pattern	*Denial*
Substance use or gambling, lack of initiative, passivity, social isolation, reports seeing no alternatives or personal control, anger, sees no meaning in life	*Hopelessness* *Isolation*

Table 12.4 **Signs and Symptoms and Patient Problems for Substance Use Disorders—cont'd**

Signs and Symptoms	Patient Problems
Substance use, edema, loss of appetite, fatigue, shortness of breath, decreased concentration, cough, decreased urine output, palpitations, irregular or rapid pulse	*Decreased cardiac output*
Blaming, broken promises, chaos, denial of problems, enabling maintenance of substance use pattern, immaturity, inability to accept help or express feelings, loneliness, lying, manipulation, rationalization, refusal to get help, social isolation, worthlessness, deterioration of family relationships	*Altered family processes*

Intervention Guidelines

1. Support the patient during detoxification.
2. Assess for feelings of hopelessness, helplessness, and suicidal thinking.
3. Determine whether the patient is being treated for a comorbid medical condition (e.g., liver disease or infections) or psychiatric condition (e.g., depression or anxiety attacks).
4. Intervene with the patient's use of denial, rationalization, projection, and other defenses that interfere with motivation for change.
5. Involve family members and support them. Be aware that they may minimize the problem or enable the patient.
6. Emphasize abstinence.
7. Refer the patient to self-help groups (e.g., AA, NA, CA) or a recovery program early in treatment.
8. Teach the patient to avoid medications that promote dependence.
9. Encourage participation in psychotherapy (e.g., cognitive–behavioral strategies, motivational interviewing, solution-focused therapy).

10. Emphasize personal responsibility, placing control within the patient's grasp.
11. Support residential treatment when appropriate, particularly for patients with multiple relapses.
12. Expect relapses.
13. Educate the patient and family on the medical and psychological consequences of substance use.
14. Educate the patient and family regarding pharmacotherapy for certain addictions (e.g., naltrexone or methadone to help prevent relapse in alcoholism and narcotic addiction).
15. Educate the patient about the physical and developmental effects taking the drug can have on future children (e.g., fetal alcohol syndrome, problems with school, social role performance).

Nursing Care for Substance Use Disorders

Potential for Injury

Due to:

- Perceptual alteration, loss, or disorientation
- Chemical toxicity (e.g., poisons, drugs, alcohol, nicotine, pharmacological agents)
- Impaired judgment (disease, drugs, reality testing, risk-taking behaviors)
- Substance withdrawal
- Severe and panic levels of anxiety and agitation
- Potential for electrolyte imbalance or seizures
- Potential for
- Presence of hallucinations (bugs, animals, snakes)
- Elevated temperature, pulse, and respirations
- Agitation, trying to escape, or climb out of bed
- Combative behaviors
- Misinterpretation of reality (illusions)

Desired Outcome:

The patient will remain free from injury while intoxicated, after overdosing, and while withdrawing from the substance.

Assessment/Interventions (Rationale)

1. Take vital signs frequently, at least every 15 minutes until stable, and then every hour for 4 to 8 hours

according to hospital protocol or care provider's order. (Withdrawal from depressants, particularly alcohol, can result in significant and dangerous autonomic hyperactivity. Pulse is the best indicator of impending DTs, signaling the need for more rigorous sedation.)

2. Provide the patient with a quiet room free from environmental stimulation, a single room near the nurse's station if possible. (Low stimulation reduces irritability and confusion.)
3. Approach the patient with a calm and reassuring manner. (Patients need to feel that others are in control and that they are safe.)
4. Use simple, concrete language and directions. (The patient is able to follow simple commands but unable to process complex or abstract ideas.)
5. Orient the patient to time, place, and person during periods of confusion; inform the patient of his or her progress during periods of lucidity. (Fluctuating levels of consciousness occur during intoxication, withdrawal, and overdose of some drugs. Orientation can help reduce anxiety.)
6. Institute seizure precautions according to hospital protocol as needed. (Seizures might occur during intoxication, overdose, and withdrawal, and precautions for patient safety are a priority.)
7. Carefully monitor intake and output. Check for dehydration or overhydration. (Dehydration can aggravate electrolyte imbalance. Overhydration can lead to congestive heart failure.)
8. If the patient is having hallucinations, reassure him or her that you do not see them but that you are there and will make sure he or she remains safe (e.g., "I don't see rats on the wall jumping on your bed. You sound frightened right now. I will stay with you for a few minutes.").
9. If the patient is experiencing illusions, correct the patient's misrepresentation in a calm and matter-of-fact manner (e.g., "This is not a snake around my neck ready to bite you, it is my stethoscope…let me show you.") (Illusions can be explained to a patient who is misinterpreting environmental cues. When the patient recognizes normal objects for what they are, anxiety is reduced.)
10. Maintain safety precautions at all times such as giving patient a private room where possible, near the nurse's

station. (During intoxication, overdose, and withdrawal, physical safety is the priority.)

11. Administer medications ordered to treat use disorders, intoxication, overdose, and withdrawal. (Medication can reverse uncomfortable responses and prevent mortality when treating use disorders.)
12. Use restraints with caution if the patient is combative and dangerous to others. Try to avoid mechanical restraints whenever possible. Always follow unit protocol. (Myocardial infarction, cardiac collapse, and death have occurred when patients have fought against restraints during experiences of terror.)
13. Keep frequent, accurate records of the patient's vital signs, behaviors, medications, interventions, and effects of interventions. (Documentation provides a record of progress, identifies what works best, and alerts for potential complications.)

Inadequate Health Behaviors

Due to:

- Inability to make appropriate judgments
- Ineffective coping skills
- Perceptual or cognitive impairment
- Focus on obtaining and using the drug
- Finances depleted because of substance use; little or none left for health care, nourishing food, or safe shelter
- Poor nutrition related to prolonged drug binges, taking drug instead of eating nourishing food, or diminished appetite related to choice of drug (e.g., cocaine)
- Malabsorption of nutrients caused by chronic alcohol misuse
- Sleep deprivation related to decreased rapid eye movement (REM) sleep as a result of use of stimulants, alcohol, or central nervous system depressants
- Inability to make or keep health care appointments (e.g., mammograms, dentist, yearly physicals) because of either being intoxicated, being hung over, or withdrawing from an illicit substance

Desired Outcome:

The patient will demonstrate a stable health status, meeting minimal requirements for sleep, nutrition, and weight, while adhering to medication and treatment regimen.

Assessment/Interventions (Rationales)

1. Encourage small feedings if appropriate. Check nutritional status (e.g., conjunctiva, body weight, eating history). (Pale conjunctiva can signal anemia. If the patient has a loss of appetite, small feedings are better tolerated. Bland foods are often more appealing.)
2. Monitor fluid intake and output. Check skin turgor and ankle edema. As ordered, perform a urine-specific gravity if skin turgor is poor. (Patients can have potentially serious electrolyte imbalances. Deficient fluid intake can cause or signal renal problems. If the patient is retaining too much fluid, congestive heart failure may result.)
3. When skin turgor is poor, encourage fluids that contain protein and vitamins (e.g., milk, malts, juices). (Proteins and vitamins help build nutritional status.)
4. Promote rest and sleep by placing the patient in a quiet environment. (It is beneficial for the patient to have long rest periods between medical interventions.)
5. Identify the patient's understanding of how the alcohol or drugs can cause future problems (e.g., fetal alcohol syndrome, hepatitis or AIDS, fertility issues). (Before teaching, the nurse must identify what the patient knows about the drugs and evaluate his or her readiness to learn.)
6. Review the patient's blood work and physical examination with him or her. (Laboratory results help the nurse identify possible causes of symptoms [e.g., infection] and initiate early counseling. Sharing this information with the patient allows him or her to assume an active role in healthcare.)
7. Set up an appointment for medical follow-up and encourage the patient to make note in his or her calendar, cell phone, or appointment book. Follow-up calls, e-mails, and texts are important reminders.(Follow-up is essential in monitoring physical status. Concrete reminders increase the likelihood of appointments being kept).

Denial

Due to:

- Misuse of the substance and a need to maintain the status quo

- Fear of giving up the substance and acknowledging its role in disrupting his or her life
- Underlying feelings of hopelessness and helplessness having to cope with life without the substance
- Ineffective coping strategies

Desired Outcome:
The patient will demonstrate acceptance or responsibility for own behavior while achieving and maintaining abstinence from substances.

Assessment/Interventions (Rationales)

1. Maintain an interested, nonjudgmental, and supportive approach. (A professional and caring approach based on medical concern is most effective.)
2. Initially, work with the patient on crisis situations and establishing a rapport. (People cannot work on issues when in crisis situations [e.g., practical living problems, family crisis].)
3. Refer the patient to appropriate social services, occupational rehabilitation, or other resources as indicated. (The patient might need help that the nurse cannot provide. If the patient is to focus on and make changes in drug-related problems and behaviors, all available assistance should be used.)
4. Avoid power struggles, defending your position, preaching, or criticizing the patient's behaviors. (These reactions will only make the patient more defensive.)
5. Continue to address defense mechanisms, especially denial. (Denial is the primary obstacle to receiving treatment.)
6. Explore initial goals and what the patient wants to change. (Initially, the patient's goal might not be total abstinence. Identifying areas the patient wants to change gives both the patient and nurse a basis for working together.)
7. Use of miracle questions can help identify what patients want to change. For example, "What if your worst problem were miraculously solved overnight. What would be different about your life the next day?" (Miracle questions help patients perceive their future without some of their problems and give direction to moving forward and identifying long- and short-term goals.)

8. Help the patient analyze specific pros and cons of substance use. (Analyzing the pros and cons helps the patient look at what substances will and will not do for them in a clear light. This can help strengthen motives for change.)
9. Discourage the patient's attempts to focus on only external problems (relationships, job-related, legal) without relating them to substance use. (This will help patients see the relationship between their problems and their drug use. It also helps break down denial.)
10. Work with the patient to identify behaviors that have contributed to life problems (e.g., family problems, social difficulties, job-related problems, legal difficulties). (When the patient takes responsibility for maladaptive behaviors, he or she is more prepared to take responsibility for learning effective and satisfying behaviors.)
11. Encourage the patient to stay in the here and now (e.g., "You can't change the fact that your mother put you down all your life" or "Let's focus on how you want to respond when you perceive that your boss puts you down"). (Dwelling on past disappointments and hurt is not useful to working on new and more adaptive coping behaviors.)
12. Refer and encourage the patient to attend a 12-step support group, recovery program, residential program, or SMART (Self-Management And Recovery Training), whichever seems to be more amenable to his or her desires and/or lifestyle. (Research shows that external supports are effective tools in beating addiction.)
13. Encourage the patient to find a sponsor within the 12-step program or another therapeutic mode. (Having a sponsor and being a sponsor support success.)
14. Work with the patient to identify times he or she might be vulnerable to substance use and strategies to use at those times. (Having thought out alternative strategies to drinking or taking drugs in vulnerable situations gives the patient a ready choice.)
15. Encourage family and friends to seek support, education, and ways to recognize and refrain from enabling the patient. (Enabling behavior supports the patient's use of drugs by taking away incentive for change.)
16. Educate the patient and his or her family regarding the physical and psychological effects of the drug, the process of treatment, and aftercare. (An addicted

family member greatly changes the dynamics and roles within families. Both the patient and family need to make decisions based on facts.)

17. Attend several open meetings in your local community. (Attending the meeting helps the nurse understand how the 12-step fellowship process works.)
18. Realize that recognition of a problem and need for treatment is a long process. (When helpers become impatient and push too hard, the patient might leave treatment before making a commitment.)

Impaired Coping

Due to:

- Inadequate resources available
- Disturbance in pattern of tension release
- Inadequate level of or perception of control
- Knowledge deficit
- Coping styles no longer adaptive in present situations
- Insufficient social support

Desired Outcome:
The patient will learn and practice effective coping skills, and participate in treatment (e.g., individual therapy, support groups) to support becoming sober and maintaining sobriety.

Assessment/Interventions (Rationales)

1. Work with the patient to keep the treatment plan simple in the beginning. (Patients with substance use problems,have mild to moderate cognitive problems while using substances, which may continue many months after sobriety.)
2. Encourage the patient to write notes and self-memos (e.g., enter them into a smartphone or computer calendar) to help keep appointments and follow the treatment plan. (Cognition usually gets better with long-term abstinence, but initially memory aids prove helpful.)
3. Encourage the patient to join relapse prevention gro. (Attending these groups helps the patient anticipate and rehearse healthy responses to stressful situations.)
4. Encourage the patient to find role models (e.g., counselors or other recovering people). (Role models serve as examples of how the patient can learn effective ways to make necessary life changes.)

5. Work with the patient on identifying triggers (people, feelings, situations) that help drive the patient's addiction. (Mastering the issues that perpetuate substance use allows for effective change and targets areas for acquiring new skills.)
6. Practice and role play alternative responses to triggers with the patient. (Increases patient confidence of handling drug triggers effectively.)
7. Give positive feedback when the patient applies new and effective responses to difficult trigger situations. (Validates the patient's positive steps toward growth and change.)
8. Continue to empathetically confront denial throughout recovery. (Denial can surface throughout recovery and can interfere with sobriety during all stages of recovery.)
9. Continue to work with patient on the following three areas: (1) personal issues (relationship issues), (2) social issues (issues of family abuse), and (3) feelings of self-worth. (These areas of human life need to find healing so that growth and change can take place.)
10. Recommend family therapy. (Enhanced strategies for dealing with conflict in the patient's family are essential to recovery.)
11. Stress the fact that substance use is a disease the entire family must conquer. (Family members also need encouragement to face their own struggles.)
12. Expect slip-ups to occur. Reaffirm that sobriety can be achieved as emotional pain becomes endurable. (Reaffirmation helps minimize shame and guilt and rebuild self-esteem.)

Nurse, Patient, and Family Resources

Addictions.com
www.addictions.com

Alcoholics Anonymous
www.aa.org

Al-Anon
www.al-anon.org

Cocaine Anonymous
www.ca.org

Center for Substance Abuse Treatment (CSAT) National Drug Helpline (bilingual)
1-800-662-HELP (4357)

Marijuana Anonymous
www.marijuana-anonymous.org

Nar-Anon Family Groups
www.nar-anon.org

Narcotics Anonymous
www.na.org

National Association for Children of Alcoholics
www.nacoa.org

National Institute on Drug Abuse (NIDA) American Self-Help Clearinghouse
www.mentalhelp.net/selfhelp

CHAPTER 13

Neurocognitive Disorders

The clarity and purpose of an individual's journey through life depends on the ability to reflect on its meaning. Unfortunately, far too many people experience profound disturbances in cognitive processing that cloud or destroy the meaning of the journey. Cognition represents a fundamental human feature that distinguishes living from existing.

Cognitive functioning involves a variety of domains. Attention and orientation are basic lower-level cognitive domains. Higher-level cognitive domains are more complex and include an ability to do the following:

- Plan and problem solve (executive function)
- Learn and retain information in long-term memory
- Use language
- Visually perceive the environment
- Read social situations (social cognition)

The three main neurocognitive classifications are delirium, mild neurocognitive disorders, and major neurocognitive disorders (American Psychiatric Association [APA], 2013). The first syndrome, delirium, tends to be short term and reversible. A mild neurocognitive disorder may or may not progress to a major disorder. Major neurocognitive disorders are commonly referred to as dementia, which is progressive and irreversible. In both mild and major neurocognitive disorders, there is a decline in cognitive functioning from a previous level, although they differ in how much they interfere with independence in everyday activities.

DELIRIUM

Delirium is an acute cognitive disturbance and often reversible condition that is common in hospitalized patients, especially older patients. It is characterized as a syndrome, that is, a constellation of symptoms rather than a disorder. The chief symptoms of delirium are an inability to direct, focus, sustain, and shift attention; an abrupt onset with clinical features that fluctuate with periods of lucidity; and disorganized thinking and poor executive functioning. Other characteristics include disorientation (often to time and place, but rarely to person), anxiety, agitation, poor memory, and delusional thinking.

Misinterpretation of the environment is evident in hallucinations, which are usually visual. Illusions are errors in perception of sensory stimuli. A person may mistake folds in the blanket for white rats or the cord of a window blind for a snake. The stimulus is a real object in the environment. Unlike delusions or hallucinations, a nurse or caregiver can explain and clarify illusions for the individual.

The prevalence of delirium in all hospitalized patients is up to 22% in general medical patients, between 11% and 35% in surgical patients, and up to 80% in patients in intensive care units (van Munster & Rooij, 2014).

Delirium is always related to underlying physiological causes. The key to helping patients avoid the consequences of delirium is recognizing and investigating potential causes as soon as possible. Some of the risk factors for developing delirium listed in Box 13.1 are modifiable.

Box 13.1 **Risk Factors for Delirium**

- Cognitive impairment
- Older age
- Severity of disease
- Infection
- Multiple comorbidities
- Polypharmacy
- Intensive care units
- Fractures
- Surgery
- Stroke
- Aphasia
- Vision impairment
- Restraint use
- Change in hospital rooms
- Unaddressed orientation, visual, or hearing issues

Assessment Guidelines

1. Assess for fluctuating levels of consciousness, which is key in delirium.
2. Interview family or other caregivers.
3. Assess for past confusional states (e.g., prior dementia diagnosis).
4. Identify other disturbances in medical status (e.g., dyspnea, edema, presence of jaundice).
5. Identify electroencephalogram (EEG), neuroimaging, or laboratory abnormalities in the patient's record.
6. Assess vital signs, level of consciousness, and neurological signs.
7. Ask the patient (if lucid) or family what they think could be responsible for the delirium (e.g., medications, withdrawal of substance, other medical condition).
8. Assess the potential for injury (is the patient safe from falls, wandering).
9. Assess the need for comfort measures (pain, cold, positioning).
10. Are immediate medical interventions available to help prevent irreversible brain damage?

Intervention Guidelines

1. Delirium is transitory when interventions are instituted and if delirium does not last a prolonged period of time. Therefore immediate intervention for the underlying cause of the delirium is needed to prevent irreversible damage to the brain. Medical interventions are the first priority.
2. When patients are confused and frightened and are having a difficult time interpreting reality, they might be prone to accidents. Therefore safety is a high priority.
3. Delirium is a terrifying experience for many patients. When some individuals recover to their premorbid cognitive function, they are left with frightening memories and images. Preventive counseling and education after recovery from acute delirium is helpful.
4. Avoid the use of restraints. Encourage one or two significant others to stay with the patient to provide orientation and comfort.

Nursing Care for Delirium

Delirium

Due to:

- Medical condition (e.g., urinary tract infection, pneumonia)
- Fluid and electrolyte imbalance
- Substance use or intoxication (illicit or prescribed)
- Substance withdrawal (illicit or prescribed)
- Toxin exposure

Desired Outcomes:

The patient will be free from injury; oriented to time, place, and person; and resume usual cognitive and physical activities.

Assessment/Interventions (Rationales)

1. Introduce self and call patient by name at the beginning of each contact. (With short-term memory impairment, the patient is often confused and needs re-introductions and orienting.)
2. Maintain face-to-face contact. (If the patient is easily distracted, he or she will need help to focus on one stimulus at a time.)
3. Use short, simple, concrete phrases. (The patient might not be able to process complex information.)
4. Briefly explain everything you are going to do before doing it. (Explanation reduces misinterpretation of actions.)
5. Encourage the patient's family and friends (one at a time) to take a quiet, supportive role. (A familiar presence lowers anxiety and increases orientation.)
6. Keep the room well lit, preferably with windows, during the day and darken the room at night if possible. (Lighting provides accurate environmental stimuli to maintain and increase orientation Lighting that mirrors the 24-hour cycle of light and darkness will help preserve circadian rhythms.)
7. Keep environmental noise to a minimum (e.g., television, visitors). (Noise interferes with rest and can be misconstrued as something frightening or threatening.)
8. Keep the head of the bed elevated. (This position can help provide important environmental cues and minimize illusions.)

9. Provide clocks and calendars. (These cues help orient the patient to time.)
10. Encourage the patient to wear prescribed eyeglasses or hearing aids. (Wearing glasses or hearing aids helps increase accurate perceptions of visual and auditory stimuli.)
11. Make an effort for the same personnel on each shift to care for patient. (Familiar faces minimize confusion and enhance nurse–patient relationships.)
12. When hallucinations are present, assure patients that they are safe (e.g., "I know you are frightened. I'll sit with you a while and make sure you are safe."). (The patient feels reassured that he or she is safe, and fear and anxiety often decrease.)
13. When illusions are present, clarify reality (e.g., "This is a coat rack, not a man with a knife…see? You seem frightened. I'll stay with you for a while."). (With illusions, misinterpreted objects or sounds can be clarified, once pointed out.)
14. Inform the patient of progress during lucid intervals. (Consciousness fluctuates: The patient feels less anxious knowing where he or she is and who you are during lucid periods.)
15. Ignore insults and name calling, and acknowledge how upset the person might be feeling. For example: **Patient:** "You incompetent jerk! Get me a real nurse, someone who knows what they are doing." **Nurse:** "What you are going through is very difficult. I'll stay with you." (Feelings of fear are often projected onto the environment. Arguing or becoming defensive only increases the patient's aggressive behaviors and defenses. Support and reassurance will decrease anxiety.)
16. If patient behavior becomes physically abusive:
    a. First, set limits on behavior (e.g., "Mr. Jones, you are not to hit me or anyone else. Tell me how you feel." "Mr. Jones, if you have difficulty controlling your actions, we will help you gain control.").
    b. Second, check orders for calming medication.
    (Clear limits need to be set to protect the patient, staff, and others. Often the patient can respond to verbal commands. Chemical and physical restraints are used as a last resort, if at all.)
17. After the patient returns to a premorbid cognitive state, educate and offer counseling for frightening memories and images. (The patient may believe that illusions or

hallucinations were real, and it may take time to come to terms with the experience.)

MILD AND MAJOR NEUROCOGNITIVE DISORDERS

The *Diagnostic and Statistical Manual of Mental Disorders, fifth edition, (DSM-5)* (APA, 2013) identifies two overall diagnostic categories for neurocognitive disorders, major and mild. When symptoms are mild, the impairments do not interfere with essential activities of daily living, although the person may need to make extra efforts. Although such impairments may be progressive, a mild cognitive impairment will not necessarily progress to a major neurocognitive disorder.

Major and mild neurocognitive disorder criteria are general. Specific disorders are more fully described in the *DSM-5* with diagnoses such as "Major or Mild Neurocognitive Disorder Due to Alzheimer's Disease." While the following paragraphs focus on Alzheimer's disease, there are many other types of neurocognitive disorders. These other disorders are listed in Table 13.1.

Table 13.1 **Types of Neurocognitive Disorders**

Type of Dementia	Symptoms
Alzheimer's disease	Early: Difficulty with recent memory, impaired learning, apathy, and depression Moderate to severe: Visuospatial and language deficits, psychotic features, agitation, and wandering Late: Gait disturbance; poor judgment; disorientation; confusion; incontinence; and difficulty speaking, swallowing, and walking
Frontotemporal dementia	Impaired social cognition, disinhibition, apathy, compulsive behavior, poor comprehension, and language difficulties

Table 13.1 **Types of Neurocognitive Disorders—cont'd**

Type of Dementia	Symptoms
Dementia with Lewy bodies	Fluctuating cognition, early changes in attention and executive function, sleep disturbance, visual hallucinations, muscle rigidity, and other parkinsonian features
Vascular	One or more documented cerebrovascular events; impaired judgment; poor decision-making, planning, and organizing (executive functions); and personality and mood changes
Traumatic brain injury	Trauma to the head with loss of consciousness, posttraumatic amnesia, disorientation and confusion, and neurological signs
Substance or medication induced	Symptoms of neurocognitive impairment persist beyond the usual duration of intoxication and acute withdrawal; substances include alcohol, inhalants, sedative, hypnotic, or antianxiety agents
HIV infection	A documented infection with HIV; impaired executive function, slowing of processing, problems with attention, difficulty learning new information, and aphasia; symptoms dependent on the area of the brain affected by HIV pathogenic processes
Prion	Insidious onset and rapid progression of impairment; motor features of such as myoclonus or ataxia; memory, coordination, and behavior changes; rapidly fatal
Parkinson's disease	Progression of Parkinson's disease results in dementia with symptoms similar to dementia with Lewy bodies or Alzheimer's disease and apathetic, depressed or anxious mood; sleep disorder
Huntington's disease	Abnormal involuntary movements, severe decline in thinking and reasoning, mood changes such as irritability and depression, related to genetic defect

ALZHEIMER'S DISEASE

The most common major neurocognitive disorder is Alzheimer's disease. Although the disease can occur at a younger age (early onset), most of those affected are 65 years of age or older (late onset). It is estimated that 5.3 million Americans have Alzheimer's disease (Alzheimer's Association, 2014). Two thirds of people with this disorder are women, most likely due to the fact that, on average, women tend to live longer.

There is an increased risk for individuals with an affected immediate family. There are three fairly rare genetic mutations that guarantee that a person will develop Alzheimer's disease.

Two processes contribute to cell death. The first is the accumulation of the protein beta-amyloid outside the neurons, which interferes with synapses. The second is an accumulation of the protein tau inside the neurons, which forms tangles that block the flow of nutrients.

Alzheimer's disease is classified according to the stage of the degenerative process. The three stages are mild, moderate, and severe. The first stage roughly corresponds to the *DSM-5* criteria for mild neurocognitive disorders. Stages two and three relate to the *DSM-5* criteria for major neurocognitive disorder. Table 13.2 describes the stages of Alzheimer's disease.

ASSESSMENT

Signs and Symptoms

- Clear evidence of memory impairment, usually short-term memory first
- Progressive decline in cognitive functions, especially with Alzheimer's disease:
  Aphasia: language disturbance, difficulty finding words, using words incorrectly
  Apraxia: inability to carry out motor activities despite motor functions being intact (e.g., putting on clothes)
  Agnosia: loss of sensory ability; inability to recognize or identify familiar objects (e.g., a toothbrush) or sounds (e.g., telephone ringing); loss of ability to problem solve, plan, organize, or abstract
- Significant gradual decline in previous level of functioning; poor judgment

Table 13.2 **Stages of Alzheimer's Disease**

Mild Alzheimer's Disease (Early Stage)

Noticeable memory lapses. May still function independently but will experience:

- Difficulties retrieving correct words or names, previously known
- Trouble remembering names when introduced to new people
- Greater difficulty performing tasks in social or work settings
- Forgetting material that one has just read
- Losing or misplacing a valuable object
- Trouble with planning or organizing

Moderate Alzheimer's Disease (Middle Stage)

Confuses words, gets frustrated or angry, or acts in unexpected ways such as refusing to bathe. Symptoms become noticeable to others and these individuals may:

- Forget events or own personal history
- Become moody or withdrawn, especially in socially or mentally challenging situations
- Be unable to recall their own address or telephone number or the high school or college from which they graduated
- Become confused about where they are or what day it is
- Need help choosing proper clothing for the season or the occasion
- Have trouble controlling bladder and bowels
- Change sleep patterns, such as sleeping during the day and becoming restless at night
- Be at risk of wandering and becoming lost
- Become suspicious and delusional or compulsive—for example, repetitive behavior like hand-wringing or tissue shredding

Severe Alzheimer Disease (Late Stage)

Loses the ability to respond to the environment, to carry on a conversation, and, eventually, to control movement. May still say words or phrases. Personality changes occur. The person may:

- Require full-time, around-the-clock assistance with daily personal care
- Lose awareness of recent experiences and of their surroundings
- Require high levels of assistance with daily activities and personal care
- Experience changes in physical abilities, including the ability to walk, sit, and, eventually, swallow
- Have increasing difficulty communicating
- Become vulnerable to infections, especially pneumonia

From Alzheimer's Association. (2016). *Stages of Alzheimer's*. Retrieved from http://www.alz.org/alzheimers_disease_stages_of_alzheimers.asp?type=alzFooter.

- Mood disturbances, anxiety, hallucinations, delusions, and impaired sleep

Assessment Tools

A variety of tools are available to measure mental status in individuals with dementia. The Montreal Cognitive Assessment (MoCA) is an evidenced-based tool to detect cognitive changes in the early stages of dementia. The tool is provided in Fig. 13.1

Assessment Guidelines

Because the symptoms of some other problems may look like neurocognitive disorders, determine whether the patient has current symptoms or a history of such problems as depression, substance use, or urinary tract infections. Box 13.2 lists potential diagnostic tests to rule out other problems.

1. Determine whether the family understands the progress of the patient's dementia.
2. How is the family coping with the patient? What are the main issues at this time?
3. What resources are available to the family? Does the family get help from other family members, friends, and community resources? Are the caregivers aware of community support groups and resources?
4. Obtain the data necessary to provide appropriate safety measures for the patient.
5. How safe is the patient's home environment (e.g., wandering, eating inedible objects, falls, provocative behaviors toward others)?
6. For what patient behaviors could the family use teaching and guidance (e.g., catastrophic reaction, lability of mood, aggressive behaviors, nocturnal delirium [increased confusion and agitation at night; sundowning])?
7. Identify family supports in the community.

Intervention Guidelines.

1. Educate the patient's family on safety features for the impaired family member living at home:
   a. Precautions for wandering (e.g., identification bracelet, "Home Safe Program," effective locks)

NAME :
Education : Date of birth :
Sex : DATE :

MONTREAL COGNITIVE ASSESSMENT (MOCA)
Version 7.1 Original Version

		POINTS
VISUOSPATIAL / EXECUTIVE	(E) End (A) (5) (B) (2) (1) Begin (D) (4) (3) (C) [ ] — Copy cube [ ] — Draw CLOCK (Ten past eleven) (3 points) [ ] Contour [ ] Numbers [ ] Hands	___/5
NAMING	[ ] [ ] [ ]	___/3

MEMORY Read list of words, subject must repeat them. Do 2 trials, even if 1st trial is successful. Do a recall after 5 minutes.

	FACE	VELVET	CHURCH	DAISY	RED	No points
1st trial						
2nd trial						

ATTENTION Read list of digits (1 digit/ sec.). Subject has to repeat them in the forward order [ ] 2 1 8 5 4
Subject has to repeat them in the backward order [ ] 7 4 2 ___/2

Read list of letters. The subject must tap with his hand at each letter A. No points if ≥ 2 errors
[ ] F B A C M N A A J K L B A F A K D E A A A J A M O F A A B ___/1

Serial 7 subtraction starting at 100 [ ] 93 [ ] 86 [ ] 79 [ ] 72 [ ] 65
4 or 5 correct subtractions: **3 pts**, 2 or 3 correct: **2 pts**, 1 correct: **1 pt**, 0 correct: **0 pt** ___/3

LANGUAGE Repeat : I only know that John is the one to help today. [ ]
The cat always hid under the couch when dogs were in the room. [ ] ___/2

Fluency / Name maximum number of words in one minute that begin with the letter F [ ] ___ (N ≥ 11 words) ___/1

ABSTRACTION Similarity between e.g. banana - orange = fruit [ ] train – bicycle [ ] watch - ruler ___/2

DELAYED RECALL	Has to recall words WITH NO CUE	FACE [ ]	VELVET [ ]	CHURCH [ ]	DAISY [ ]	RED [ ]	Points for UNCUED recall only	___/5
Optional	Category cue							
	Multiple choice cue							

ORIENTATION [ ] Date [ ] Month [ ] Year [ ] Day [ ] Place [ ] City ___/6

© Z.Nasreddine MD **www.mocatest.org** Normal ≥26 / 30 TOTAL ___/30
Administered by:___ Add 1 point if ≤ 12 yr edu

Fig. 13.1 Montreal Cognitive Assessment (MOCA). Nasreddine, Z.S., Phillips, N.A., Bedirian, V., Charbonneau, S., Whitehead, V., Collin, I. … Chertkow, H. (2005).The Montreal Cognitive Assessment, MoCA: A brief screening tool for mild cognitive impairment. *Journal of the American Geriatric Society, 53*(4), 695-9.

Box 13.2 **Diagnostic Tests to Rule Out Other Problems**

- Chest x-ray
- Electrocardiograph
- Urinalysis
- Basic metabolic panel
- Complete blood count
- Sequential multiple analyzer: 13-test serum profile
- Liver panel
- B12 and folate levels
- Thyroid function studies
- Venereal disease research laboratories (VDRL)
- Human immunodeficiency (HIV) tests
- Serum creatinine assay
- Electrolyte assessment
- Vision and hearing evaluation
- Neuroimaging (computed tomography [CT] head without contrast, magnetic resonance imaging [MRI] with and without contrast)

b. Home safety features (e.g., eliminating slippery rugs, labeling of rooms and drawers, installing complex locks on top of doors)
c. Self-care guidelines on maintaining optimal nutrition, bowel and bladder training, optimal sleep patterns, and working to optimal ability in activities of daily living

2. Educate the family (and staff) on effective communication strategies with a confused patient:
   a. Alternative modes of communication when a patient is aphasic
   b. Basic communication techniques for confused patients (e.g., introduce self each time; use simple, short sentences; maintain eye contact; focus on one topic at a time; talk about familiar and simple topics)
3. Family and caregiver support is a priority. Provide names and telephone numbers of support groups, respite care, day care, protective services, recreational services, Meals On Wheels, hospice services, and so on that are within the family or caregivers' community. Encourage the use of support groups for caregivers.

4. Provide the family with information on all medications the patient is taking (use for each, potential side effects and toxic effects, interactions that could occur) and the name and number of whom to call with future questions.

Patient Problems

Because the symptoms of delirium and major neurocognitive disorders are quite similar, the following patient problems can be individualized and applied to patients with either diagnosis. Table 13.3 identifies signs and symptoms along with potential patient problems for both delirium and major neurocognitive disorders.

Nursing Care for Major Neurocognitive Disorders

Potential for Injury

Due to:

- Alzheimer's disease
- Sensory dysfunction
- Cognitive or emotional difficulties
- Confusion, disorientation
- Faulty judgment
- Loss of short-term memory

Desired Outcomes:
Patient will remain free of injury with the aid of environmental precautions and interventions.

Assessment/Interventions (Rationales)

1. Restrict driving. (Impaired judgment can lead to accidents.)
2. Remove throw rugs and other objects that could lead to falls. (Removing these hazards minimizes tripping and falling.)
3. Minimize sensory stimulation. (Minimizing sensory stimulation decreases sensory overload [which can increase anxiety and confusion].)
4. If patients become verbally upset, listen, give support, and then change the topic. (When attention span is short, patients can be briefly distracted to more productive topics and activities.)
5. Label all rooms and drawers with pictures. Label often-used objects (e.g., hairbrushes and toothbrushes).

Table 13.3 **Signs and Symptoms and Patient Problems for Delirium and Dementia**

Signs and Symptoms	Patient Problems
Wanders, has unsteady gait, acts out fear from hallucinations or illusions, forgets things (leaves stove on, doors open), falls	*Potential for injury*
Awake and disoriented during the night (sundowning), frightened at night	*Sleep pattern disturbance*
Unable to take care of basic needs, incontinence, imbalanced nutrition, insufficient fluid intake	*Impaired activities of daily living*
Sees frightening things that are not there (hallucinations), mistakes everyday objects for something frightening (illusions), may become paranoid and think that others are doing bad things (delusions)	*Anxiety (severe/panic)* *Impaired social functioning*
Does not recognize familiar people or places, has difficulty with short- and/or long-term memory, forgetful, confused	*Altered thought processes*
Difficulty with communication, cannot find words, has difficulty in recognizing objects and/or people, incoherent	*Impaired verbal communication*
Devastated over losing place in life (during lucid moments), fearful and overwhelmed by what is happening	*Hopelessness* *Grieving*
Family and loved ones overburdened and overwhelmed, unable to care for patient's needs	*Caregiver burden*

(Labeling can keep the patient from wandering into other patients' rooms and increases environmental clues to familiar objects.)

6. Install safety bars in the bathroom. (Use of a safety bar can prevent falls.)
7. Supervise patients when they smoke. (The danger of burns is always present.)
8. If the patient wanders during the night, put a mattress on the floor. (Putting a mattress on the floor prevents falls when the patient is confused.)

9. Have the patient wear an identification bracelet that cannot be removed (with a name, address, and telephone number). Provide the police department with recent pictures. (The patient can be identified easily by police, neighbors, or hospital personnel.)
10. Alert local police and neighbors about the wanderer. (This can reduce the time necessary to return the patient to home or hospital.)
11. Put complex locks on the door. (This reduces the opportunity to wander.)
12. Place locks at the top of the door. (In moderate and late neurocognitive disorders, the ability to look up and reach upward is lost.)
13. Encourage physical activity during the day. (Physical activity during the day helps to decrease wandering at night.)
14. Explore the feasibility of installing sensor devices. (Sensor devices can provide a warning if the patient wanders.)
15. Enroll the patient in the Alzheimer's Association's Safe Return program (www.alz.org). (This program helps track individuals with dementia who wander and are at risk for getting lost or injured.)

Impaired Activities of Daily Living

Due to:

- Alzheimer's disease
- Perceptual or cognitive impairment
- Neuromuscular impairment
- Decreased strength and endurance
- Confusion
- Apraxia (inability to perform tasks that were once routine)
- Severe memory impairment

Desired Outcome:

The patient will participate in self-care at an optimal level with supervision and guidance.

Assessment/Interventions (Rationales)

Dressing and Bathing

1. Encourage patients to perform all tasks of which they are capable. (Maintains self-esteem, uses muscle groups, and minimizes further regression.)

2. Patients should wear their own clothes, even if in the hospital. (Helps maintain the patient's identity and dignity.)
3. Use clothing with elastic, and substitute fastening tape (Velcro) for buttons and zippers. (Minimizes the patient's confusion and increases independence of functioning.)
4. Label clothing items with the patient's name and the name of the item. (Helps identify patients if they wander, and gives caregivers additional clues when aphasia or agnosia occurs.)
5. Give step-by-step instructions whenever necessary (e.g., "Take this blouse…put in one arm…now the other arm…pull it together in the front…now…"). (Patient can focus on small pieces of information more easily; allows the patient to perform at optimal level.)

Eating and Drinking

6. Monitor food and fluid intake. (The patient might have limited appetite or be too confused to eat.)
7. Offer finger foods that the patient can walk around with. (Increases intake throughout the day; the patient might eat only small amounts at meals.)
8. During periods of hyperorality, ensure that the patient does not eat nonfood items (e.g., ceramic fruit or food-shaped soaps). (The patient puts everything into the mouth during these periods and may be at risk for choking or being poisoned.)

Elimination

9. Begin a bowel and bladder program early using a regular schedule for toileting. For example, direct the patient to the toilet early in the morning, after meals and snacks, and before bedtime. (A toileting routine will reduce episodes of incontinence and help to maintain dignity.)
10. Evaluate the need for adult disposable undergarments. (Prevents embarrassment if incontinent.)
11. Label the bathroom door, as well as doors to other rooms, with a picture. (Additional environmental clues can maximize independent toileting. Pictures may be more easily interpreted than words.)

Sleep Hygiene

12. Because the patient might awaken frightened and disoriented at night, keep the area well lit. (Reinforces orientation, minimizes possible illusions.)

13. Monitor for side effects if using sleep-promoting medications. (Because of metabolic changes, older adults experience more severe side effects.)

Impaired Verbal Communication

Due to:

- Alzheimer's disease
- Deterioration or damage to neurological centers that regulate speech and language
- Biochemical changes in the brain
- Decreased circulation to the brain
- Severe memory impairment
- Escalating anxiety

Desired Outcomes:

The patient will communicate basic needs optimally with the use of visual and verbal clues as needed.

Assessment/Interventions (Rationales)

In addition to the interventions for delirium in the first half of this chapter, communication techniques specific to neurocognitive disorders follow.

1. Use a variety of nonverbal techniques to enhance communication:
   a. Point, touch, or demonstrate an action while talking about it.
   b. Ask patients to point to parts of their body or things they want to communicate about.
   c. When the patient is searching for a particular word, guess at what is being said and ask whether you are correct (e.g., "You are pointing to your mouth, saying pain. Is it your dentures? No. Is your mouth sore? Yes. Okay, let me take a look to see if I can tell what is hurting you."). Always ask patient to confirm whether your guess is correct.
   d. The use of cue cards, flash cards, alphabet letters, signs, and pictures on doors to various rooms is often helpful for many patients and their families (e.g., bathroom, "Charles's bedroom"). Use of pictures is helpful when ability to read decreases.
   (Both delirium and dementia can pose huge communication problems, and often alternative nonverbal or verbal methods must be used.)
2. Encourage reminiscing about happy times in life. (Remembering accomplishments and shared joys helps

distract the patient from deficits and gives meaning to existence.)

3. If a patient gets into an argument with another patient, stop the argument and remove them from each other's presence. After a short time (5 minutes), explain to each patient matter-of-factly why you had to intervene. (This prevents escalation to physical acting out and shows respect for the patient's right to know. Explaining in an adult manner helps maintain self-esteem.)
4. Reinforce the patient's speech through pictures, nonverbal gestures, Xs on calendars, and other methods used to anchor the patient in reality. (When aphasia starts to hinder communication, alternate methods of communication must be instituted.)

Refer to useful guidelines for implementing nursing interventions or teaching a patient with severe cognitive impairment (Box 13.3).

Caregiver Burden

Due to:

- Complexity of activities and severity of the illness
- 24-hour care responsibility
- Years of caregiving
- Lack of support
- Caregiver's isolation
- Inadequate community support (e.g., respite and recreation for the caregiver)
- Inadequate physical environment (transportation, housing) for providing care

Box 13.3 Teaching Patients With Severe Cognitive Impairment

Provide only one visual clue (object) at a time.
Know that the patient might not understand the task assigned.
Remember that relevant information is remembered longer than irrelevant information.
Break tasks into very small steps.
Give only one instruction at a time.
Report, record, and document all data.

Desired Outcomes:
Caregivers will demonstrate adaptive coping strategies for dealing with the stress of the caregiver role.

Assessment/Interventions (Rationales)

1. Assess what caregivers know about the patient's illness, and provide education. (Empowering caregivers with knowledge of the illness promotes patience, reduces the tendency to view the patient's actions as simply bad behavior, and helps them to anticipate further deterioration and plan accordingly.)
2. Provide a list of community agencies and support groups where the family and primary caregiver can receive support, further education, and information regarding how to arrange respite care. (This support helps diminish a sense of hopelessness and increase a sense of empowerment.)
3. Help the caregiver and family identify areas that need intervention and areas that are presently stable. (This identifies specific areas needing assistance and those that will need assistance in the future.)
4. Teach the caregiver and family specific interventions to use in response to behavioral or social problems brought on by the dementia. (Caregivers need to learn many new ways to intervene in situations that are common with demented patients, such as agitation, catastrophic reactions, sleep–wake disturbances, and wandering.)
5. Safety is a major concern. Box 13.4 identifies some steps the caregiver and family can take to make the home a safer place. (These steps, prepared by the Alzheimer's Association, can help make the home safe for the person with dementia.)
6. Encourage spending nonstressful time with the patient at his or her present level of functioning (e.g., watching a favorite movie together; reading a simple book with pictures together; performing simple tasks like setting the table, washing dishes, washing the car). (Encourages the patient to participate as much as possible in family life. Helps diminish feelings of isolation and alienation temporarily.)
7. Encourage the caregiver or family to follow family traditions (church activities, holidays, and vacations). (This helps the family maintain their family rituals and increases the patient's sense of belonging.)

Box 13.4 Home Safety for Individuals With Cognitive Impairment

Avoid Injury During Daily Activities

Avoid serving food and beverages that are too hot. The person with dementia may not remember to check the temperature.

Install walk-in showers.

Add grab bars to the shower or tub and at the edge of the vanity to allow for independent, safe movement.

Add textured stickers to slippery surfaces.

Apply adhesives to keep throw rugs and carpeting in place, or remove rugs completely.

Monitor the hot water temperature in the shower or bath. Consider installing an automatic thermometer.

Adapt to Vision Limitations

Changes in levels of lights can be disorienting. Create an even level by adding extra lights in entries; outside landings; and in areas between rooms, stairways, and bathrooms.

Use nightlights in hallways, bedrooms, and bathrooms.

Beware of Dangerous Objects and Substances

Use appliances that have an automatic shut-off feature. Keep them away from water sources such as sinks.

Install a hidden gas valve or circuit breaker on the stove so a person with dementia cannot turn it on. Consider removing the knobs.

Store grills, lawn mowers, power tools, knives, and cleaning products in a secure place.

Discard toxic plants and decorative fruits that may be mistaken for real food.

Remove vitamins, prescription drugs, sugar substitutes, and seasonings from the kitchen table and counters. Medications should be kept in a locked area at all times.

Supervise the use of tobacco and alcohol. Both may have harmful side effects and may interact dangerously with some medications.

Consider removing guns and firearms from the home.

From Alzheimer's Association. Alz.org®. (n.d.). Home safety and Alzheimer's. Retrieved from www.alz.org/care/alzheimers-dementia-home-safety.asp

8. Encourage the caregiver or family to use respite care during regular intervals (e.g., vacations). (Regular periods of respite can help prevent burnout, can allow caregivers to continue participating in their life, and can help minimize feelings of resentment.)
9. Identify financial burdens placed on the caregiver and family. Refer to community, national associations, or other resources that can help. (Any kind of long-term illness within a family can place devastating financial burdens on all members.)
10. Point out areas that will benefit from planning and preparation such as legal and financial issues and make suggestions for resources in the community. (Advanced planning for eventual deterioration and death will make these transitions less difficult.)

TREATMENT FOR ALZHEIMER'S DISEASE

Biological Approaches

Pharmacological Therapy

The U.S. Food and Drug Administration (FDA) has approved several medications for the treatment of Alzheimer's disease. Although these medications are used widely and have shown statistically significant effects compared with placebos, they produce only a marginal clinical improvement on cognition and functioning. The benefits of these medications wane after 1 to 2 years, so patients should weigh the potential side effects against the potential benefits. See Chapter 28 for a discussion of neurocognitive medications.

Psychotherapeutic Approaches

Health Teaching and Health Promotion

Educating families who have a cognitively impaired member is one of the most important health-teaching duties nurses encounter. Families who are caring for a member in the home need to know about communication strategies. Their caregiving responsibilities should be balanced with self-care activities.

Community Supports

The Alzheimer's Association is a national agency that provides various forms of assistance to individuals with the disease and their families. The Alzheimer's Association has a Community Resource Finder that is useful in locating local resources.

Some families manage the care of their loved one until death. Other families eventually find that they can no longer deal with the labile and aggressive behavior, incontinence, wandering, unsafe habits, or disruptive nighttime activity. Families need information, support, and legal and financial guidance at this time. Include information regarding advance directives, durable power of attorney, guardianship, and conservatorship in the communication with the family.

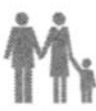

Nurse, Patient, and Family Resources

AlzConnected
www.alzconnected.org

Alzheimer's Association
www.alz.org

Alzheimer Society of Canada
www.alzheimer.ca

Association for Frontotemporal Degeneration
www.theaftd.org

Cruetzfeldt-Jakob's Disease Foundation, Inc. (Prion Disease)
cjdfoundation.org

Huntington's Disease Society of America
hdsa.org

Lewy Body Dementia Association
www.lbda.org

National Institute on Aging
www.nia.nih.gov

National Parkinson's Foundation
www.parkinson.org

CHAPTER 14

Personality Disorders

Personality disorders are among the most challenging and complex group of disorders to treat. Individuals who meet criteria for these disorders display significant challenges in self-identity or self-direction. Relationships are always affected because these individuals have problems with empathy or intimacy.

Personality can be described operationally in terms of functioning. Personality is an individual's characteristic patterns of relatively permanent thoughts, feelings, and behaviors that define the quality of their experiences and relationships. A personality is considered unhealthy when interpersonal and social relationships and functioning are consistently maladaptive, complicated, or dysphoric. Personality can be protective for a person in times of difficulty but may also be a liability if one's personality results in ongoing relationship problems or leads to emotional distress on a regular basis.

People with personality disorders have difficulty recognizing or owning that their difficulties are problems of their personality. Some individuals truly believe the problems originate outside of themselves. Still others may be unaware that their behavior is unusual, and they may not experience any distress. It is unusual for people to seek health care for a personality disorder, although they may seek treatment for comorbid conditions such as major depressive disorder or generalized anxiety disorder.

EPIDEMIOLOGY

Although studies vary in their estimates of prevalence depending on methodologies, personality disorders affect about 6% of the global population (Huang et al., 2009). In the U.S. population, the overall prevalence rate of personality disorders among community samples is higher—around 10% (Sansone & Sansone, 2011).

Risk Factors

Personality disorders represent extreme variations of normal personality traits in four areas: anxious-dependency traits, psychopathy-antisocial, social withdrawal, and compulsivity. These traits are probably inherited and reflect a genetic transmission. The expression of these characteristics is influenced by the environment, including family life (e.g., stability and abuse), cultural expectations, and social determinants (e.g., poverty, education, and violence). Childhood neglect or trauma has been established as a risk factor for personality disorders. This association has been linked to possible biological mechanisms involving corticotropin-releasing hormones in response to early life stress and emotional reactivity.

TYPES OF PERSONALITY DISORDERS

According to the American Psychiatric Association (APA, 2013), there are 10 personality disorders. These 10 disorders are grouped into clusters of similar behavior patterns and personality traits:

Cluster A: Behaviors described as odd or eccentric
- Paranoid personality disorder
- Schizoid personality disorder
- Schizotypal personality disorder

Cluster B: Behaviors described as dramatic, emotional, or erratic
- Borderline personality disorder
- Narcissistic personality disorder
- Histrionic personality disorder
- Antisocial personality disorder

Cluster C: Behaviors described as anxious or fearful
- Avoidant
- Dependent
- Obsessive–compulsive

The following sections discuss the personality disorders, provide guidelines for care, and briefly describe treatments for each of the 10 personality disorders.

CLUSTER A PERSONALITY DISORDERS

Disorders within Cluster A are considered the odd or eccentric personality problems. The common features within this cluster are social awkwardness and social withdrawal.

Paranoid Personality Disorder

Paranoid personality disorder is characterized by a distrust and suspiciousness of others based on the belief, which is unsupported by evidence, that others want to exploit, harm, or deceive the person. Relationships are difficult because of jealousy, controlling behaviors, and grudge-holding.

The prevalence of paranoid personality disorder is about 2% to 4% (APA, 2013). Slightly more men than women are diagnosed with this disorder. Relatives of patients with schizophrenia are more commonly affected. Symptoms may be apparent in childhood or adolescence.

Nursing Guidelines

- Due to mistrust, promises, appointments, and schedules should be strictly adhered to.
- Being too friendly may be met with suspicion. Give clear and straightforward explanations of tests and procedures beforehand.
- Fears may result in threats; setting limits may be necessary.

Treatment

If the patient ends up in treatment, he or she will be suspicious about why this is happening. Paranoia makes communication difficult. The establishment of a professional and trusting relationship is essential. Although threatening, group therapy may be useful in improving social skills. Role playing and group feedback can help reduce suspiciousness.

Antianxiety agents such as diazepam (Valium) may be considered to reduce anxiety and agitation (Sadock et al., 2015). Short-term use of antipsychotic medication such as haloperidol (Haldol) in small doses may manage delusional thinking or severe agitation. Another first-generation antipsychotic medication, pimozide (Orap), may be useful in reducing paranoid thoughts.

Schizoid Personality Disorder

People with schizoid personality disorder exhibit a lifelong pattern of social withdrawal. They operate with a restricted range of emotional expression. Others tend to view them as odd or eccentric. People with this disorder do not seek out or enjoy close relationships. Neither approval nor rejection from others seems to have much effect.

Individuals with this disorder may be able to function well in a solitary occupation such as being a security guard on the night shift. They often express feelings of being an observer rather than a participant in life. They may describe feelings of depersonalization or detachment from themselves and the world.

The prevalence rate for schizoid personality disorder may be as high as 5% of the population (APA, 2013). Males are more commonly affected. Symptoms of schizoid personality disorder appear before adulthood. There is an increased prevalence of the disorder in families with a history of schizophrenia or schizotypal personality disorder.

Nursing Guidelines

- Nurses should avoid being too "nice" or "friendly."
- Do not try to increase socialization.
- Perform a thorough diagnostic assessment as needed to identify symptoms or disorders the patient is reluctant to discuss.
- Protect the patient from ridicule from group members, which may be provoked by the patient's distinctive interests or ideas.

Treatment

Because patients with schizoid personality disorder tend to be introspective, they may be good, but distant, candidates for talk therapy. As trust develops, these patients may describe a fantasy life and fears, particularly of dependence. Group therapy may also be helpful, even though the patient may frequently be silent. Group members may become quite important to the person with schizoid personality disorder and may make up the only form of socialization he or she has.

Antidepressants such as bupropion (Wellbutrin) may increase pleasure in life. Second-generation antipsychotics, such as risperidone (Risperdal) or olanzapine (Zyprexa), are used to improve emotional expressiveness.

Schizotypal Personality Disorder

Schizotypal personality disorder is both a personality disorder and the first of the schizophrenia spectrum disorders (APA, 2013). Characteristics of this disorder include magical thinking, odd beliefs, strange speech patterns, and inappropriate affect.

These individuals have severe social and interpersonal deficits and tend to ramble with lengthy, unclear, and overly detailed content. As a result of suspiciousness, they tend to misinterpret the motives of others as being out to get them. Odd beliefs (e.g., being overly superstitious) or magical thinking (e.g., "He caught a cold because I wanted him to") are also common. Psychotic symptoms such as hallucinations and delusions might also exist with schizotypal personality disorder, but to a lesser degree and only briefly. As opposed to schizophrenia, people with this disorder can be made aware of their suspiciousness, magical thinking, and odd beliefs.

The prevalence of schizotypal personality disorder ranges from 0.6% to 4.6% (APA, 2013). It is more common in men. Symptoms are evident in young people. Having a first-degree relative with schizophrenia increases the risk.

Nursing Guidelines

- Respect the patient's need for social isolation.
- Perform careful diagnostic assessment as needed to uncover other medical or psychological symptoms that may need intervention (e.g., suicidal thoughts).
- Monitor personal responses to the patient's strange beliefs and activities.

Treatment

The principles of psychotherapy are similar to those for schizoid personality disorder (Sadock et al., 2015). Clinicians should be aware that therapy may be impacted by involvement in groups such as cults and unusual religious groups and engagement in occult activities.

People with schizotypal personality disorder may benefit from low-dose antipsychotic agents for psychotic-like symptoms and day-to-day functioning. These agents help with such symptoms as ideas of reference or illusions. Comorbid depression and anxiety may be treated.

CLUSTER B PERSONALITY DISORDERS

Four disorders share dramatic, erratic, or flamboyant behavior as symptoms. They share a high degree of overlapping symptoms as well as comorbidity with disorders such as substance use, mood and anxiety disorders, and other personality disorders.

Antisocial Personality Disorder

Antisocial personality disorder is characterized by a pattern of disregard for, and violation of, the rights of others. The main pathological traits that characterize antisocial personality disorder are antagonistic behaviors such as being deceitful and manipulative for personal gain or hostile if needs are blocked. People with disorder also exhibit disinhibited behaviors such as high risk taking, disregard for responsibility, and impulsivity. Criminal misconduct and substance use are common.

One of the most disturbing qualities associated with antisocial personality disorder is a lack of empathy, also known as callousness. This callousness results in a lack of concern about the feelings of others; an absence of remorse or guilt except when facing punishment; and a disregard for meeting school, family, and other obligations. They may seem concerned and caring if these attributes help them manipulate and exploit others. Wittiness, charm, and flattery may accompany manipulation and exploitation.

The prevalence of antisocial personality disorder is about 1.1% in community studies (Skodol et al., 2011). The disorder is much more common in men than women (3% versus 1%). Symptoms are evident by the midteen and tend to peak during the late teenage years. By 40 years of age the symptoms may improve even without treatment.

Nursing Guidelines

- Recognize attempts to manipulate (e.g., flattery, seductiveness, and instilling guilt).
- Set clear and realistic limits for specific behaviors.
- All staff involved should be aware of and adhere to the treatment plan.
- Know that having wishes prevented may result in aggression.

- Document behaviors objectively (i.e., provide times, dates, circumstances).
- Establish and communicate clear boundaries and consequences.

Treatment

The most useful approach is to target specific problem behaviors that can be changed in individual therapy. Other approaches such as family therapy are useful. Some positive results have been obtained through milieu programs (e.g., token economy systems and therapeutic communities).

There are no medications specifically approved by the FDA for antisocial personality disorder. However, mood-stabilizing medications such as lithium or valproic acid (Depakote) may help with aggression, depression, and impulsivity. Selective serotonin reuptake inhibitors (SSRIs) such as fluoxetine (Prozac) and sertraline (Zoloft) may be used to decrease irritability and help with anxiety and depression. Benzodiazepines may reduce anxiety but should be used with caution because they are addictive agents. Methylphenidate (Ritalin) may help if there is a comorbidity of attention- deficit/hyperactivity disorder.

Borderline Personality Disorder

People with borderline personality disorder exhibit patterns of marked instability in emotional regulation (dysregulation), impulsivity, identity, unstable mood, and unstable interpersonal relationships. Emotional lability results in moving from one emotional extreme to another, usually in response to a pathological fear of separation and intense sensitivity rejection.

Another disruptive trait is impulsivity. Impulsivity is manifested in acting quickly in response to emotions without considering the consequences. This impulsivity results in damaged relationships and even in suicide attempts. Self-destructive behaviors such as cutting, promiscuous sexual behavior, and numbing with substances are common. Suicidal ideation is common and increases the likelihood of accidental deaths. Co-occurring mood, anxiety, or substance disorders complicate the treatment and prognosis of the condition. Antagonism is manifested in hostility, anger, and irritability in relationships. Violence may occur in relationships and against property.

Splitting, a primitive defense mechanism, refers to the inability to view both positive and negative aspects of others as part of a whole. This results in seeing someone as either a wonderful person or a horrible person. Initially, the individual tends to idealize another person. At the first disappointment or frustration, the individual's status quickly shifts to one of devaluation, and the other person is despised.

Nursing Guidelines

- Set realistic goals, using clear action words.
- Be aware of manipulative behaviors (flattery, seductiveness, guilt instilling).
- Provide clear and consistent boundaries and limits.
- Use clear and straightforward communication.
- When behavioral problems emerge, calmly review the therapeutic goals and boundaries of treatment.
- Avoid rejecting or rescuing.
- Assess for suicidal and self-mutilating behaviors, especially during times of stress.

Treatment

A person with borderline personality disorder may seek repeated hospitalizations. Although hospitalization may decrease self-destructive risk, it is not an effective long-term solution.

There are three essential therapies for borderline personality disorder. Cognitive–behavioral therapy (CBT) helps individuals to identify and change inaccurate core perceptions of themselves and others and problems interacting with others. Dialectical behavior therapy (DBT) combines cognitive and behavioral techniques with mindfulness, which emphasizes being aware of thoughts and actively shaping them. Schema-focused therapy combines parts of CBT with other forms of therapy that focus on the ways that individuals view themselves. These three therapies are discussed in Chapter 29.

Pharmacology is geared toward maintaining patients' cognitive function, symptom relief, and improved quality of life. People with borderline personality disorder may respond to anticonvulsant mood-stabilizing medications, lithium, antidepressants, and omega-3 fatty acid supplementation for mood and emotion dysregulation symptoms. Naltrexone, an opioid receptor antagonist, has been found to reduce self-injurious behaviors. Second-generation antipsychotics may assist with anger control and brief psychosis.

Histrionic Personality Disorder

Though often high functioning, people with histrionic personality disorder are excitable and dramatic. Characteristics include being overly dramatic, extroverted, flamboyant, and colorful. Despite this bold exterior, they tend to have a limited ability to develop meaningful relationships.

Histrionic personality disorder occurs at a rate of nearly 2% (APA, 2013). It tends to be diagnosed more frequently in women than men. Symptoms begin by early adulthood. Inborn character traits such as emotional expressiveness and egocentricity have been identified as predisposing an individual to this disorder.

Nursing Guidelines

- Encourage and model the use of concrete and descriptive rather than vague and dramatic language.
- Assist the patient to clarify inner feelings; patients with this personality disorder often have difficulty identifying their own real feelings.
- Teach and role model assertiveness.

Treatment

In general, individuals with histrionic personality disorder do not think they need psychiatric help. They may go into treatment for associated problems such as depression that may be precipitated by losses such as loss of a relationship.

Individuals with histrionic personality disorder may be out of touch with their feelings. Psychotherapy may promote clarification of inner feelings and appropriate expression. Both individual and group therapy are useful in this population.

There are no specific treatments targeted at people with histrionic personality disorder. Medications such as antidepressants can be used for depressive or somatic symptoms.

Antianxiety agents may be helpful in treating anxiety. Antipsychotics may be used if the patient exhibits derealization or illusions.

Narcissistic Personality Disorder

Narcissistic personality disorder is characterized by feelings of being entitled, an exaggerated belief in one's own importance, and a lack of empathy. In reality, people with this disorder suffer from a weak self-esteem and hypersensitivity to criticism. Narcissistic personality disorder is associated with less impairment in individual functioning and quality of life than the other personality-based disorders.

The prevalence of narcissistic personality disorder ranges from 0% to about 6% (APA, 2013). It tends to be more common in males than females. Age of onset is difficult to determine because of the narcissistic traits that are commonly found in adolescents. There may be a familial pattern; parents with narcissism may attribute an unrealistic sense of talent, importance, and beauty to their children. These attributions put the children at higher risk.

Nursing Guidelines

- Nurses should remain neutral.
- Avoid engaging in power struggles or becoming defensive in response to the patient's disparaging remarks.
- Convey self-confidence.
- Role model empathy.

Treatment

If a person with this narcissistic personality disorder seeks treatment, individual CBT helps to deconstruct faulty thinking and promote realistic thoughts. Group therapy can also assist the person in sharing with others, seeing their own qualities in others, and learning empathy. In family-oriented approaches, narcissistic individuals are likely to deny that they contribute to family problems and will instead blame others.

Lithium (Eskalith, Lithobid) has been used in patients with narcissism who demonstrate mood swings. Antidepressants can also be used if the person has symptoms of depression.

CLUSTER C PERSONALITY DISORDERS

High levels of anxiety and the outward signs of fear characterize cluster C personality disorders. These personality types also exhibit social inhibitions.

Avoidant Personality Disorder

People with avoidant personality disorder avoid interpersonal contact because of fears of rejection or criticism. These individuals are extremely sensitive to rejection, feel inadequate, and are socially inhibited. They are especially sensitive to and preoccupied with rejection, humiliation, and failure.

Avoidant personality disorder occurs in 2.4% of the population (APA, 2013). It occurs equally in men and women. Early symptoms include shyness and avoidance in childhood that increases during adolescence and early adulthood.

Guidelines for Nursing Care

- Nurses should use a friendly, accepting, reassuring approach.
- Remember that social situations can cause extreme and severe anxiety.
- Convey an attitude of acceptance toward patient fears.
- Though anxiety-provoking, group therapy may help the person understand the fear of rejection and how it affects personal relationships.
- Provide the exercises to enhance new social skills with caution, because failure can increase feelings of poor self-worth.
- Assertiveness training can assist the person to learn to express his or her needs.

Treatment

Individual and group therapy is useful in processing anxiety-provoking symptoms and in planning methods to approach and handle anxiety-provoking situations. Psychotherapy focuses on trust and assertiveness training.

Antianxiety agents can help. Beta-adrenergic receptor antagonists (e.g., atenolol) reduce autonomic nervous system hyperactivity. Antidepressants such as SSRIs such as citalopram (Celexa) and serotonin norepinephrine reuptake inhibitors (SNRIs) such as venlafaxine (Effexor) may reduce social anxiety. Serotonergic agents may help individuals with avoidant personalities feel less sensitive to rejection.

Dependent Personality Disorder

Dependent personality disorder is characterized by a pattern of submissive and clinging behavior related to an overwhelming need to be cared for. This results in intense fears of separation. These individuals may experience intense anxiety when left alone for even brief periods of time (APA, 2013).

The prevalence is estimated at about 0.5% (APA, 2013). The inherited trait of submissiveness may be a factor in the development of this disorder.

Guidelines for Nursing Care

- Help the patient identify and address current stressors.
- Be aware that strong countertransference often develops in clinicians because of the patient's excessive clinging (demands of extra time, nighttime calls, crisis before vacations).
- The therapeutic relationship can provide a testing ground for increased assertiveness through role modeling and teaching of assertive skills.

Treatment

Psychotherapy is the treatment of choice for dependent personality disorder. CBT can help in the development of new perspectives and attitudes about other people.

There are no specific medications indicated for this disorder, but symptoms of depression and anxiety may be treated with appropriate antidepressant and antianxiety agents. Panic attacks can be alleviated with the tricyclic antidepressant imipramine (Tofranil).

Obsessive–Compulsive Personality Disorder

Obsessive–compulsive personality disorder is characterized by limited emotional expression, stubbornness, perseverance, and indecisiveness. Preoccupation with orderliness, perfectionism, and control are the hallmarks of this disorder. Rigidity and inflexible standards of self and others persist even if they are self-defeating or relationship defeating. Preoccupation with the activity often results in losing the major point of the activity. Projects are often incomplete because of overly strict standards.

A distinction should be made: Obsessive–compulsive *disorder* is characterized by repetition or adherence to rituals. Obsessive–compulsive *personality disorder* is characterized more by an unhealthy focus on perfectionism.

Obsessive–compulsive personality disorder is one of the most prevalent personality disorders. Prevalence rates range from about 2% to 8% (APA, 2013). It is more common in men than women. Risk factors for this disorder include a background of harsh discipline and having a first-degree relative with the disorder.

Nursing Guidelines

- Nurses should guard against power struggles with patients, because their need for control is very high.
- Remember that patients with this disorder have difficulty dealing with unexpected changes.

Treatment

Typically, patients do seek help for obsessive–compulsive personality disorder, because they are aware of their own suffering. Treatments are often long and complicated. Group therapy can help the person learn new coping skills, manage anxiety, and receive feedback from the group.

Clomipramine (Anafranil) may help reduce the obsessions, anxiety, and depression associated with this disorder. Other serotonergic agents such as fluoxetine (Prozac) may also be helpful.

ASSESSMENT

Signs and Symptoms

When assessing an individual with a personality disorder, the patient's history will reveal persistent traits. These traits cause distress or impairment in functioning. Does the patient:

- Suspect others of exploiting or deceiving him or her? Bear grudges and not forget insults?
- Detach self from social relationships? Not desire close relationships or being part of a family? Take pleasure in few if any activities?
- Have a history of social and interpersonal deficits marked by acute discomfort? Have any cognitive or perceptual distortions?
- Have a pervasive pattern of disregard for and violation of the rights of others? Act deceitfully (repeated lying, use others for own needs)? Act consistently irresponsible toward others?
- Have a pattern of unstable and chaotic personal relationships? Have a history of suicide attempts or self-mutilation? Have chronic feelings of emptiness, or show intense anger, intense anxiety, and dysphoria?
- Have a pattern of excessive emotionality and attention-seeking behaviors (e.g., sexually seductive or provocative)? Have self-dramatic, theatrical, and exaggerated expressions of emotion?
- Act grandiose, need admiration, and lack empathy for others? Have unreasonable expectations of favored treatment? Act interpersonally exploitive?

Does the patient do the following:

- Persistently avoid social situations because of feelings of inadequacy and hypersensitivity to negative evaluation? View self as socially inept or inferior to others?
- Have an excessive need to be taken care of, show clinging behaviors within relationships, or have an intense fear of separation? Have difficulty making everyday decisions without an excessive amount of advice and reassurance from others?
- Have a preoccupation with neatness, perfectionism, and mental and interpersonal control? Show rigidity and stubbornness?

Assessment Tools

The Personality Inventory (Krueger et al., 2013) is a useful tool for assessing for personality disorders (Fig. 14.1). This 25-item scale measures traits found in these conditions, including negative affect, detachment, antagonism, disinhibition, and psychoticism.

The Personality Inventory for DSM-5—Brief Form (PID-5-BF)—Adult

Name: ____________________ Age: ____ Sex: ☐ Male ☐ Female Date: __________

Instructions: This is a list of things different people might say about themselves. We are interested in how you would describe yourself. There are no right or wrong answers. So you can describe yourself as honestly as possible, we will keep your responses confidential. We'd like you to take your time and read each statement carefully, selecting the response that best describes you.						**Clinician Use**
		Very False or Often False	**Sometimes or Somewhat False**	**Sometimes or Somewhat True**	**Very True or Often True**	**Item score**
1	People would describe me as reckless.	0	1	2	3	
2	I feel like I act totally on impulse.	0	1	2	3	
3	Even though I know better, I can't stop making rash decisions.	0	1	2	3	
4	I often feel like nothing I do really matters.	0	1	2	3	
5	Others see me as irresponsible.	0	1	2	3	
6	I'm not good at planning ahead.	0	1	2	3	
7	My thoughts often don't make sense to others.	0	1	2	3	
8	I worry about almost everything.	0	1	2	3	
9	I get emotional easily, often for very little reason.	0	1	2	3	
10	I fear being alone in life more than anything else.	0	1	2	3	
11	I get stuck on one way of doing things, even when it's clear it won't work.	0	1	2	3	
12	I have seen things that weren't really there.	0	1	2	3	
13	I steer clear of romantic relationships.	0	1	2	3	
14	I'm not interested in making friends.	0	1	2	3	
15	I get irritated easily by all sorts of things.	0	1	2	3	
16	I don't like to get too close to people.	0	1	2	3	
17	It's no big deal if I hurt other peoples' feelings.	0	1	2	3	
18	I rarely get enthusiastic about anything.	0	1	2	3	
19	I crave attention.	0	1	2	3	
20	I often have to deal with people who are less important than me.	0	1	2	3	
21	I often have thoughts that make sense to me but that other people say are strange.	0	1	2	3	
22	I use people to get what I want.	0	1	2	3	
23	I often "zone out" and then suddenly come to and realize that a lot of time has passed.	0	1	2	3	
24	Things around me often feel unreal, or more real than usual.	0	1	2	3	
25	It is easy for me to take advantage of others.	0	1	2	3	
					Total/Partial Raw Score:	
					Prorated Total Score: (if 1-6 items left unanswered)	
					Average Total Score:	

Krueger RF, Derringer J, Markon KE, Watson D, Skodol AE.

Fig. 14.1 Reprinted with permission from The Personality Inventory for DSM-5, (Copyright ©2013). American Psychiatric Association. All Rights Reserved.

Assessment Guidelines

Assessment about personality functioning needs to be viewed within the individual's ethnic, cultural, and social background. Personality disorders are often exacerbated after the loss of significant supporting people or in a disruptive social situation.

A change in personality in middle adulthood or later signals the need for a thorough medical workup or assessment for unrecognized substance use disorder. Be cognizant that social stereotypes can influence the clinician's judgment in that a particular diagnosis can be overdiagnosed or underdiagnosed (e.g., for males or females because of sexual bias; because of social class or immigrant status).

Patient Problems

Patients with personality disorders often act impulsively. The nurse may be asked to intervene during acting-out behaviors. These behaviors are often marked by impulsivity, such as self-mutilation or suicide attempts, anger and hostility toward the staff, paranoia, blaming others for problems, manipulation and splitting, and intense anxiety.

Four common patient problems are presented here: *potential for self-mutilation* (scratching, burning, cutting), *decreased self-esteem, impaired social functioning,* and *impaired coping.*

Intervention Guidelines

Creating a therapeutic relationship with patients who have personality disorders is challenging. A history of interrupted therapeutic connections can be a setup for failure.

Because these patients often require a sense of control, giving them choices (e.g., setting up times for appointments) might enhance adherence. A feeling of being threatened and vulnerable might lead to blaming or verbally attacking others. Patients with personality disorders are hypersensitive to criticism. One of the most effective methods of teaching new behaviors is to build on the patient's existing skills.

Setting limits is essential in working with patients with personality disorders. It is important for the nurse to take time to set clear boundaries (nurse and patient responsibilities) and repeat the limits frequently when working with patients with personality disorders.

Nursing Care for Personality Disorders

Potential for Self-Mutilation

Due to:

- Personality disorder
- History of self-mutilation
- Impulsivity
- Poor self-esteem
- Unstable self-image
- Feelings of emptiness

- Impaired problem-solving abilities
- Culture of self-mutilation
- Efforts to avoid abandonment
- Intense anger

Desired Outcomes:
Patient will adopt more positive coping skills and refrain from self-injurious behaviors.

Assessment/Interventions (Rationales)

1. Assess the patient's history of self-mutilation including:
   a. Types of mutilation
   b. Frequency of self-mutilation
   c. Stressors preceding behavior
   (Identifying patterns and circumstances surrounding self-injury helps the nurse plan interventions and teaching strategies to fit the individual.)
2. Identify feelings experienced around the time of self-mutilation. (Feelings are a guideline for future intervention [e.g., rage at feeling left out or abandoned].)
3. Explore with the patient what these feelings might mean. (Self-mutilation might be a way to relieve anxiety, feel alive through pain, or an expression of guilt or self-hate.)
4. Identify specific steps (e.g., persons to call upon) when feeling the urge to self-mutilate. (The patient is encouraged to take responsibility for healthier behavior. Talking to others and learning alternative coping skills can reduce the frequency and severity until the behavior ceases.)
5. Use a matter-of-fact approach when self-mutilation occurs. Avoid criticizing or giving sympathy. (A neutral approach prevents blaming, which increases anxiety, giving special attention that encourages acting out.)
6. After treatment of the wound, discuss what happened right before and the thoughts and feelings the patient had immediately before self-mutilating. (Identifies dynamics for both the patient and nurse clinician. Allows the identification of less harmful responses to help relieve intense tensions.)
7. Develop alternatives to self-mutilating behaviors.
   a. Anticipate certain situations that might lead to increased stress (e.g., anger or frustration).
   b. Identify actions that might modify the intensity of such situations.

c. Identify two or three people whom the patient can contact to discuss and examine intense feelings (e.g., rage, self-hate) when they arise.

(Planning for stressful situations provides the patient with increasing self-agency rather than relying on external controls.)

8. Set and maintain limits on acceptable behavior and make clear the patient's responsibilities. If patient is hospitalized, be clear regarding unit rules. (Clear and nonpunitive limit setting is essential for decreasing negative behaviors.)

Decreased Self-Esteem

Due to:

- Personality disorder
- Repeated failures
- Childhood abuse and/or neglect
- Avoidant and dependent patterns
- Lack of integrated self-view
- Shame and guilt
- Inconsistent affection and discipline in family of origin

Desired Outcomes:

The patient will demonstrate the ability to reframe negative self-thoughts into more realistic appraisals and identify positive aspects of self.

Assessment/Interventions (Rationales)

1. Maintain a neutral, calm, and respectful manner. (Helps the patient see himself or herself as respected as a person, even when behavior might not be appropriate.)
2. Keep in mind that patients with personality disorders might defend against feelings of low self-esteem through blaming, projection, anger, passivity, and demanding behaviors. (Many behaviors seen in patients with personality disorders cover a fragile sense of self. Often these behaviors are the crux of the patient's interpersonal difficulties in all of his or her relationships.)
3. Assess the patient's self-perception. Target a variety of aspects in the patient's life:
   a. Strengths and weaknesses in performance at work, school, and daily life tasks
   b. Strengths and weaknesses in relation to physical appearance, sexuality, and personality

(After identifying realistic areas of strengths and weaknesses, the patient and nurse can work on the realities of the self-appraisal and target the areas that seem inaccurate.)

4. Review the types of cognitive distortions that affect self-esteem (e.g., self-blame, mind reading, overgeneralization, selective inattention, all-or-none thinking). (These are the most common cognitive distortions individuals use. Identifying them is the first step to correcting false thoughts.)
5. Help the patient recognize cognitive distortions, their impact on emotion, and influence on behavior. Encourage the patient to keep a log. (Cognitive distortions are automatic. Keeping a log helps make automatic, unconscious thinking clear.)
6. Teach the patient to reframe and dispute cognitive distortions. Disputes need to be strong, specific, and nonjudgmental. (Practice and belief in the disputes over time help patients gain a more realistic appraisal of events, the world, and themselves.)
7. Discourage the patient from dwelling on and reliving past mistakes. (The past cannot be changed. Dwelling on past mistakes prevents the patient from appraising the present and planning for the future.)
8. Discourage the patient from making repetitive self-blaming and negative remarks. (Unacceptable behavior does not make the patient a bad person; it means that the patient made some poor choices in the past.)
9. Focus questions in a positive and active way to help the patient refocus on the present and look to the future. For example: "What could you do differently now?" or "What have you learned from that experience?" (Focusing questions in an active light allows the patient to look at past behaviors differently and a sense of control over the future.)
10. Provide honest and genuine feedback regarding your observations as to his or her strengths and areas that could use additional skills. (Feedback helps give the patient a more accurate view of self, strengths, areas to work on, as well as a sense that someone is trying to understand him or her.)
11. Set goals realistically, and revise goals as needed. Improvement generally occurs in small steps. (The patient's negative self-view and distrust of the world took years to develop. Unrealistic goals can set up hopelessness in patients and frustration in staff.)

12. Help the patient to set realistic short-term goals for the future. Identify skills the patient will need to reach his or her goals. (Looking toward the future minimizes dwelling on the past and negative self-rumination. When realistic short-term goals are met, the patient gains a sense of accomplishment, direction, and purpose in life. Accomplishing goals can bolster a sense of control and enhance self-perception.)

Impaired Social Functioning

Due to:

- Inability to engage in mature interactions
- Manipulative behavior
- Self-concept disturbance
- Unacceptable social behavior or values
- Immature interests
- Biochemical changes in the brain
- Disruptive or abusive early family background

Desired Outcomes:

The patient will voluntarily interact with others and derive satisfaction from the interactions.

Assessment/Interventions (Rationales)

1. Encourage the patient to recognize maladaptive patterns of social interaction. (The patient does not recognize patterns of maladaptive behaviors. Change cannot happen until this recognition occurs.)
2. Identify alternative social interaction methods. (Once maladaptive behavior is eliminated, new methods of social interaction must be identified and adopted.)
3. Role-play to practice successful social interaction. (The nurse–patient relationship is an ideal testing ground for developing relationship skills.)
4. Encourage attendance at group therapy and group work. (Group member influence, confrontation, altruistic learning, and recognition of own behaviors in others are often more valuable than one-to-one encounters.)

Impaired Coping

Due to:

- Disturbance in patterns of tension relief
- Intense emotional state

- Failure to intend to change behavior
- Lack of motivation to change behaviors
- Negative attitudes toward health behavior
- Neurobiological factors

Desired Outcomes:
The patient will demonstrate the use of newly learned coping skills to modify anxiety and frustration.

Assessment/Interventions (Rationales)

1. Assess for self-mutilating or suicidal thoughts or behaviors. (Maintaining safety by monitoring for urges or acts of self-mutilation and suicidal thoughts is a priority.)
2. Intervene in times of intense and labile mood swings, anxiety, depression, and irritability. (Many of these dysfunctional behaviors of patients [e.g., parasuicidal, anger, manipulation, substance use] are used as behavioral solutions to intense pain.)
   a. Anxiety: Teach stress-reduction techniques such as deep breathing, relaxation, meditation, and exercise. (Patients experience intense anxiety and fear of abandonment. Stress-reduction techniques help the patient focus more clearly.)
   b. Depression: The patient might need medications to improve mood. Assess for side effects. (Medication combined with talk therapy and exercise is effective in decreasing depression. Side effects should be managed or medication changed to promote adherence.)
   c. Irritability, anger: Use interventions early before anxiety and anger escalate. (Intervening early can help reduce or eliminate escalation.)
3. Reduce manipulation through consistency, limit setting, and unit or community rules. (External structure will decrease negative behaviors while patients develop internal control.)
4. Be assertive when setting limits on the patient's unreasonable demands for time and attention. (Firm, clear, nonjudgmental limits give the patient structure.)
5. Be nonjudgmental and respectful when listening to the patient's thoughts, feelings, or complaints. (Developing a trusting relationship with the nurse lays the groundwork for future relationships.)

6. Encourage the patient to explore feelings and concerns (e.g., identify fears, loneliness, self-hate). (The patient is used to acting out feelings rather than expressing them verbally. Appropriate self-expression is an essential new skill.)
7. When the patient is ready and interested, teach coping skills to help diffuse tension and troubling feelings (e.g., anxiety reduction, assertiveness skills). (Increasing skills helps the patient to use healthier ways to diffuse tensions and get needs met.)
8. Patients with personality disorders often benefit from additional training (e.g., dialectical behavioral therapy, interpersonal skills, anger management skills, emotional regulation skills). Provide referrals or involve professional experts. (This training teaches the patient to refine skills in changing behaviors, emotions, and thinking patterns associated with problems in living that are causing misery and distress.)
9. Treatment of substance use is best handled by well-organized treatment systems, not by an individual nurse clinician. (Keeping detailed records and having a team involved with each patient can minimize manipulation.)
10. Provide and encourage the patient to use professionals in other disciplines such as social services, vocational rehabilitation, social work, or the law. (Patients with personality disorders often have multiple social problems and do not know how to obtain these services.)

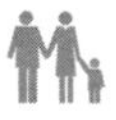

Nurse, Patient, and Family Resources

Borderline Personality Disorder Central
www.bpdcentral.com

Internet Mental Health
www.mentalhealth.com

Dialectical Behavior Therapy
www.dbtncaa.com

MedlinePlus
medlineplus.gov/personalitydisorders.html

National Alliance on Mentally Illness (NAMI)
www.nami.org

Self-Injury Outreach and Support
sioutreach.org

PART III
Psychiatric Crises

CHAPTER 15

Grieving

Loss is part of the human experience, and grieving is the response that enables people to accept and reconcile with the loss and adapt to change. We grieve the commonplace losses in our lives—loss of a relationship, health, a friendship, status or prestige, security, or a dream. Other normal losses include changes in circumstances such as retirement, promotion, marriage, and aging. These losses can promote growth through adaptation or may result in apathy, anger, and resentment.

Losing a significant person through death is a major life crisis. Long-term relationships bond us to each other deeply, shaping our world and our identity in it. The loss of a significant other can diminish aspects of our own self-concept. Grief is experienced holistically, affecting us emotionally, cognitively, spiritually, and physically. Those who grieve sometimes describe the death of a loved one feeling like an amputation.

Bereavement, derived from the Old English word *berafian,* poignantly meaning, "to rob," is the period of grieving after a death. Mourning refers to things people do to cope with grief, including shared social expressions of grief such as calling hours, funerals, and bereavement groups. Everyone grieves, but not everyone engages in the work of mourning. The length of time, degree, and ritual for mourning are often typically determined by cultural, religious, and familial factors.

The goals of mourning have evolved from doing the grief work, getting over it, and moving on with life. Mourning is a complex, individual, culturally embedded process of accepting the death. It involves confronting the painful experience of grief, constructing an identity and a life in a transformed environment, and finding an enduring relationship with the deceased based not on physical presence but on accurate memory.

Depending on many factors, this process can take months to a number of years. Losses transform lives. After a loss we are never quite the same person again. Yet, over time, people move on from pain defining who they are to living with the residual pain and forever carrying the memory of the loved one.

THEORY

Kübler-Ross's (1969) groundbreaking work provides a framework for understanding reactions to dying. Her stage theory was eventually applied to the grieving process as well. Denial, anger, bargaining, depression, and acceptance are used to explain responses to loss.

Although viewing the grieving process as linear—from denial to eventual acceptance—is appealing, grieving is not that simple. In reality, these stages overlap and may be nonsequential. Strobe (1998) incorporates the stage–phase models of loss-oriented processes with the restoration of a new lifestyle. This process involves coping with everyday life, building a new identity, and developing new relationships. Table 15.1 summarizes the dual process model.

ANTICIPATORY GRIEF

Once a life-threatening diagnosis has been received or curative efforts are stopped, people begin a period of grieving called *anticipatory grief* or *anticipatory mourning*. This type of grief is anticipatory in the sense that a future loss is being mourned in advance. It happens as people acknowledge the importance of the dying person, adjust their lives to

Table 15.1 **Dual Process Model of Coping**

Loss-Oriented Processes	Restoration-Oriented Process
Grief work	Attending to life changes
Intrusion of grief	Distraction from grief
Denial or avoidance of restoration changes	Doing new things
Breaking bonds or ties	Establishing new roles, identities, and relationships

accommodate the intervening time, and foresee how their futures will be altered by the loss.

The experience of anticipatory grief varies by individual, family, and culture. Aspects of finalizing the connection include spending time together, talking, making memories, life review, saying goodbye (often indirectly or metaphorically), touch, communication, taking care of business, and detaching from one another. A common emotional experience is anger—at the disease, the medical community, others, life—in addition to sadness, hurt, fear, anxiety, and hidden grief. Table 15.2 summarizes nursing interventions for families who are grieving in a hospital setting.

GRIEVING

Grieving is the painful experience after a loss. Grieving is a normal response that involves the emotional, spiritual, physical, social, and intellectual responses that occur as a loss is incorporated into one's daily life.

Symptoms of grieving may mirror those of major depressive disorder. Feelings of intense sadness, constant thinking about the loss, insomnia, lack of appetite, and weight loss may be understandable in light of the loss (American Psychiatric Association [APA], 2013). In grief the predominant feelings are emptiness and loss that occur in waves, sometimes alternating with feelings of acceptance. Depression, on the other hand, results in a global inability to experience joy and feelings of guilt and self-loathing. Table 15.3 identifies common expressions of grieving.

There is no clear ending for grieving. Gradually the sadness diminishes, the pain subsides, and the individual moves on. Signs that grief is subsiding include the following:

- Accepting that the loved one has died.
- Distressing memories of the deceased are under control.
- Anger over the loss is no longer present.
- Adaptive appraisals of oneself in relation to the deceased are experienced.
- Reminders of the loss are no longer avoided.
- Belief that life is worth living without the deceased develops.
- An increased sense of identity apart from the lost relationship emerges.
- Engaging in activities, pursuing relationships, or planning for the future are evident.

Table 15.2 Nursing Interventions for Grieving Families in a Hospital Setting

At the death or imminent death of a family member:
1. Communicate the news to the family in an area of privacy. (Family members can support each other in an atmosphere in which they can behave naturally.)
2. The individual or family will need support, answers to questions, and guidance as to immediate tasks and information. (Nurses are the constant members of the health care team who have the experience and expertise to provide support during this difficult period.)
3. If only one family member is available, stay with that member until clergy, a family member, or a friend arrives. (The presence and comfort of the nurse during the initial stage of shock can help minimize feelings of acute isolation and anxiety.)

If the family requests to see the dying or dead person:
1. Support this request. (Individuals may need to say goodbye, ask for forgiveness, or take a lock of hair. This helps people face the reality of death.)

If angry family members accuse the nurse or doctor of mismanaging the care of the deceased:
1. Continue to provide the best care for the dying or final care to the dead. Avoid becoming involved in angry and painful arguments and power struggles. (Complaints are not directed toward the nurse personally. The anger may serve the purpose of keeping grieving relatives from falling apart. Projected anger may be an attempt to deal with aggression and guilt toward the dying person.)

If relatives behave in a grossly disturbed manner (e.g., refuse to acknowledge the truth, collapse, or lose control):
1. Show patience and tact, and offer sympathy and warmth. (Shock and disbelief are the first responses to the news of death, and the bereaved need ways to protect themselves from the overwhelming reality of loss.)
2. Encourage the bereaved to cry. (Crying helps provide relief from feelings of acute pain and tension.)
3. Provide a place of privacy for grieving. (Privacy facilitates the natural expression of grief.)

If the family requests specific religious, cultural, or social customs that are strange or unknown to the nurse:
1. Help facilitate the steps necessary for the family to carry out the desired arrangements. (Institutional mourning rituals of various cultures provide important external supports for the grief-stricken individual.)

Table 15.3 **Common Expressions of Grieving**

Yearnings	Survivors repeatedly want to reunite with the person who died in some way, and may even want to die themselves to be with their loved one.
Deep sadness	People often experience waves of deep sadness and regret about the loved one; crying and even sobbing jags are also normal.
Other negative emotions	Anger, remorse, and guilt are all often present in painful ways.
Somatic disturbances	Grief affects people physically as well as mentally. It is normal for people to have sleep problems, changes in appetite, digestive difficulties, dry mouth, or fatigue after a loss. Occasional bouts of restlessness and agitation also may occur.
Disbelief	It takes people a long time to truly accept that the loved one has died. People often forget at times the loved one is gone until some reminder brings the searing reality back.
Apathy	It is typical for people to withdraw or disengage at times when grieving. People may become irritable toward others.
Emotional surges	Although the worst emotions and disturbances diminish with time, the grieving process also involves surges of emotions. Holidays, anniversaries, birthdays, and other significant events can trigger bouts of grief.
Vivid memories	Recalling vivid memories of times with the deceased is common. Images of the deceased—or even the sound of a loved one's voice—may emerge without warning.

COMPLICATED GRIEVING

The APA (2013) has proposed a condition for further study called *persistent complex bereavement disorder.* This disorder would apply to individuals whose bereavement persists beyond 12 months in adults and 6 months in children. In addition to the timing, interference with normal functioning is the hallmark symptom that distinguishes grieving from a disorder. Suicidal ideation and disinterest in living make this bereavement disorder particularly dangerous.

Symptoms of complicated grieving include preoccupation with thoughts of the deceased person, feelings of emptiness, anger, depression, disbelief, detachment, and rumination. Self-blame may be a prominent symptom. For example, a widow may obsessively blame herself for her spouse not seeking help for chest pain.

Assessment

Signs and Symptoms of Complicated Grieving

- Prolonged, severe symptoms beyond 12 months in adults and 6 months in children
- Limited response to support
- Profound feelings of hopelessness
- Excessive withdrawal
- Fears of being alone
- Inability to work
- Inability to feel emotion
- Panic attacks
- Self-neglect
- Maladaptive behaviors:
    - Alcohol or drug misuse
    - Promiscuity
    - Fugue states
    - Feeling dead or unreal
    - Suicidal ideation
    - Aggressive behaviors
    - Compulsive spending
- Recurrent nightmares, night terrors, or compulsive reenactments

Assessment Guidelines

Grieving and Complicated Grieving

1. Identify whether the individual is at risk for complicated grieving.
2. Evaluate for psychotic symptoms, agitation, increased activity, alcohol or drug abuse, and extreme vegetative symptoms (anorexia, weight loss, not sleeping).
3. Do not overlook people who do not express significant grief in the context of a major loss. Those individuals might have an increased risk of impaired grief reaction.

4. Always assess for suicide with signs of depression or other dysfunctional signs or symptoms.
5. Assess support systems. If support systems are limited, find bereavement groups in the bereaved individual's community.
6. When grieving is stalled or complicated, a variety of therapeutic approaches have proved extremely beneficial (e.g., cognitive-behavioral interventions). Provide referrals.
7. Grieving can bring with it severe spiritual anguish. Determine whether spiritual counseling or counseling would be useful for the bereaved.

Patient Problems

Three specific patient problems relate to loss: *grieving, complicated grieving,* and *potential for complicated grieving*. In this chapter, nursing care is presented for *grieving* and *complicated grieving*. The patient problem *potential for complicated grieving* can be addressed with interventions from the first two plans of care.

Because nurses are in constant contact with people and their families experiencing painful losses, other responses may also be the focus of treatment. During this time, the nurse might need to intervene for impaired individual coping, impaired family coping, sleep pattern disturbance, potential for spiritual distress, or spiritual distress.

Intervention Guidelines

Grieving

1. Listening is the best nursing intervention that a nurse can use. People need to tell their stories, usually over and over, and move through the storyline in their own time.
2. Sincere expression of sympathy such as "I am so sorry for your loss. You must be devastated," shows engagement, interest, and empathy.
3. Avoid clichés and minimizing expressions, which may actually be damaging. Saying "Have you considered having another child?" or "She is no longer suffering"

suggest that the patient should move on or wanted the loved one to suffer.

4. Spiritual care is important to people with spiritual convictions and religious beliefs. Offer support and referrals to pastoral counseling (when available) or community resources.
5. Grief support groups are available for every type of loss (e.g., spouse, child, pet), age group, and special conditions (e.g., disease, suicide, casualty of war). Hearing from others in various stages of grief, sharing the story of loss with others and receiving feedback, and being part of a group who really understands are powerful tools for healing.

Complicated Grieving

1. Nursing care for complicated grieving includes the care previously discussed for grieving. Protection from self-harm is an additional nursing intervention for this population.
2. Encouraging the patient to talk and helping him or her integrate the good and bad aspects of the deceased into a unified whole is an important aspect of care.
3. Assisting with aspects of everyday life, such as encouraging adequate nutrition and hydration, monitoring sleep, and encouraging physical activity, may be required.

Nursing Care for Grieving

Grieving

Due to:

- Anticipatory loss of significant object (e.g., possession, job, status, home, parts and processes of body)
- Anticipatory loss of a significant other
- Death of significant other
- Loss of a significant object (e.g., possession, job, status, home, parts and processes of body)

Desired Outcome:
The patient will express positive expectations for the future and report a successful life reorganization.

Assessment/Interventions (Rationales)

1. Provide your full presence: Use appropriate eye contact, listen attentively, and use appropriate touch.

(Appropriate eye contact helps the patient know you are there. Listening supports the patient's processing of the loss. Suitable touch can express warmth and nurturance.)

2. Be patient with the bereaved in times of silence. Do not fill the silence. (Sharing painful feelings followed by periods of silence allows the patient to process thoughts and feelings without be rushed. Listening patiently helps the bereaved express feelings, even ones he or she thinks are negative.).
3. Avoid euphemisms such as, "I am sorry that James has *passed away*" or "You lost your husband." Instead, say something like, "I am so sorry to hear that James died." (Euphemisms can do harm by making the bereaved think we have do not understand the gravity of the situation.)
4. Avoid trite and philosophical statements such as "He's no longer suffering"; "You can always have another child"; or "It's better this way." Table 15.4 provides recommendations for communicating with grieving individuals. (Making these statements gives the bereaved the impression that his or her experience is not understood and that you are minimizing the feelings and pain.)
5. It is helpful to acknowledge the bereaved individual's painful feelings:
   a. "His death will be a terrible loss."
   b. "No one can replace her."
   c. "He will be missed for a long time."
   d. "Your relationship was complicated."

   (Verbalizing painful feelings reduces feelings of isolation in the bereaved.)

Table 15.4 **Communication and Grief**

What Not To Say	What To Say	Rationale
"I know how you feel."	"Your loss must be devastating. I can't imagine how you must be feeling right now."	Unfortunately, you cannot really know how that person feels.

Continued

Table 15.4 **Communication and Grief—cont'd**

What Not To Say	What To Say	Rationale
"When my mother died, I cried for months and could hardly eat… [*and proceed with long story*]."	"When I lost my mother, I was in a fog for days. This must be difficult for you right now."	Although it is helpful to know that others have experienced loss, during the acute grief period the focus should be on the griever. Sharing lengthy stories is not helpful.
After a sudden and unexpected death: "At least he didn't suffer."	"It must have been so shocking to lose your husband so suddenly. Did he have any symptoms?"	No one wants suffering for a loved one, yet sudden deaths are also highly traumatizing. Chances to prepare and say goodbye are lost.
"Have you thought about getting another ____ [wife, pet, job]?"	"Your loved one was irreplaceably special."	The griever is not interested in a replacement; they want their loved one back.
"She is with [God, a messiah] now."	"I can only imagine how much you are missing her now."	Implying that the loss is a high power's doing may make the griever feel betrayed or punished by God. This statement also assumes that the griever believes in God.
"You can be grateful for the time you had together."	"You were married for 36 years."	This implies that the griever is ungracious. The griever is probably gracious but still wants the loved one back.
"Let me know if there is anything I can do for you."	"I would like to take the flowers from the funeral home to your house."	The grieving person is overwhelmed. Suggesting that they find something for you to do is an additional burden. Make a concrete offer of assistance.

6. Encourage the support of family and friends for the following:
   a. Getting food to the house
   b. Making telephone calls
   c. Driving to the funeral home
   d. Taking care of children or other family members

   (Friends can help with routine matters that may be overwhelming to the grieving individual.)
7. Refer the bereaved individual to a community bereavement group. (Bereavement groups are helpful, even when the bereaved individual has many friends or family support.)
8. Offer spiritual support and referrals when needed. (Dealing with an illness or catastrophic loss can cause the most profound spiritual pain.)
9. When intense emotions are present, provide understanding and support. (Empathetic words that reflect acceptance of a bereaved individual's feelings are healing.)

Complicated Grieving

Due to:

- Lack of support systems
- Emotional instability
- Death of a significant other
- Presence of factors identified in history (e.g., substance abuse, multiple losses, poor physical health, other mental health risks)
- Violent death of loved one
- Death of child
- Death of a non-socially sanctioned significant other

Desired Outcome:

Patient will have a realistic appraisal, both good and bad, of the deceased and resume normal functioning.

Assessment/Interventions (Rationales)

1. Assess for suicidal thoughts or ideation. (Severely depressed or suicidal individuals might require hospitalization and protection from self-harm and severe self-neglect.)
2. Talk with the bereaved in realistic terms. Discuss concrete changes that have occurred and how they may affect the bereaved individual's future. (Discussing the death and how it has and will continue to affect the

person's life can help the death become more concrete and real.)

3. If the bereaved cannot talk about the death initially, encourage other means of expression (e.g., keeping a journal, drawing, reading about the experience of grief). (Talking is usually the most important tool for resolving initial pain; however, any avenue for the expression of feelings can help the bereaved identify, accept, and work through the feelings.)
4. Explore negative (even hate) toward the deceased, feelings of guilt, or feelings of resentment. (Understanding that negative feelings are normal and experienced by most people can make the bereaved aware of such feelings and then work through them.)
5. Encourage the person to recall memories (happy ones, sad ones, difficult ones); listen actively; and stay silent when appropriate. (Reviewing memories is an important stage in mourning. Being with the bereaved and sharing painful feelings can be healing.)
6. Encourage the bereaved to talk to others individually, in small groups, or in community bereavement groups. (Talking and listening are the most important activities that can help resolve grief and reactivate the mourning process.)
7. Avoid false reassurances that everything will be okay as time passes. (For some, separation through death is never okay; even when the grieving process is complete, the person might be deeply missed.)
8. Provide referrals for complicated grief treatment or traumatic grief therapy. (Complicated grief treatment includes both interpersonal and cognitive–behavior approaches to mitigate the effects of trauma and relieve stress.)
9. Identify the person's religious or spiritual background, and determine whether the bereaved would be receptive to a spiritual counselor. (For many people, spiritual needs and support are extremely comforting at this time, and sharing feelings with a trusted and empathetic religious figure might be comforting.)
10. Offer written guidelines for coping with overwhelming grief. (When one is grieving, even simple tasks can become monumental, life becomes confusing, and normal routines are often interrupted.)

These guidelines offer simple reminders and help validate the bereaved individual's experience. Box 15.1 provides guidelines to help people who are grieving.

Box 15.1 **Guidelines to Help the Bereaved**

Take the time you need to grieve. The hard work of grief uses psychological energy. Resolution of the "numb state" that occurs after loss requires a few weeks at least. A minimum of 1 year—to cover all the birthdays, anniversaries, and other important dates without your loved one—is required before you can "learn to live" with your loss.

Express your feelings. Remember that anger, anxiety, loneliness, and even guilt are normal reactions, and that everyone needs a safe place to express them. Tell your personal story of loss as many times as you need to—this repetition is a helpful and necessary part of the grieving process.

Make a daily structure, and stick to it. Although it is hard to do, keeping to some semblance of structure makes the first few weeks after a loss easier. Getting through each day helps restore the confidence you need to accept the reality of loss.

Don't feel that you have to answer all the questions asked of you. Although most people try to be kind, they might be unaware of their insensitivity. At some point, you might want to read books about how others have dealt with similar circumstances. They often have helpful suggestions for a person in your situation.

As hard as it is, try to take good care of yourself. Eat well, talk with friends, and get plenty of rest. Be sure to let your primary care clinician know if you are having trouble eating or sleeping. Make use of exercise. It can help you let out pent-up frustrations. If you are losing weight, sleeping excessively or intermittently, or still experiencing deep depression after 3 months, be sure to seek professional assistance.

Expect the unexpected. You may begin to feel a bit better, only to have a brief "emotional collapse." These are expected reactions. You also might dream, visualize, think about, or search for your loved one. This too is a part of the grief process.

Give yourself time. Do not feel that you have to resume all of life's duties right away.

Make use of rituals. Those who take the time to "say goodbye" at a funeral or a viewing tend to find that it helps the bereavement process.

If you do not begin to feel better within a few weeks, at least for a few hours every day, be sure to tell your primary

Continued

Box 15.1 Guidelines to Help the Bereaved—cont'd

care clinician. If you have had an emotional problem in the past (e.g., depression, substance use), be sure to get the additional support you need. Losing a loved one puts you at higher risk for relapse of these disorders.

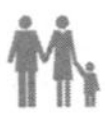

NURSE, PATIENT, AND FAMILY RESOURCES

American Academy of Hospice and Palliative Medicine
www.aahpm.org

American Association of Retired People (AARP)
www.aarp.org

GriefShare (Support Groups)
www.griefshare.org

Hospice Foundation of America
www.hospicefoundation.org

National Hospice Foundation
www.hospiceinfo.org

National Institute on Aging
www.nia.nih.gov

CHAPTER 16

Suicide

Suicide is a serious problem that can have long-lasting and devastating effects on family, friends, and communities. Yet, suicide is largely a preventable problem. In fact, a recent study found that in the year before their deaths by suicide, 83% received healthcare services (Ahmedani et al., 2014). This finding highlights the need for mental health screening in all settings, not just psychiatric settings. In fact, the same study found that about half of those who died by suicide did not have a mental health diagnosis.

This chapter focuses on self-harm and interventions to keep people safe. Terms associated with self-harm are suicidal ideation, suicide attempts, and completed suicide. Suicidal ideation is thinking about personal death, including the wish to be dead; considering methods of accomplishing death; and formulating plans to carry the act out. A suicide attempt is actually carrying out an act or acts with the intention of death, which may or may not prove fatal. A completed suicide is one in which self-injurious acts committed by an individual result in death.

EPIDEMIOLOGY

According to the Centers for Disease Control and Prevention (2016) nearly 43,000 people died by suicide in 2014, making it the tenth-leading cause of death in the United States. In 2014 suicide was the second-leading cause of death for 10 to 34 year olds, the fourth-leading cause of death in 35 to 54 year olds, and the eighth-leading cause of death among 55 to 64 year olds. Males are far more likely than females (4:1) to commit suicide, but women are more likely to attempt suicide (3:1). The rate of suicide per 100,000 people is about 18 for whites, American Indians, and Alaska Natives, and nearly 6 for both blacks and Hispanics.

RISK FACTORS

Twin and adoption studies suggest genetic factors in suicide since concordance rates are higher among monozygotic (identical) twins than among dizygotic (fraternal) twins. Low serotonin levels are related to depressed mood. Postmortem examinations of individuals who complete suicide reveal low levels of serotonin in the brainstem and/or the frontal cortex.

The central emotional factor underlying suicide intent is hopelessness. Cognitive styles that contribute to higher risk are rigid all-or-nothing thinking, inability to see different options, and perfectionism. Adolescents are at especially high risk because of their immature prefrontal cortex, the portion of the brain that controls the executive functions involving judgment, frustration tolerance, and impulse control.

ASSESSMENT

Assessing History

- Past history of suicide attempts or self-mutilation
- Family history of suicide attempts or completion
- History of being bullied and/or victimized in any fashion
- History of a mood disorder, drug or alcohol abuse, or schizophrenia
- History of chronic pain, recent surgery, or chronic physical illness
- History of personality disorder (borderline, paranoid, antisocial)
- Bereavement or experiencing another significant loss (divorce, job, home)
- Legal or discipline problems

Signs and Symptoms

- Suicidal ideation: thoughts of harming self
- Suicidal threat: communicates desire to harm or kill self
- Suicide attempt: attempted to reach the state of completed suicide
- High degree of hopelessness, helplessness, and anhedonia
- Has a plan for how to kill self

Assessment Tools

There are a variety of assessment tools to measure suicide risk. The Columbia-Suicide Severity Rating Scale (C-SSRS) assesses patients through a series of simple questions that anyone can ask. These answers can assist in identifying suicide risk, decide the severity and immediacy of that risk, and determine the level of support that the person needs. Box 16.1 contains the scale.

Assessment Guidelines

Suicide

1. Assess risk factors:
   - History of suicide (family, patient, friends)
   - Degree of hopelessness, helplessness, and anhedonia
   - Lethality of plan
2. Determine the appropriate level of suicide precautions for the patient (physician or nurse clinician), even in the emergency department. If the patient is at a high risk, hospitalization may be necessary. For example, if individuals state they have a plan for how to kill themselves, it is important to ascertain concrete behavioral information to assess the measure of lethality. Some guidelines include the following:
   - Find out what plans have been contemplated.
   - Determine how far the individual took suicidal actions or made plans to take action.
   - Determine how much of the individual's time is spent on these plans and accompanying ruminations about suicide.
   - Determine how accessible and lethal the mode of action is.
3. Assess for sudden mood improvement. Often a decision to commit suicide gives a way out of severe emotional pain.

Patient Problems

A sound assessment provides the framework for determining the level of protection the patient warrants at the time. Therefore *potential for suicide* is the first area of concern. Believing that one's situation or problem is intolerable,

Box 16.1 **Columbia-Suicide Severity Rating Scale (C-SSRS)**

Suicide Ideation Definitions and Prompts	*Past Month*	
Ask Questions That Are Bolded and Underlined	*Yes*	*No*

Ask Questions 1 and 2

1) Wish to be Dead:

Have you wished you were dead or wished you could go to sleep and not wake up?

2) Suicidal Thoughts:

Have you actually had any thoughts of killing yourself?

If YES to 2, Ask Questions 3, 4, 5, and 6. If NO to 2, go Directly to Question 6

3) Suicidal Thoughts with Method (without Specific Plan or Intent to Act):

E.g. *"I thought about taking an overdose but I never made a specific plan as to when where or how I would actually do it….and I would never go through with it."*

Have you been thinking about how you might do this?

4) Suicidal Intent (without Specific Plan):

As opposed to *"I have the thoughts but I definitely will not do anything about them."*

Have you had these thoughts and had some intention of acting on them?

5) Suicide Intent with Specific Plan:

Have you started to work out or worked out the details of how to kill yourself? Do you intend to carry out this plan?

6) Suicide Behavior Question:

Have you ever done anything, started to do anything, or prepared to do anything to end your life?

Examples: Collected pills, obtained a gun, gave away valuables, wrote a will or suicide note, took out pills but didn't swallow any, held a gun but changed your mind or it was grabbed from your hand, went to the roof but didn't jump; or actually took pills, tried to shoot yourself, cut yourself, tried to hang yourself, etc.

If YES, ask: **Was this within the past three months?**

Box 16.1 Columbia-Suicide Severity Rating Scale (C-SSRS)—cont'd

Suicide Ideation Definitions and Prompts	*Past Month*	
Ask Questions That Are Bolded and Underlined	*Yes*	*No*
Response Protocol to C-SSRS Screening (linked to last item marked Yes) Item 1: Behavioral health referral Item 2: Behavioral health referral Item 3: Behavioral health consult and consider patient safety precautions Item 4: Immediate notification of physician and/or behavioral health and safety precautions Item 5: Immediate notification of physician and/or behavioral health and safety precautions Item 6 (over 3 months ago): Behavior health consult and consider patient safety precautions Item 6 (3 months ago or less): Immediate notification of physician and/or behavioral health and safety precautions		

From Posner, K., Brent, D., Lucas, C., Gould, M., Stanley, B., Brown, G. … Mann, J.et al. (2009). Columbia-Suicide Severity Rating Scale. Retrieved from http://www.integration.samhsa.gov/clinical-practice/Columbia_Suicide_Severity_Rating_Scale.pdf

inescapable, and interminable leads to feelings of hopelessness. Therefore *hopelessness* is most often a crucial phenomenon requiring intervention.

A third area of intervention is to tackle the phenomenon of the "tunnel vision" suicidal patients have during times of acute stress and pain. That is, problem-solving skills are poor, and suicidal people have difficulty performing flexible cognitive operations. Teaching the patient or reinforcing the patient's own effective problem-solving skills and helping him or her reframe life difficulties as events that can be controlled is a strategic part of the counseling process with suicidal patients. Therefore *impaired coping* can be viewed as the third point of intervention. Other potential patient problems include decreased self-esteem, isolation, impaired social functioning, spiritual distress, and altered family processes.

Nursing Care for Suicidal Patients

Potential for Suicide

Due to:

- History of prior suicide attempt
- Family history of suicide
- Suicidal ideation
- Suicide gesture
- Suicide plan
- Alcohol and substance use
- Adverse childhood experiences
- At-risk demographics (older adult, young adult male, adolescent, widowed, white, Native American)
- Physical illness, chronic pain, terminal illness
- Grief, bereavement, loss of important relationship, job, home
- Psychiatric disorder (e.g., major depressive disorder, schizophrenia, bipolar disorder)
- Despair, hopelessness, helplessness, and nothing left to live for
- Legal or disciplinary problems
- Poor support system, loneliness
- Hopelessness or helplessness

Desired Outcomes:
The patient will express an interest in living and identify realistic goals for the future.

Assessment/Interventions (Rationales)
Hospitalized

1. Follow agency protocol for suicide regarding creating a safe environment (taking away potential weapons such as belts and sharp objects, checking what visitors bring into the patient's room). (While suicidal, the availability of means of harming oneself could bring about death.)
2. Suicide precautions range from one-on-one with a staff member at arm's length at all times to less frequent checks. (Close contact with health care workers not only provides safety for a suicidal patient, but also improves socialization and self-esteem.)
3. If there is fear of imminent harm to self, seclusion or restraint may be required. (For the most severely suicidal patients, temporary seclusion or restraint may be the safest option.)

4. Follow unit protocol, and document the patient's behavior and statements along with nursing interventions. (Documentation provides for continuity of care with other health care workers, tracks progress, and provides a legal record of nursing care.)
5. Encourage the patient to talk about his or her feelings and stressors. (Talking about feelings and looking at alternatives can reduce the chances for suicidal thinking.)

Outside the Hospital

6. If a patient is managed outside the hospital, the family, significant other, or friends should be alerted to the risk and treatment plan and informed of signs of deepening depression, such as a return or worsening of hopelessness. (Family and friends can support the individual and also facilitate access to health care should suicidal ideation increase.)
7. Be sure that the patient is being treated with appropriate pharmacotherapy, counseling, and/or psychotherapy. (Antidepressants and a mood stabilizer should be initiated rapidly, because there is a significant lag time before they take effect. Counseling and psychotherapy will provide immediate support.)
8. Provide the patient and his or her family and friends the psychiatric care provider's contact number as well as that of a backup emergency department or crisis care unit.
9. Schedule a return visit (as early as the next day) if decisions concerning hospitalization need to be reconsidered. (During a crisis period, individuals should be monitored carefully for increasing suicidal ideation.)
10. Alert friends and family to signs such as increasing withdrawal, preoccupation, silence, remorse, and sudden change from sad to happy and worry-free. (Friends and family can intervene and get the patient into more acute care.)
11. Identify social supports and encourage the patient to initiate contact. (Social connections reduce self-absorption. Talking with other people is one of the best activities for improving mood and reducing suicidal thoughts.)
12. List support people and agencies to use as outpatient and crisis hotline numbers for the patient and his or her

family and friends. (Suicide attempts are often impulsive. Immediate access to another person can be life saving.)

Hopelessness

Due to:

- Deteriorating physical condition
- Social isolation
- Long-term stress
- Lost beliefs and spiritual power
- Severe losses (financial reversals, ending relationship, loss of job)
- Chronic pain
- Perceiving the future as bleak and wasted

Desired Outcomes:

The patient will demonstrate a positive future orientation and identify concrete goals.

Assessment/Interventions (Rationales)

1. Teach the patient steps in the problem-solving process. (Stress that it is not so much people who are ineffective, but rather strategies they are using that are ineffective.)
2. Encourage the patient to look into his or her negative thinking, and reframe negative thinking into neutral objective thinking. (Cognitive reframing helps a person look at situations in ways that allow for alternative approaches.)
3. Point out unrealistic and perfectionistic thinking. (Constructive interpretations of events and behavior open up more realistic and satisfying options for the future.)
4. Work with the patient to identify strengths. (When people are feeling overwhelmed, they no longer view their lives or behavior objectively.)
5. Spend time discussing the patient's dreams and wishes for the future. Identify short-term goals he or she can set for the future. (Renewing realistic dreams and hopes can give promise to the future and meaning to life.)
6. Identify things that have given meaning and joy to life in the past. Discuss how these things can be reincorporated into the present lifestyle (e.g., religious or spiritual beliefs, group activities, creative endeavors). (Reawakens in the patient abilities and experiences that tapped areas of strength and creativity. Creative activities give

people intrinsic pleasure and joy and a great deal of life satisfaction.)

7. Encourage contact with religious or spiritual persons or groups that have supplied comfort and support in the patient's past. (During times of hopelessness, people might feel abandoned and too paralyzed to reach out to caring people or groups.)

Impaired Coping

Due to:

- Situational or maturational crises
- Disturbance in pattern of tension release
- Inadequate opportunity to prepare for stressor
- Inadequate social support created by characteristics of a relationship
- Inadequate or poorly developed coping skills
- Impulsive use of extreme solutions
- Inadequate resources available

Desired Outcome:

The patient will replace destructive coping methods with new and adaptive coping strategies.

Assessment/Interventions (Rationales)

1. Identify situations that trigger suicidal thoughts. (This helps to identify targets for learning more adaptive coping skills.)
2. Assess the patient's strengths and positive coping skills (e.g., talking to others, creative outlets, social activities, problem-solving abilities). (Use these strengths and skills to build on and draw from in planning alternatives to self-defeating behaviors.)
3. Assess the patient's coping behaviors (e.g., drinking, angry outbursts, withdrawal, denial, procrastination) that are not effective and result in negative emotional sequelae. (This helps to identify areas to target for teaching and planning strategies for supplanting more effective and self-enhancing behaviors.)
4. Role-play with the patient adaptive coping strategies that can be used when situations that lead to suicidal thinking begin to emerge. (Not all new coping strategies are effective. The idea is that the nurse and patient work together to find what does work, and that there is no one right way to behave.)

5. Assess the need for assertiveness training. (Assertiveness skills can help the patient develop a sense of control and balance.)
6. Clarify things that are not under the patient's control. Such as one cannot control another's actions, likes, choices, or health status. (Recognizing one's limitations in controlling others is, paradoxically, a beginning to finding one's strength.)
7. Assess the patient's social supports. (Social supports reduce isolation, thereby reducing the possibility of suicide attempts.)
8. Encourage the patient to identify two potential social activities such as local groups of people who share mutual interests such as walking, books, or dining. Such groups are easily searchable online. (Involvement in outside activities reduces introspection and self-absorption.)

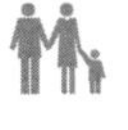

Nurse, Patient, And Family Resources

Alliance of Hope for Suicide Survivors
www.allianceofhope.org

American Association of Suicidology
www.suicidology.org

American Foundation for Suicide Prevention
www.afsp.org

American Suicide Foundation
www.afsp.org

Crisis Text Line
www.crisistextline.org

Friends for Survival, Inc.
www.friendsforsurvival.org

(If You Are Thinking About) Suicide... Read This First
www.metanoia.org/suicide

National Suicide Prevention Lifeline
1-800-273-8255

Samaritans
www.samaritans.org

Suicide Awareness Voices of Education
www.save.org

CHAPTER 17

Crisis Intervention

The human organism's internal environment maintains a relatively stable state while interacting with external forces. This stable state is referred to as *homeostasis* or *equilibrium.* A crisis, which is a major disturbance caused by a stressful event or threat, disrupts this homeostasis. In a crisis normal coping mechanisms fail, resulting in an inability to function as usual. Equilibrium is replaced by disequilibrium.

A successful outcome for a crisis depends on (1) a realistic perception of the event, (2) adequate situational supports, and (3) adequate coping skills.

Perception of the Event

Perception of a crisis may range from realistic to distorted. People vary in the way they absorb, process, and use information from the environment. Some people may respond to a minor event as if it were life threatening, whereas others may calmly assess a life-threatening event.

Situational Support

Situational support includes all the people who are available and who can be depended upon to help during the time of a crisis. Nurses and other health professionals who use crisis intervention are providing situational support.

Coping Skills

The quality and quantity of a person's usual coping skills affect a person's ability to cope with a crisis situation. Other factors may compromise a person's ability to cope with a crisis event. These include the number of other stressful life events with which the person is currently coping, other unresolved losses, the presence of psychiatric disorders or other medical problems, and excessive fatigue or pain.

Crisis by definition is self-limiting and is resolved within 4 to 6 weeks. The overall goal of crisis intervention is to regain the precrisis level of functioning. However, an individual can emerge from the crisis at a lower or higher level of functioning. This variation in functional outcome is why crisis intervention and community services are so vital.

TYPES OF CRISES

There are three basic types of crisis situations: (1) maturational (or developmental) crises, (2) situational crises, and (3) adventitious crises. Identifying which type of crisis the individual is experiencing or has experienced helps in the development of a patient-centered plan of care.

Maturational

Erikson (1963) identified eight stages of growth and development that must be completed to reach maturity. Each stage is associated with a specific task that must be successfully mastered to progress through the growth process. When an individual reaches a new stage, former coping styles may no longer be age appropriate, and new coping mechanisms have yet to be developed.

A maturational crisis occurs when former coping mechanisms are inadequate in dealing with a stress common to a particular stage in the life cycle. This life crisis may also be caused by the transition from one stage to the next. This temporary disequilibrium might affect interpersonal relationships, body image, and social and work roles.

Situational

A situational crisis is a serious life and unanticipated event where disequilibrium results that threatens the integrity of an individual. Examples of situations that could precipitate a crisis include loss of a job, death of a loved one, witnessing a crime, abortion, change of job, change in financial status, revealing homosexual orientation, divorce, and school problems. These situations are often referred to as *life events* or *crucial life problems,* because most people encounter some of these problems during the course of their lives.

Adventitious

An adventitious crisis is not a part of everyday life and tends to impact an extensive number of people, entire communities, or populations. This type of crisis results from such events as (1) a natural disaster (e.g., flood, fire, earthquake), (2) a national disaster (e.g., acts of terrorism, war, riots, airplane crashes), or (3) an extreme act of violence (e.g., workplace or school shootings, bombing in crowded areas). In addition to injury and loss of life, adventitious crises result in long-term psychological trauma.

PHASES OF CRISIS

Through extensive study of individuals experiencing crisis, Caplan (1964) identified behaviors that followed a fairly distinct path. Caplan categorized these behaviors as four distinct phases of a crisis.

Phase 1

When a person is confronted by a threatening stressor, conflict, or problem, the person responds with feelings of anxiety. The increase in anxiety stimulates the use of problem-solving techniques and defense mechanisms in an effort to solve the problem and lower anxiety.

Phase 2

If the usual defense response fails and the threat persists, anxiety continues to rise and produce mounting levels of discomfort. Individual functioning becomes disorganized. Trial-and-error attempts at solving the problem and restoring balance begin.

Phase 3

If the trial-and-error attempts fail, anxiety can escalate to severe and panic levels. The person mobilizes automatic relief behaviors, such as withdrawal and flight. The individual may make some form of resolution (e.g., compromising needs or redefining the situation to reach an acceptable solution) in this stage.

Phase 4

If the problem is not solved and new coping skills are ineffective, anxiety can overwhelm the person and lead to serious personality disorganization, depression, confusion, violence against others, or suicidal behavior.

ASSESSMENT

Assessing History

A positive history for potential crises might include the following:

- Overwhelming life event (maturational, situational, or adventitious)
- History of violent behavior
- History of suicidal behavior
- History of a psychiatric problem (e.g., major depressive disorder, personality disorder, bipolar disorder, schizophrenia, anxiety disorder)
- History of or concurrent medical condition (cancer, ongoing cardiac problems, uncontrolled diabetes, lupus, multiple sclerosis)

Signs and Symptoms

People in crisis exhibit a variety of behaviors, such as the following:

- Confusion, disorganized thinking
- Immobilization, social withdrawal
- Violence against others, suicidal thoughts or attempts
- Agitation, increased psychomotor activity
- Crying, sadness
- Flashbacks, intrusive thoughts, nightmares
- Forgetfulness, poor concentration

Sample Questions

Nurses use a variety of therapeutic techniques to obtain the answers to the following questions. The nurse assesses three main areas during a crisis: (1) perception of the event, (2) support system, and (3) coping skills.

Perception of the Event

"What happened in your life before you started to feel this way?"

"What does this event/problem mean to you?"
"How does this event/problem affect your life?"
"How do you see this event/problem affecting your future?"

Support System

"Who is available to help you?"
"Are these people available now?"
"Is religion an important part of your life?"
"Where do you go to school? Are you involved in any community-based activities?"

Coping Skills

"What do you usually do when you feel stressed or overwhelmed?"
"What has helped you get through difficult times in the past?"
"What have you done so far to cope with this situation?"
"Have you thought of killing yourself or someone else?"

Assessment Guidelines

- Determine whether individuals who have a preexisting psychiatric disorder are decompensating in the event of a crisis. *Decompensation* refers to deterioration of the mental health of an individual who, up until the crisis, was in recovery from mental illness.
- Assess whether the patient has a clear understanding of the precipitating event.
- Assess the patient's situational supports.
- Consider the coping styles the patient usually uses. What coping mechanisms might help the present situation?
- Consider the patient's religious beliefs and cultural determinants when intervening in the patient's crisis.
- Determine whether the situation is one in which the patient needs primary (education, environmental manipulation, or new coping skills), secondary (crisis intervention), or tertiary (rehabilitation) intervention.

Patient Problems

When anxiety levels escalate to moderate, severe, or panic levels, the ability to problem solve is impaired to varying degrees. In an acute crisis an individual's usual coping skills are not effective in meeting the challenges of the crisis situation. For individuals with already compromised coping skills, this situation is compounded. *Impaired coping* is evidenced by the inability to meet basic needs, use of inappropriate defense mechanisms, or alteration in social participation. In this chapter, *impaired coping* is addressed in the context of acute crisis intervention and separately with the rehabilitation phase.

Other patient problems that are essential targets of nursing intervention are anxiety and family coping. *Anxiety (moderate, severe, panic)* is always present at various levels in crisis situations. Reducing anxiety so that patients can start problem solving on their own is key in crisis management. Since a crisis in a family member results in stress to the whole family, *altered family processes* is an important area to address. Family members might have difficulty responding to each other in a helping manner. Communications become disorganized and the ability to express feelings appropriately may be problematic. Interventions support the individual and family in engaging in healthy interactions.

Interventions Guidelines

Levels of Crisis Intervention

Psychotherapeutic crisis interventions are directed toward three levels of care: (1) primary, (2) secondary, and (3) tertiary.

Primary Care (Prevention). The goals of primary care are to assist the individual to cope with stress and to reduce stressors. On this level the nurse can do the following:

- Work with a patient to recognize potential problems by evaluating the patient's experience of stressful life events.
- Teach the patient specific coping skills, such as decision making, problem solving, assertiveness skills, meditation, and relaxation skills.

- Assist the patient to evaluate the timing or reduction of life changes to decrease the negative effects of stress as much as possible. This may involve working with a patient to plan environmental changes, make important interpersonal decisions, and rethink changes in occupational roles.

Secondary Care (Intervention). Secondary care happens during an acute crisis to *prevent* prolonged anxiety and personality disorganization. The nurse's initial focus is ensuring the safety of the patient. After safety issues are dealt with, the nurse works with the patient to assess the patient's problem, support systems, and coping styles. Goals are explored and interventions planned. Secondary care is provided in hospital units, emergency departments, clinics, or mental health centers.

Tertiary Care (Rehabilitation). Tertiary care provides support after a severe crisis. Tertiary care occurs in day treatment programs, rehabilitation centers, sheltered workshops, and outpatient clinics. The goals are to facilitate optimal levels of functioning and prevent further emotional disruptions. People with severe and persistent psychiatric problems are more susceptible to crisis, and community facilities provide the structured environment that can help prevent problem situations. Table 17.1 describes the impact of a crisis based on mental health and mental illness.

Acute Crisis

- Safety is the first consideration: Assess for suicidal or homicidal thoughts or plans.
- Initial steps focus on increasing feelings of safety and decreasing anxiety.
- At this stage, the nurse should take an active and directive approach (e.g., make telephone calls, set up and mobilize social supports).
- Along with the patient plan interventions that are acceptable to both the patient and you.
- Monitor the patient's progress.

Crisis Stabilization and Rehabilitation

- Individuals with severe and long-term mental health problems are more susceptible to crises.

Table 17.1 **Responses to Crisis in Mental Health and Mental Illness**

Mental Health	Mental Illness
Able to adapt to day-to-day disappointments and changes	May respond to a mild disruption as a crisis situation (e.g., a cancellation in a nurse practitioner appointment).
Has a healthy sense of self, place, and purpose in life; good problem-solving abilities.	Inadequate sense of self and purpose or abilities. Inadequate problem-solving abilities.
Usually has adequate situational supports and is able to activate them during stressful times	Often has no family or friends, might be living in isolation, and may be homeless.
Usually has adequate coping skills with a number of techniques that can be used to lower anxiety and adapt to the situation	Coping ability tends to be compromised, and more support is required.

- Adapting the crisis model to this group includes focusing on the patient's strengths, modifying and setting realistic goals, and taking a more active role.

After Crisis Stabilization

- Assess and provide for the patient's and family's educational needs.
- Assess and provide for social skills training as needed.
- Assess and refer to a vocational rehabilitation program when appropriate.
- Evaluate and refer to supportive group therapy.
- Teach or refer patients to cognitive–behavioral therapy programs, where they can learn to manage their psychotic symptoms.

Nursing Care for Crisis

The following sections apply *impaired coping* to the acute crisis intervention period and then to the rehabilitation period.

Acute Crisis Intervention

Impaired Coping

Due to:

- Maturational crisis
- Situational crisis
- Adventitious crisis
- Inadequate social support
- Inadequate level of perceived control
- Inadequate resources available
- High degree of threat
- Lack of opportunity to prepare for stressors
- Disturbance in pattern of appraisal of threat
- Disturbance in pattern of tension release

Desired Outcome:

Within 4-6 weeks, the patient will return to precrisis level of functioning or higher.

Assessment/Interventions (Rationales)

1. Provide a liaison (e.g., social worker) to agencies to take care of emergency needs. (The patient's physical needs (e.g., shelter, food, protection from abuser) must be handled immediately.)
2. Make appointments for medical or other health care providers. (A integrative approach to care will reduce the potential for missing other health problems.)
3. Document the appointments and provide directions. (A written reminder for follow-up is essential since anxiety reduces the capacity for attention and memory formation.)
4. Assess for patient safety. Examples of questions to ask include the following: Are there suicidal thoughts? Is there child or spouse abuse? Are you living in unsafe living conditions? (Patient safety is the first consideration.)
5. Identify the patient's perception of the event. Reframe this perception of the event if the event is seen as overwhelming or hopeless or patient views himself or herself as helpless. (The patient's distorted perception raises anxiety. Help the patient experience the event as a problem that can be solved.)
6. Assess stressors and the precipitating cause of the crisis. (Assessing for these stressors helps identify areas for change and intervention.)

7. Identify the patient's current skills, resources, and knowledge to deal with problems. (This encourages the patient to use strengths and usual coping skills.)
8. Identify other skills the patient might need to develop (e.g., decision-making skills, problem-solving skills, communication skills, relaxation techniques). (Teaching the patient about additional skills helps minimize crisis situations in the future and helps the patient regain more control over the present situation.)
9. Assess the patient's support systems. Rally existing supports (with the patient's permission) if the patient is overwhelmed. (The patient might be immobilized initially. The nurse often takes an active role during a crisis intervention.)
10. Identify and arrange for extra supports if the patient's current support system is unavailable or insufficient. (The patient might have lost important supports because of death, divorce, or distance, for example, or simply may not have sufficient supports in place.)
11. Take an active role in crisis intervention (e.g., make telephone calls; arrange temporary child care; arrange for shelters, emergency food, or first aid). (Patients in crisis are often temporarily immobilized by anxiety and unable to problem solve. The nurse can organize the situation so the patient sees it as solvable and controllable.)
12. Give only small amounts of information at a time. (Only small pieces of information can be understood when a patient's anxiety level is high.)
13. Encourage the patient to stay in the present to deal with the immediate situation only. (Crisis intervention deals with the immediate problem disrupting the patient's present situation.)
14. Listen to the patient's story. Avoid interrupting. (Telling the story can in itself be healing.)
15. Help the patient set achievable goals. (Working in small, achievable steps helps the patient gain a sense of control and mastery.)
16. Work with the patient on devising a plan to meet goals. (A realistic and specific plan helps decrease anxiety and promote hopefulness.)
17. Identify and contact other members of the health care team who can work with the patient to solve the

crisis event. (This provides a broad base of support to intervene with the problem and enlarges the patient's network for future problems.)

18. Provide debriefing to patients and family members after a crisis and to staff after a serious unit event such as a suicide attempt). (Survivors, family members, and staff all need to discuss the effects of a disaster, and debriefing provides the structure in which to do so.)

Tertiary Prevention (Rehabilitation)

Sometimes a crisis may be so severe and prolonged that individuals cannot reestablish equilibrium. This is especially true when support is not available. In this type of situation, some individuals may experience a lower level of functioning once the crisis is over. This may happen to veterans who return from war after prolonged exposure to traumatic events in the absence of adequate support. At other times, individuals with limited coping skills are faced with overwhelming situations. For example, individuals with severe psychiatric disorders such as schizophrenia can experience an exacerbation (worsening) of symptoms that can negatively affect their functioning.

The patient problem *impaired coping* applies to people with severe and persistent mental illness. Severe mental illness usually impacts multiple areas, including activities of daily living (e.g., cooking, hygiene), relationships, social interaction, task completion, leisure activities, safe movement about the community, finances and budgeting, health maintenance, vocational and academic activities, and coping with stressors. Associated issues for these individuals include poverty, stigma, isolation, unemployment, and inadequate housing.

Impaired Coping

Due to:

- Situational crisis
- Maturational crisis
- Severe and persistent mental illness
- Inadequate social supports
- Impaired ability to reduce anxiety
- Impaired ability to accurately appraise threat

- Poor coping skills
- Inability to problem solve
- Inadequate level of personal resources

Desired Outcomes:
Within 4-6 weeks, the patient will function in the community with minimal use of inpatient services and maintain stable functioning between episodes of exacerbation.

Assessment/Interventions (Rationales)

1. Nurses and trained health care workers meet with the patient and family to assess the patient's various needs. (Patients with psychiatric disabilities have a wide range of needs.)
2. Identify the patient's highest level of functioning in terms of:
   a. Living skills
   b. Learning skills
   c. Working skills
   Table 17.2 lists skills that promote psychiatric rehabilitation.
   (This provides a baseline and helps evaluate whether interventions help maintain or improve the patient's level of functioning.)
3. Identify the social supports available to the family:
   a. Education about the disease, treatment, prognosis, and medications
   b. Community supports to help the patient function optimally
   c. Community supports that offer family support, groups, and ongoing psychoeducation
   (Family members need a variety of supports to prevent family deterioration.)
4. Identify specific community supports that can provide individuals to help the patient and family with continuity of care, such as:
   a. Residential support services
   b. Transportation support services
   c. Intensive case management
   d. Psychosocial rehabilitation
   e. Peer support
   f. Consumer-run services
   g. Around-the-clock crisis services
   h. Outpatient services with mobile capabilities

Table 17.2 **Living, Learning, and Working Skills for Patients With Psychiatric Disability**

Physical	Emotional	Intellectual
Living Skills		
Personal hygiene	Human relations	Money management
Physical fitness resources	Self-control	Use of community resources
	Selective reward	Goal setting
Use of public transportation	Stigma reduction	
	Problem solving	
Cooking	Conversational skills	Problem development
Shopping		
Cleaning		
Participating in sports		
Using recreational facilities		
Learning Skills		
Being quiet	Making speeches	Reading
Paying attention	Asking questions	Writing
Staying seated	Volunteering answers	Arithmetic
Observing	Following directions	Study skills
Being punctual	Asking for directions	Hobby activities
	Listing	Typing
Working Skills		
Punctuality	Job interviewing	Job qualifying
Use of job tools	Job decision making	Job seeking
Job strength	Human relations	Specific job tasks
Job transportation	Self-control	
Specific job tasks	Job keeping	
	Specific job tasks	

(Comprehensive community support services are available to help people function at optimal levels and slow their relapse rate.)

5. Obtain a referral for social skills training, especially if the patient is living with family. (Some studies have shown that social skills training decreases relapse over time, especially for those living with families.)
6. Work with the patient and family to identify the patient's prodromal (early) signs of impending relapse. (The patient and family can secure professional help before exacerbation of illness occurs.)

7. Work with the patient and family to identify an appropriate vocational rehabilitation service for the patient. (Employment makes a significant contribution to relapse prevention, improved clinical outcomes, and improved self-image.)
8. Teach patient and family about psychotropic medications:
   a. Side effects
   b. Toxic effects
   c. What medication can do
   d. What medication cannot do
   e. Who or where to call with questions or in emergencies (Medication teaching reduces relapse rates, prolongs the time between relapses, and increases self-advocacy.)

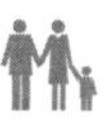

NURSE, PATIENT, AND FAMILY RESOURCES

Crisis Call Center
www.crisiscallcenter.org/crisisservices-html

Crisis Text Line
www.crisistextline.org

Emotions Anonymous
www.emotionsanonymous.org

Lifeline Crisis Chat
www.crisischat.org

Mental Help Net
www.mentalhelp.net

NAMI (National Alliance on Mental Illness)
www.nami.org

Red Cross Disaster Mental Health Services (DMHS)
www.redcross.org
(Contact local Red Cross for information)

Teenline Online
www.teenlineonline.org/talk-now

CHAPTER 18

Anger, Aggression, and Violence

Anger is a primal—and not always logical—human emotion. It can range from mild annoyance to intense fury and rage. Aggression may be appropriate or self-protective, as in protecting oneself, one's family, or another individual who is being bullied. If it is characterized by initiating hostilities directed at others, it can result in verbal or physical violence.

Some patients are more prone toward angry and aggressive behaviors than others. Individuals who might at times be at risk for violent behaviors are those who use substances or have poor coping skills; are psychotic or have antisocial, borderline, or narcissistic traits; or suffer from cognitive disorders, paranoia, or mania.

Control of anger, aggression, and violence in the health care setting is a top priority. Fortunately, patients most often demonstrate signs of increasing anxiety before it escalates to destructive levels. The most useful nursing interventions would be instituted during the initial phases, before a patient's anger starts to escalate out of control. However, there are times when anger has already escalated, and the threat of violence is imminent. At this time, different intervention strategies are needed.

RESPONSES TO ANGER, AGGRESSION, AND VIOLENT BEHAVIOR

Guidelines for working with angry and aggressive patients follow the least restrictive means of helping a patient gain control. Least restrictive usually starts with verbal interventions, pharmacological interventions, and finally physical seclusion and restraints.

Verbal Interventions

If you can attempt to determine what the patient is feeling, you have already begun to intervene. Typically you can accomplish this by telling the patient that you are concerned and want to listen. It is equally as important to clearly state your expectations for the patient's behavior: "I expect that you will stay in control."

Approach the patient in a controlled, nonthreatening, and caring manner. Allow the patient enough personal space so that you are not perceived as threatening. Stay about 1 foot farther than the patient can reach with arms or legs. Make sure that the patient is not between you and the door. Choose a quiet place to talk to the patient but one that is visible to staff. Staff should know you are working with the patient, keep an eye on the interaction, and be prepared to intervene if the situation escalates.

When anger is escalating, a patient's ability to process decreases. It is important to speak to the patient slowly and in short sentences, using a low and calm voice. Use open-ended statements and questions such as "You think people are treating you unfairly?" Find out what is behind the angry feelings and behaviors. You may want to give two options such as, "Do you want to go to your room or to the quiet room for a while?" This approach decreases the sense of powerlessness that often precipitates violence.

Pharmacological Interventions

When a patient is showing increased signs or symptoms of anxiety or agitation, it is appropriate to offer the patient an as-needed medication to alleviate symptoms. When used in conjunction with psychosocial interventions and deescalation techniques, this can prevent an aggressive or violent incident.

The use of second-generation antipsychotics, olanzapine (Zyprexa) and ziprasidone (Geodon), has become more widespread because of the side effects of first-generation antipsychotics such as haloperidol (Haldol). Inhaled loxapine (Adasuve) is an alternative to injectable medication, with effects being seen within 10 minutes of administration. A combination of an antipsychotic and a benzodiazepine can be administered intramuscularly. Diphenhydramine or benztropine added to the injection reduces extrapyramidal side effects. Table 18.1 lists medications that have been found useful in managing aggression.

Table 18.1 **Drugs Used for Acute Management of Violent Behavior**

Generic (Trade)	Forms	Considerations
Antianxiety Agents (Benzodiazepines)		
Lorazepam (Ativan)	PO, SL, IM, IV	Drug of choice in this class. Use with caution with hepatic dysfunction.
Alprazolam (Xanax)	PO	Paradoxical (opposite response) with personality disorders and the elderly.
Diazepam (Valium)	PO, IM, IV	FDA approved for alcohol withdrawal agitation. Rapid onset of calming and sedating. Long half-life; use with caution in elderly.
First-Generation Antipsychotics		
Haloperidol (Haldol)	PO, IM, IV	Favorable side effect profile. Because of risk of neuroleptic malignant syndrome, keep hydrated, check vital signs, and test for muscle rigidity.
Loxapine (Adasuve)	Inhaled	FDA approved for schizophrenia and bipolar I agitation in adults. Common side effects of dysgeusia (altered sense of taste), sedation, and throat irritation; can cause fatal bronchospasm.
Perphenazine	PO	Risk of neuroleptic malignant syndrome increases; keep hydrated. Frequent vital sign checks and testing for muscular rigidity are recommended.
Chlorpromazine (Thorazine)	PO, PR, IM	Very sedating. Injections can cause pain; watch for hypotension.

Continued

Table 18.1 **Drugs Used for Acute Management of Violent Behavior—cont'd**

Generic (Trade)	Forms	Considerations
Second-Generation Antipsychotics		
Risperidone (Risperdal)	PO, disintegrating tablet	Calms while treating the underlying condition. Watch for hypotension with reflex tachycardia. Increased risk of stroke in the elderly.
Olanzapine (Zyprexa)	PO, IM, disintegrating tablet	IM is FDA approved for agitation with schizophrenia or bipolar I in adults. Useful in patients unresponsive to haloperidol. Calms while treating underlying condition. Avoid IM combination with lorazepam. Increased risk of stroke in the elderly.
Ziprasidone (Geodon)	PO, IM	IM is FDA approved for agitation with schizophrenia in adults. Use cautiously with QT prolongation. Less sedating.
Combinations		
Haloperidol (Haldol), lorazepam (Ativan), and diphenhydramine (Benadryl) or benztropine (Cogentin)	IM	Commonly used in the acute setting. Men who are young and athletic are at increased risk of dystonia. Consider akathisia if agitation increases.
Perphenazine, lorazepam (Ativan), and diphenhydramine (Benadryl) or benztropine (Cogentin)	IM	Consider this combination if the patient has difficulty taking haloperidol.

IM, Intramuscularly; *IV*, intravenously; *PO*, orally; *SL*, sublingually.
From US Food and Drug Administration. (2017). Online label repository. Retrieved from https://labels.fda.gov/; Gerken, A. T., Gross, A. F., & Sanders, K. M. (2016). Aggression and violence. In T. A. Stern, M. Fava, T. E. Wilens, & J. F. Rosenbaum, (Eds.), *Massachusetts General Hospital comprehensive clinical psychiatry*, (2nd ed.) (p. 716.). St. Louis, MO: Elsevier, 2016.

Seclusion or Restraints

Occasionally, a patient will become violent and require seclusion or restraint. The goal is to maintain the safety of the patient and others. Seclusion is confinement in a room that is not within the control of the person to leave. Restraint is any method that immobilizes or reduces the ability of a patient to move his or her arms, legs, body, or head freely. Seclusion or restraint is used only if the patient presents a clear and present danger to self or others. These interventions require an order from a licensed practitioner, although the order may happen after an emergency event. Licensing and accreditation agencies mandate how frequently patients in seclusion and restraint should be observed and assessed.

Each team member should be trained in the correct use of seclusion and physical restraining. There should be a clear leader who does the talking. The leader informs the patient of the team's intent to either seclude or restrain and the reason for the actions. Once the patient is secluded or restrained, the nurse may get an order for medication and administer it. Box 18.1 provides guidelines for the use of seclusion and restraints.

Nursing Care for Anger, Aggression, and Violence

The following sections offer nursing guidelines for assessing (1) anger and potential aggression when a patient's behavior is escalating and (2) interventions when a patient's anger has escalated to physical abuse and staff intervention is required, sometimes in the form of restraints or seclusion. Hospital protocols that follow legal and ethical guidelines should always be followed when restraining or secluding patients.

Assessment

- History of violence (the best predictor of future behavior is past behavior)
- Paranoia
- Alcohol or drug use
- Mania or agitated depression
- Patients with a personality disorder who are prone to rage, violence, or impulse dysregulation (antisocial, borderline, and narcissistic)
- Oppositional defiant disorder or conduct disorder

Box 18.1 **Guidelines for the Use of Seclusion and Restraint**

Indications for Use
- To protect the patient from self-harm
- To prevent the patient from assaulting others

Legal Requirements
- Multidisciplinary involvement
- Appropriate health care provider's signature according to state law
- Patient advocate or relative notification
- Restraint or seclusion discontinued as soon as possible

Documentation
- Behaviors leading to restraint or seclusion
- Least-restrictive interventions used before restraint
- Response to interventions
- Plan of care for seclusion or restraint use implemented
- Ongoing evaluations by appropriate health care providers

Clinical Assessments
- Patient's mental status at time of restraint
- Physical examination for medical problems that may contribute to behaviors
- Need for restraints

Observation
- Have staff in constant attendance
- Document every 15 minutes
- Range of movement
- Monitor vital signs
- If restrained, observe blood flow in the hands and feet and chafing
- Provide for nutrition, hydration, and elimination

Release Procedure
- Patient must be able to follow instructions and stay in control
- Terminate seclusion or restraints
- Debrief with the patient

Other Tips
- Physical holding of a patient against will is a restraint
- Four side rails up is a restraint except in seizure precautions
- Tucking sheets in so tightly patient cannot move is a restraint
- Orders for seclusion or restraint cannot be PRN

- Psychosis (hallucinations, delusions, illusions)
- Experiencing command hallucinations
- Neurocognitive disorder
- Intermittent explosive disorder (e.g., domestic violence)
- Medical conditions (e.g., chronic illness or loss of body function) that can strain a person's coping abilities and lead to uncharacteristic anger

Important questions:
- Have you ever thought of harming someone else?
- Have you ever seriously injured another person?
- What is the most violent thing you have ever done?

Signs and Symptoms

Violence is usually preceded by the following:
- Hyperactivity is the most important predictor of imminent violence (e.g., pacing, restlessness)
- Increasing anxiety and tension: clenched jaw or fist, rigid posture, fixed or tense facial expression, mumbling to self, shortness of breath, sweating, rapid pulse
- Verbal abuse (e.g., uses profanity, is argumentative, makes intrusive demands)
- Loud voice, change of pitch, or very soft voice, forcing others to strain to hear
- Changes in level of consciousness (e.g., confusion, disorientation, memory impairment)
- Intense eye contact or avoidance of eye contact
- Recent acts of violence, including property violence
- Stony silence
- Alcohol or drug intoxication
- Carrying a weapon or object that might be used as a weapon (e.g., fork, knife, rock)
- Milieu conducive to violence:
  - Overcrowding
  - Inexperienced staff
  - Confrontational/controlling staff
  - Poor limit setting
  - Unfairly taking away privileges

Assessment Tools

Assessment Guidelines: Violence and Aggression

- History of violence is the single best predictor of violence.

- Does patient have a violent wish or intention to harm another?
- Does patient have a plan?
- Does patient have the availability or means to carry out a plan?
- Consider demographics: sex (male), age (14–24 years), socioeconomic status (low), and support systems (few).

Self-Assessment

Assess yourself for defensive response or taking the patient's anger personally, which may accelerate the anger cycle. For example, are you:

- Responding aggressively toward the patient?
- Avoiding the patient?
- Suppressing or denying either your own or the patient's anger?

Assess your level of comfort in the situation and the prudence of enlisting other staff to work with you to deal with a potentially explosive situation.

Patient Problems

Impaired coping is an appropriate patient problem for patients who have angry and aggressive responses to stressful, frustrating, or threatening situations. When a patient's anxiety and anger escalate to levels at which there is a threat of harm to others, *potential for violence is the priority problem.* During this time, talking-down skills are used first. Offering as needed medication is the next step. If pharmacology is ineffective, restraint or seclusion of an aggressive patient may be necessary.

The following text discusses two patient problems: one for intervening with patients who are angry and hostile, and a second for intervening with patients whose anger has escalated to threats of violence.

Patients Who Are Angry and Hostile

Impaired Coping

Due to:

- Inadequate perception of control
- Perception of being threatened

- Impaired tension management
- Misperception of others' motives
- Inappropriate or ineffective use of defense mechanisms
- Knowledge deficit
- Overwhelming crisis situations
- Impaired reality testing
- Excessive anxiety
- Substance use, intoxication, or withdrawal
- Ineffective problem-solving strategies or skills
- Chemical or biological brain changes
- Personal vulnerability

Desired Outcome:
The patient will recognize when anger begins to escalate and use tension-reducing behaviors.

Assessment/Interventions (Rationales)

1. Assess your own feelings in the situation; guard against taking the patient's abusive statements personally or becoming defensive. (Although patients are often skillful at making personal and pointed statements, they do not know nurses personally and have no basis on which they can make accurate judgments.)
2. Avoid angry responses, no matter how threatened or angry you feel. (Confrontational responses by an authority figure will increase hostility.)
3. Monitor anger and aggressive behavior; do not minimize such behavior in the hope that it will go away. (Minimizing angry behaviors and ineffective limit setting are the most common factors contributing to the escalation to violence.)
4. Set clear, consistent, and enforceable limits on behavior, and stress the consequences of not adhering to those behaviors. (Behavioral limits provide structure for the patient and promote consistent responses from the staff.)
5. Emphasize that cognitively-aware patients are responsible for the consequences of their aggressive behavior, including legal charges. (Patients may believe that behaviors in the hospital are immune from legal ramification. The majority of states have statutes addressing assaults on healthcare providers and 32 states have made such assaults felonies.)

6. Emphasize that you are setting limits on specific behaviors, not feelings (e.g., "It is okay to be angry with Tom, but it is not okay to threaten him or verbally abuse him"). (Patients can learn to express feelings safely while recognizing that acting on feelings is not acceptable.)
7. Use a matter-of-fact, neutral approach. Remain calm using a moderate, firm voice and calming hand gestures. (A matter-of-fact approach can help interrupt the cycle of escalating anger.)
8. If anger threatens to escalate, inform the patient that you will leave the room for a period of time and will be back when the situation is calmer. Return when the time is up. (When this response is given in a neutral, matter-of-fact manner, the patient's anger is not rewarded. Always return at the time specified, and focus communication on neutral topics.)
9. Provide positive feedback for interactive communication, such as nonillness-related topics, by responding to requests and by providing emotional support. (This reinforces appropriate communication and behaviors and gives the patient and nurse time to share healthier communication and build a sounder working relationship.)
10. Avoid power struggles. (Power struggles are perceived as a challenge and generally lead to escalation of the conflict.)
11. Respond to patient anxiety or anger with active listening and validation of distress. (Active listening and validation build trust and allow the patient to feel heard and understood.)
12. Work with the patient to identify triggers for aggression. (Recognizing triggers is the first step in a structured violence-prevention strategy.)
13. Identify risk factors for perpetuating violence (family chaos, other mental or environmental risk factors). (Treating the risk factors (e.g., getting family counseling, finding a job) reduces the family cycle of violence. This is the second step in a structured violence-prevention strategy.)
14. Work with the patient to identify what supports are lacking, and problem-solve ways to attain support. (Advocacy with support is the third step in a structured violence-prevention strategy.)

15. Teach the patient (and family) the steps in the problem-solving process. (Many people have never learned a systematic and effective approach to dealing with and mastering tough life situations or problems.)
16. Role play with the patient alternative behaviors he or she can use in stressful and overwhelming situations when anger threatens. (Role playing allows the patient to rehearse alternative ways of handling stressful and angry feelings in a safe environment.)
17. Work with the patient to set behavioral goals. Give positive feedback when goals are reached. (Setting goals and giving positive feedback allow the patient a sense of control while learning goal-setting skills. Achieving self-set goals can enhance a person's sense of self and foster new and more effective approaches to frustrating feelings.)
18. Provide the patient with other outlets for stress and anxiety such as exercising, listening to music, reading, talking to others, attending support groups, and participating in a sport. (Alternative means of channeling aggression and angry feelings can help patients decrease their anxiety and stress and allow for more cognitive approaches to their situation (e.g., using a problem-solving approach).)
19. Provide the patient and family with community resources that teach assertiveness training, anger management, and stress-reduction techniques. (Patients and families will need continued support in the community.)

Patients Who Threaten Harm to Self or Others

Potential for Violence

Due to:

- History of violent behavior
- History of childhood abuse or witnessing family violence
- History of violence against others
- Psychosis (hallucinations, delusions, illogical thought processes)
- Impulsivity
- Rage
- Mania
- Cognitive impairment
- Substance use, intoxication, or withdrawal
- Excitement, irritability, agitation

Desired Outcomes:
The patient will refrain from violent behavior.

Assessment/Interventions (Rationales)

1. Keep environmental stimulation at a minimum (e.g., lower lights, keep stereos down, ask patients and visitors to leave the area, or have staff take the patient to another area). (Over-stimulation can increase the patient's anxiety level, leading to increased agitation or aggressive behaviors.)
2. Keep your voice calm, and speak in a low tone. (A high-pitched rapid voice can increase anxiety levels in others; the opposite is true when the tone of voice is low and calm and the words are spoken slowly.)
3. Call the patient by name, and introduce yourself. Orient the patient when necessary, and explain beforehand what you are going to do. (Calling the patient by name helps to establish contact. Orienting and giving information can minimize misrepresentation of nurses' intentions.)
4. Use personal safety precautions:
   a. Leave the door open in the interview room or use a hallway to talk.
   b. If you feel uncertain of patient's potential for violence, other staff should be nearby.
   c. Never turn your back on an angry patient.
   d. Have a quick exit available.
   e. For home visits, go with a colleague if there is concern regarding aggression.
   f. Leave the home immediately if there are signs that the patient's behavior is escalating.

   (Your safety is always first. Always call in colleagues or other staff if you feel threatened or in physical danger.)
5. Nursing and security staff should receive frequent training in managing disruptive behavior, including anger de-escalation and seclusion and restraint procedures. (Professional training increases safe responses and reduces negative outcomes such as injury.)
6. Document the patient's behaviors and staff interventions during each level of intervention. (Documentation provides direction for future episodes and is essential from a legal standpoint.)
7. When interventions are needed to reduce escalating anger, always use the least restrictive first and move to more restrictive methods if necessary:

a. Verbal
b. Pharmacological
c. Physical—seclusion or restraint
(Human dignity and autonomy are supported through the least restrictive approach. Seclusion or restraint should be used only when there is no less-restrictive alternative.)

8. Verbal interventions: Encourage the patient to talk about angry feelings and find ways to tolerate or reduce angry and aggressive feelings. (When the patient feels heard and understood and has help with problem-solving alternative options, de-escalation of anger and aggression is often possible.)
9. Use empathetic verbal interventions (e.g., "It must be frightening to be here and to be feeling out of control"). (Empathetic verbal intervention is the most effective method of calming an agitated, fearful, panicky patient.)
10. When interpersonal interventions fail to decrease the patient's anger, consider the need for medication. Assessment includes determining whether aggression is acute or chronic. (Often pharmacological interventions can help patients gain control of their behavior and prevent continued escalation of anger and hostile impulses.)
11. Alert other staff and hospital security before violent behavior escalates for additional support if needed. (Hospital staff and security should have frequent training in restraining or secluding patients. Alerting staff and security beforehand best ensures that the restraint or seclusion process will be handled safely for the patient, staff, and other patients on the unit.)
12. When interpersonal and pharmacological interventions fail, physical intervention (seclusion or restraint) is the final resort. Follow organization protocol. Refer to Box 18.1 for guidelines for the use of restraints. (Protocol tells staff when to restrain, how to restrain, how long before a physician's order is needed, nursing interventions for the patient during the period of restraint or seclusion, how often to check restraints or the patient in seclusion, whom to call, and how often the need for restraints or seclusion must be reevaluated by physician.)

Nurse, Patient, and Family Resources

Anger Busters.com
www.angerbusters.com

Anger Management
www.mentalhelp.net
Search for "anger management."

Centers for Disease Control and Prevention
www.cdc.gov
Search for "anger" to find multiple articles.

Centers for Medicare and Medicaid Services
www.cms.gov
Search for "seclusion and restraint" for national guidelines

National Anger Management Association
www.manageanger.com/guidelines.htm

CHAPTER 19

Family Violence

Family violence can take the form of emotional, physical, or sexual abuse or neglect. Emotional abuse kills the spirit and may impair the ability to succeed later in life, to feel deeply, or to make emotional contact with others. Physical abuse includes emotional abuse in addition to the potential for long-term physical injuries, scarring, pain and, in some cases, death. The consequences of being sexually abused as a child are devastating. Survivors of sexual abuse experience low self-esteem, self-hatred, emotional instability, and anger and aggression, Interpersonal relationships are impaired by an inability to trust and difficulty in protecting themselves.

ASSESSMENT

Sensitivity is required of a nurse who suspects family violence. Interview guidelines are suggested in Box 19.1. A person who feels judged or accused of wrongdoing will become defensive. This defensiveness will undermine attempts to change coping strategies in the family. It is better for the nurse to ask about ways of solving disagreements or methods of disciplining children rather than using the word abuse or violence, which appear judgmental and therefore are threatening to the family.

Does the child have a history of unexplained "accidents" and physical injuries?

Does the child appear well nourished, appropriately dressed, clean, and appropriately groomed?

Does the woman have a history of abuse as a child?

Does the man have a history of abuse as a child?

Does the older adult have a history of unexplained "accidents" or physical injuries?

Does the older adult have a history of being abused as a child or abusing his or her children?

Is there a history of alcohol or drug use within the family system?

Box 19.1 Interview Guidelines

Do

- Conduct the interview in private.
- Be direct, honest, and professional.
- Use language the patient understands.
- Ask the patient to clarify words not understood.
- Be understanding.
- Be attentive.
- Inform the patient if you must make a referral to child or adult protective services, and explain the process.
- Assess safety, and help reduce danger (at discharge).

Do Not

- Try to "prove" abuse by accusations or demands.
- Display horror, anger, shock, or disapproval of the perpetrator or situation.
- Place blame or make judgments.
- Allow the patient to feel "at fault" or "in trouble."
- Probe or press for responses or answers the patient is not willing to give.
- Conduct the interview with a group of interviewers.

Does the patient re-experience the abuse through flashbacks, dreams or nightmares, or intrusive thoughts?

Does the patient or other family member state that he or she has had suicidal or homicidal thoughts in the past?

Signs and Symptoms

- Feelings of helplessness or powerlessness
- Repeated emergency room or hospital visits
- Vague complaints, including insomnia, abdominal pain, hyperventilation, headache, or menstrual problems
- Poorly explained bruises in various stages of healing
- Injuries (bruises, fractures, scrapes, lacerations) that do not seem to fit the description of the "accident"
- Frightened, withdrawn, depressed, and/or despondent appearance

Assessment Questions

The nurse uses a variety of therapeutic techniques to obtain the answers to the following questions. Use your discretion, and decide which questions are appropriate to complete your assessment.

"Tell me about what happened to you."

"Who takes care of you?" (for children or dependent older adult)

"What happens when you do something wrong?" (for children)

"How do you and your partner/caregiver resolve disagreements?" (for women and older adults)

"What do you do for fun?"

"Who helps you with your children [parent]?"

"How much time do you have for yourself?"

For Partner

"Have you been hit, kicked, or otherwise hurt by someone in the past year? By whom?"

"Do you feel safe in your current relationship?"

"Is there a partner from a previous relationship who is making you feel unsafe now?"

For Parents

"What arrangement do you make when you have to leave your child alone?"

"How do you discipline your child?"

"When your infant cries for a long time, how do you get him or her to stop?"

"What about your child's behavior bothers you the most?"

Assessment Tools

Assessment Guidelines

Family Violence. During your assessment and counseling, maintain an interested and empathetic manner. Retain self-awareness and avoid displaying horror, anger, shock, or disapproval of the perpetrator or the situation. Assess for the following:

- Signs and symptoms of survivors of family violence
- Indicators of vulnerable parents who might benefit from education and the effective coping techniques listed in Box 19.2.

Box 19.2 Assessing for Parents Who Are Vulnerable for Child Abuse

- New parents whose behavior toward the infant is rejecting, hostile, or indifferent.
- Teenage parents, most of whom are children themselves, require special help and guidance in handling the baby and discussing their expectations of the baby and their support systems.
- Parents with intellectual disability, for whom careful, explicit, and repeated instructions on caring for the child and recognizing the infant's needs are indicated.
- People who grew up in abusive homes. This is the biggest risk factor for perpetuation of family violence.

- Physical, sexual, or emotional abuse and neglect and economic maltreatment in the case of older adults
- Family coping patterns
- Patient's support system
- Drug or alcohol use
- Suicidal or homicidal ideas
- Posttrauma syndrome

If the patient is a child or an older adult, identify the protection agency in your state that will need to be notified.

SELF-ASSESSMENT

Working with those who experience violence may arouse intense and overwhelming feelings in the nurse, especially in new nurses. Strong negative feelings toward abuse may cloud your judgment and interfere with objective assessment and intervention. A personal history of abuse may also cause a nurse to identify too closely with the victim Sharing perceptions and feelings with other professionals can moderate feelings of anger, frustration, and the need to rescue.

Patient Problems

Violence brings with it pain, psychological and physical injury and anguish, the potential for disfigurement, and the potential for death. Therefore *potential for injury* is a major concern for nurses and other members of the health care team.

Within all families in which violence occurs, severe communication problems are evident. Coping skills are not adequate to handle the emotional and environmental events that trigger the crisis situation. Inadequate coping skills among family members result in family members not having their needs met, including the need for safety, security, and sense of self. Therefore there exists *impaired role performance* within the family.

This chapter discusses *potential for injury* for the child, adult, and older adult and *impaired role performance* geared toward the perpetrator.

There are many other patient problems the nurse can address in caring for children and adults who are suffering from abuse at the hands of others. Problems include *anxiety, fear, impaired family coping, post-trauma syndrome, powerlessness, caregiver burden, body image alteration, decreased self-esteem,* and *parenting problems.*

Intervention Guidelines

Child, Adult, and Older Adult

- Establish rapport before focusing on the details of the violent experience.
- Reassure the patient that he or she did nothing wrong.
- Allow the patient to tell his or her story without interruptions.
- If the patient is an adult, assure him or her of confidentiality, and that any changes are his or hers to make.
- If the patient is a child, report abuse to appropriate authorities designated in your state.
- If the patient is an older adult, check with state laws for reporting information.
- Establish a safety plan in situations of partner abuse.

Forensic Issues

- Follow hospital protocol. Keep your charting detailed, accurate, and up to date.
- The sexual assault nurse examiner (SANE) has specialized training to carry out evidentiary examinations of victims of sexual assault. The SANE nurse:
  - Documents verbatim statements of who caused the injury and when it occurred

- Draws a body map to indicate size, color, shape, areas, and types of injuries with explanation
- Gathers physical evidence, when possible, of sexual abuse (e.g., vaginal and anal swabs, fingernail scrapings)
- Obtains permission to take photos

Nursing Care for Family Violence

Survivors of Abuse
Potential for Injury

Due to:
- History of rage reaction
- Poor coping skills
- History of or current substance use
- Limited impulse control
- Pathological family dynamics
- History violence, neglect, or emotional deprivation as a child
- Psychiatric disorders

Abused Child

Desired Outcomes:
The child will be free from emotional, physical, and injury

Assessment/Interventions (Rationales)
1. Use a nonthreatening, nonjudgmental relationship with the parents. (If the parents feel judged or blamed or become defensive, they may take the child and either seek help elsewhere or not seek help at all.)
2. Understand that children do not want to betray their parents. (Even in an intolerable situation, the parents are the most important security the child knows.)
3. Provide for a complete physical assessment of the child. (A complete physical assessment will support essential care and substantiate reporting to the child welfare agency if required.)
4. Use dolls to help child tell his or her story. (The child might not know how to articulate what happened or might be afraid of punishment. Using dolls can be an easier way for the child to act out what happened.)

Forensic Issues with Child Sexual Assault
1. Be aware of your agency and state policy on reporting child abuse. Contact the supervisor or social worker to

implement appropriate reporting. (Health care workers are mandated to report cases of suspected or actual child abuse.)

2. Ensure that proper procedures are followed and evidence is collected. (If the child is temporarily taken to a safe environment, appropriate evidence helps protect the child's future welfare.)
3. Keep accurate and detailed records of the incident:
   a. Verbatim statements of who caused the injury and when it occurred
   b. Body map to indicate size, color, shape, areas, and types of injuries, along with an explanation
   c. Physical evidence, when possible, of sexual abuse
   d. Photographs(check hospital policy; e.g., permissions) (Accurate records can help ensure the child's future safety and court presentation.)
   4. Conduct a forensic examination of a sexually assaulted child according to specific protocols provided by law enforcement agencies and particular medical facilities. Ideally, SANE nurses, or nurses who have advanced training will conduct the examination. (The proper collection, handling, and storage of forensic specimens is crucial to the court presentation.)

Abused Partner

Desired Outcome:

The abused partner will be free from emotional, physical, and sexual injury.

Assessment/Interventions (Rationales)

1. Ensure that medical attention is provided to the patient. Ask permission to take photographs. (If the patient wants to file charges, photographs will support the case.)
2. Set up an interview in private, and ensure confidentiality. (The patient might be terrified of retribution and further attacks from the partner for telling someone about the abuse.)
3. In a nonthreatening manner, assess the following areas:
   a. Sexual abuse
   b. Substance use
   c. Suicidal or homicidal thoughts

   (These are all vital issues in planning care. Sexual abuse often accompanies physical abuse. Survivors of abuse may self-medicate. Self-directed or other-directed violence may seem like the only way out.)

Box 19.3 Partner Abuse—Assessing the Level of Violence in the Home

Does the patient feel safe?
Has there been a recent increase in violence?
Has the patient been choked?
Is there a weapon in the house?
Has the perpetrator used or threatened to use a weapon?
Has the perpetrator threatened to harm the children?
Has the perpetrator threatened to kill the patient?

4. Encourage the patient to talk about the battering incident without interruptions. (Listening, along with attending behaviors, will facilitate full sharing.)
5. Assess for the level of violence in the home (Box 19.3). (Each cycle of violence can become more intense. Danger for the life of the survivor and children increases over time.)
6. Ask about the welfare of the children in the home. (Intimate partner abuse is often accompanied by child abuse.)
7. Assess whether the patient has a safe place to go when violence is escalating. If not, include a list of shelters or safe houses with other written information. (When an abused partner makes the decision to leave, the risk of homicide dramatically increases. An emergency shelter can make the difference between life and death.)

Forensic Issues with Abused Partners

1. Identify whether the patient is interested in pressing charges. If yes, give information on:
   a. Attorneys who specialize in abuse
   b. Nonprofit law firms for low-income individuals and families
   c. Community advocates
   (Legal support and advocates who can direct the abused partner to community resources are essential in helping to establish independence.)
2. Be aware of your state laws for documenting and reporting suspected partner abuse. (State laws vary on the process for documenting and reporting domestic violence.)
3. Provide a written plan that includes shelter and referral numbers that can be used during the escalation of

anxiety, before actual violence erupts. (A sense of emergency may be the motivation to leave and a plan must be in place to keep the patient safe.)

4. Emphasize the following messages:
   a. "No one deserves to be beaten."
   b. "You cannot make anyone hurt you."
   c. "It is not your fault."

   (When self-esteem is eroded, people often buy into the myth that they deserved the abuse because they did something wrong, and if they had not done it, then it would not have happened.)
5. Encourage patients to reach out to family and friends whom they might have been avoiding. (Often survivors of violence are isolated from family and friends due to shame and/or control on the part of their partners who want to isolate them. Rallying support will strengthen the patient's resolve.)
6. Become familiar with therapists in your community with experience working with battered partners. (Psychotherapy with survivors of trauma requires special skills on the part of even an experienced therapist.)
7. If the patient is not ready to take action at this time, provide a list of community resources available:
   a. Hotlines
   b. Shelters
   c. Support groups
   d. Community advocates
   e. Social services

      (It can take time for patients to make decisions to change their life situation. Survivors of abuse need appropriate information.)

See Box 19.4 for a personalized safety plan for when the abused partner is in a relationship and when the relationship is over.

Abused Older Adult

Desired Outcome:

The older adult will be free from emotional, physical, and sexual injury.

Assessment/Interventions (Rationales)

1. Assess the severity of signs and symptoms of abuse and potential for further abuse on a weekly level. (Determines the need for further intervention.)

Box 19.4 **Personalized Safety Plan**

Suggestions for Increasing Safety—In the Relationship

I will have important phone numbers available to my children and myself.

I can tell _____ and _____ about the violence and ask them to call the police if they hear suspicious noises coming from my home.

If I leave my home, I can go (list four places) _____, _____, _____, or _____.

I can leave extra money, car keys, clothes, and copies of documents with _____.

If I leave, I will bring _____ (see checklist below).

To ensure safety and independence, I can: keep change for phone calls with me at all times; open my own savings account; rehearse my escape route with a support person; and review my safety plan on _____ (date).

Suggestions for Increasing Safety—When the Relationship Is Over

I can change the locks; I can install steel or metal doors, a security system, smoke detectors, and an outside lighting system.

I will inform _____ and _____ that my partner no longer lives with me and ask them to call the police if he or she is observed near my home or my children.

I will tell people who take care of my children the names of those who have permission to pick them up. The people who have permission are: _____, _____, and _____.

I can tell _____ at work about my situation and ask _____ to screen my calls.

I can avoid stores, banks, and _____ that I used when living with my battering partner.

I can obtain a protective order from _____. I can keep it on or near me at all times, as well as have a copy with _____.

If I feel down and ready to return to a potentially abusive situation, I can call _____ for support or attend workshops and support groups to gain support and strengthen my relationships with other people.

Important Telephone Numbers

Police ____________

Hotline ____________

Friends ____________

Shelter ____________

Continued

Box 19.4 **Personalized Safety Plan—cont'd**

Items to Take Checklist
Identification
Birth certificates for me and my children
Social Security cards
School and medical records
Money, bankbooks, credit cards
Keys (house/car/office)
Driver's license and registration
Medications
Change of clothes
Welfare identification
Passports, Green Cards, work permits
Divorce papers
Lease/rental agreement, house deed
Mortgage payment book, current unpaid bills
Insurance papers
Address book
Pictures, jewelry, items of sentimental value
Children's favorite toys and/or blankets

2. Assess environmental conditions as factors in the abuse or neglect (Box 19.5). (Assessment identifies the areas in need of intervention and the degree of abuse or neglect.)
3. If abuse is suspected, discuss it with the older adult and caregiver separately. (Talking separately helps attain a better understanding of what is happening and minimizes friction among the parties involved.)
4. Discuss with the older adult factors leading to abuse. (Discussing these factors identifies triggers to abusive behaviors and areas for teaching for the perpetrator.)
5. Stress concern for physical safety. (Stressing concern validates that the situation is serious.)

Forensic Issues with Abused Older Adults

1. Know your state laws regarding older adult abuse. Notify your supervisor, physicians, and social services when a suspected abuse is reported. (Knowing the laws keeps the channels of communication open and emphasizes the need for accurate and detailed records.)
2. If undue influence is suspected, consult with an expert who is experienced in geriatric or forensic psychiatry. (Consulting with an expert can help determine whether the older adult is making medical, legal, or financial decisions based on coercion and manipulations of others

Box 19.5 Older Adult Abuse/Neglect— Home Assessment

- House in poor repair
- Inadequate heat, lighting, furniture, cooking utensils
- Presence of garbage or rodents
- Old food in kitchen
- Lack of assistive devices
- Locks on refrigerator
- Blocked stairways
- Older adult lying in urine, feces, or food
- Unpleasant odors

to gain control of the older adult's finances, home, or decision making.)

3. Stress that no one has the right to abuse another person. (Often individuals who have been abused begin to believe they deserve the abuse.)
4. Discuss the following with the patient:
   a. Hotline
   b. Crisis unit
   c. Emergency numbers

   (Discussing these options with the patient maximize older adult safety through the use of support systems.)
5. Explore with the older adult ways to make changes. (Exploring the various ways to make changes directs the assessment to positive areas.)
6. Assist the older adult in making decisions for future action. (Assisting the older adult lowers feelings of helplessness and identifies realistic options to an abusive situation.)
7. Involve community supports to help monitor and support the older adult. (It is best to involve as many agencies as can take a legitimate role in maintaining the older adult's safety.)

Perpetrators of Abuse

Impaired Role Performance

Due to:

- Domestic violence
- Inadequate support system
- Family conflict
- Young age, developmental level
- Low socioeconomic status

- Substance use
- Psychiatric disorders
- Neurological condition
- Lack of resources
- Lack of knowledge about role skills

Parents Who Abuse

Desired Outcome:

Parents will cease battering behavior and adopt adaptive parenting skills.

Assessment/Interventions (Rationales)

1. Identify whether the child needs the following:
   a. Hospitalization for treatment and observation
   b. Referral to child protective services
   (Immediate safety of the child is foremost. Temporary removal of the child in a volatile situation gives the nurse or counselor time to assess the family situation and coping skills and to rally community resources to decrease family stress.)
2. Discuss with parents any stresses the family unit is currently facing. Contact the appropriate agencies to help reduce stress:
   a. Economic aid
   b. Job opportunities
   c. Social services
   d. Family service agencies
   e. Social supports
   f. Public health nurse
   g. Day care teacher
   h. School teacher
   i. Social worker
   j. Respite worker
   k. Anger management therapy
   l. Encourage and give referrals for family therapy; family therapy is very complex and hopes to teach family members how to develop new strategies and requires a specialist in family therapy
   (With the help of outside resources, family stress can be lowered, leading to an improved ability to problem solve.)
3. Reinforce the parents' strengths, and acknowledge the importance of continued medical care for the child. (Giving parents credit and support for positive parenting skills will encourage positive growth.)

4. Work with the parents to try safe methods to effectively discipline the child. (Understanding alternatives to abuse increases healthy family functioning while minimizing feelings of frustration and helplessness.)
5. Encourage parents to join a self-help group (e.g. Parents Anonymous, family counseling, group counseling). (Learning new ways of dealing with stress takes time, and support from others acts as an important incentive to change.)
6. Provide written information on hotlines, community supports, and agencies. (External resources reduces isolation and increases support during crisis periods.)

Partners Who Abuse

Desired Outcome:

The abuser will cease abusive behavior and demonstrate alternative ways to deal with anger and frustration.

Assessment/Interventions (Rationales)

1. If the partner who abuses is motivated, make arrangements for participation in an anger management program. (Some evidence suggests that a 6- to 8-week structural program that trains patients with anger issues may help to deactivate angry emotional states.)
2. Work with the perpetrator to recognize signs of escalating anger. (Often the perpetrator is unaware of the process leading up to the rage reaction.)
3. Work with the perpetrator to learn ways of channeling anger nonviolently. (Violence is often a learned coping skill. Adaptive skills for dealing with anger must be learned.)
4. Encourage the perpetrator to discuss thoughts and feelings with others who have similar problems. (Discussing these thoughts and feelings minimizes isolation and encourages problem solving.)
5. Refer to self-help groups in the community (e.g., Batterers Anonymous). (Self-help groups help patients look at their own behaviors among those who have similar problems.)

Older Adult Caregivers who Abuse

Desired Outcome:

The perpetrator of older adult abuse will refrain from abusive behavior and will demonstrate appropriate methods of dealing with frustration.

Assessment/Interventions (Rationales)

1. Research your state laws regarding older adult abuse. (State laws vary regarding documenting and reporting abuse of older adults.)
2. Encourage the perpetrator to verbalize feelings about the older adult and the abusive situation. (The abused might feel overwhelmed, isolated, and unsupported.)
3. Encourage problem solving when identifying stressful areas. (Encouragement assesses the perpetrator's approach to problem-solving skills and explores alternatives.)
4. Meet with the entire family, and identify stressors and problem areas. (Other family members might not be aware of the strain the perpetrator is under or the lack of safety to the abused family member.)
5. If there are no other family members, notify other community agencies that might help the perpetrator and older adult stabilize the situation:
   a. Support group for the older adult
   b. Support group for the perpetrator
   c. Meals On Wheels
   d. Day care for seniors
   e. Respite services
   f. Visiting nurse service

   (Support minimizes family stress and isolation and increases safety.)
6. Initiate referrals for available support services. (This rallies needed support for the abusive situation.)
7. Encourage the perpetrator to undergo counseling. (Encouraging the use of counseling will increase coping skills and social supports.)
8. Suggest that family members meet together on a regular basis for problem solving and support. (Meeting will encourage the family to learn to solve problems together.)

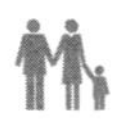

Nurse, Patient, and Family Resources

Adult Survivors of Childhood Abuse Anonymous
www.asca12step.org

Child Abuse Prevention—KidsPeace
(800) 334-4KID.
www.kidspeace.org

Child Abuse Prevention Network
www.child-abuse.com

Childhelp USA
(800) 4-A-CHILD—(800) 422-4453 (hotline)
www.childhelp.org

Institute on Violence, Abuse, and Trauma
www.fvsai.org

National Coalition Against Domestic Violence
www.ncadv.org

National Domestic Violence Hotline
www.thehotline.org
(800) 799-SAFE (hotline)

Rape, Abuse, and Incest National Network (RAINN)
www.rainn.org

Survivors of Incest Anonymous
www.siawso.org

Teen Line
teenlineonline.org
(800) TLC-TEEN

CHAPTER 20

Sexual Violence

Sexual assault is a violent crime. It is an act of violence, power, and hate, and sex is the weapon used by the perpetrator. Sexual violence typically results in devastating severe and long-term trauma. The official U.S. Department of Justice (2012) definition of rape is, "The penetration, no matter how slight, of the vagina or anus with any body part or object, or oral penetration by a sex organ of another person, without the consent of the victim."

It is usually men who rape, and most individuals who are raped are women. However, women may also sexually assault other women. Male-on-male sexual assault is also more prevalent in prisons and in the military than in the general population. A male who is sexually assaulted is more likely to have physical trauma and to have been victimized by several assailants than is a female. Males experience the same devastating severe and long-lasting trauma as females.

Long-term psychological effects of sexual assault include depression, dysfunction, and somatic complaints in many survivors. Victims of incest might experience a negative self-image, self-destructive behavior, and substance abuse.

Rape-trauma syndrome is closely related to posttraumatic stress disorder (PTSD) and consists of two phases: (1) the acute phase and (2) the long-term reorganization phase. Nurses may encounter a patient right after the sexual assault or weeks, months, or even years after the assault. In either case, the individual will benefit from compassionate and effective nursing interventions.

When available, special care for this population is provided by sexual assault nurse examiners (SANEs). They are forensic nurses who have been certified to work with victims of sexual violence. Functions of the SANE are to perform a physical examination of the survivor, collect forensic evidence, provide expert testimony regarding forensic evidence collected, and support the psychological needs of the survivor.

ASSESSMENT

Signs and Symptoms

Acute Phase of Rape-Trauma Syndrome (0–2 weeks)

- Shock, numbness, and disbelief
- Calm and composed
- Severe anxiety
- Tearful, sobbing
- Smiling, laughing
- Disorganization
- Somatic symptoms

Long-Term Reorganization Phase (2 weeks or more)

- Intrusive thoughts of the rape throughout the day and night
- Flashbacks of the incident (reexperiencing the traumatic event)
- Dreams with violent content
- Insomnia
- Increased motor activity (moving, taking trips, changing telephone numbers, staying with friends)
- Mood swings, crying spells, depression
- Fears and phobias:
  - Fear of indoors (if rape occurred indoors)
  - Fear of outdoors (if rape occurred outdoors)
  - Fear of being alone
  - Fear of crowds
  - Fear of sexual encounters

Assessment Guidelines

Assessment should be done in a nonthreatening manner. Use open-ended questions, broad openings, and general leads. For example, "It must have been very frightening to know that you had no control over what was happening."

1. Assess:
   a. Physical trauma: Document using a body map, and ask permission to take photographs.

   b. Psychological trauma: Write down verbatim statements of the patient.
   c. Level of anxiety: If patients are in severe to panic levels of anxiety, they will not be able to problem solve or process information.
   d. Support system: Often partners or family members do not understand about rape and might not be the best supports to rally at this time.
   e. Community supports (e.g., attorneys, support groups, therapists) who work in the area of sexual assault.
2. Encourage patients to tell their story. Do not press them to do so.

Intervention Guidelines

1. Follow your institution's protocol for sexual assault.
2. Do not leave the patient alone.
3. Maintain a nonjudgmental attitude.
4. Ensure confidentiality.
5. Encourage the patient to talk; listen empathetically.
6. Emphasize that the patient did the right thing to save his or her life.

Nursing Care Plan for Sexual Assault

Rape-Trauma Syndrome

Due to:

- Sexual assault

Desired Outcome:
The patient will return to pre-crisis level of functioning.

Assessment/Interventions (Rationales)

1. Ideally, someone should stay with the patient (friend, neighbor, or staff member) while he or she is waiting to be treated in the emergency department. (Individuals who are experiencing high levels of anxiety need someone with them until the anxiety level is reduced to moderate.)
2. Approach the patient in a nonjudgmental manner. (Nurses' attitudes can have an important therapeutic effect.)

3. The patient's situation should not be discussed with anyone other than medical personnel involved, unless the patient gives consent. (Confidentiality is crucial.)
4. Explain to the patient the signs and symptoms many patients experience during the long-term phase, such as nightmares, phobias, anxiety, depression, insomnia, and somatic symptoms. (Many patients think they are going crazy as time goes on and are unaware that this is a process that many individuals in their situation have experienced.)
5. Listen and let the patient talk. Do not press the patient to talk. (When the patient feels understood, he or she feels more in control of the situation.)
6. Stress that the patient did the right thing to save his or her life. (Rape patients might feel guilt or shame. Reinforcing that they did what they had to do to stay alive can reduce guilt and maintain self-esteem.)
7. Avoid judgmental language. For example, use the following words: reported rather than alleged, declined rather than refused, penetration rather than intercourse. (Sensitive word choices support the patient during the crisis phase and as the patient recovers.)

Forensic Issues for Sexual Assault Survivors

1. Assess the patient for signs and symptoms of physical trauma. (The most common injuries are to the face, head, neck, and extremities.)
2. Make a body map to identify the size, color, and location of injuries.
3. Ask permission to take photographs. (Accurate records and photos can be used as medicolegal evidence for the future.)
4. Carefully explain all procedures before doing them (e.g., "We would like to do a vaginal examination and do a swab. Have you had a vaginal (rectal) examination before?"). (The patient is experiencing high levels of anxiety. Matter-of-fact explanations of what you plan to do and why you are doing it can help reduce fear and anxiety.)
5. Explain the forensic specimens you plan to collect. Inform the patient that they can be used for identification and prosecution of the perpetrator:
   a. Pubic hair
   b. Skin from underneath nails

   c. Semen samples
   d. Blood
   (Collecting body fluids and swabs [DNA] is essential for identifying the perpetrator.)
6. Encourage the patient to consider treatment and evaluation for sexually transmitted diseases before leaving the emergency department. (Many survivors are lost to follow-up after being seen in the emergency department or crisis center and will not otherwise get protection.)
7. Offer emergency contraception to women who have been assaulted. (Women are at risk for pregnancy; about 5% of women who are raped become pregnant without contraception.)
8. All data should be carefully documented.
   a. Verbatim statements
   b. Detailed observations of physical trauma
   c. Detailed observations of emotional status
   d. Results from the physical examination
9. All laboratory tests should be noted. (Accurate and detailed documentation is crucial legal evidence.)
10. Arrange for follow-up support:
    a. Rape counselor
    b. Support group
    c. Group therapy
    d. Individual therapy
    e. Crisis counseling

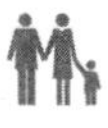

NURSE, PATIENT, AND FAMILY RESOURCES

Institute on Violence, Abuse, and Trauma
www.ivatcenters.org

Rape, Abuse, and Incest National Network (RAINN)
(800) 656-HOPE (4673)
www.rainn.org
Online chat: online.rainn.org

Survivors of Incest Anonymous (SIA)
www.siawso.org

David Baldwin's Trauma Information Pages
www.trauma-pages.com
Focuses on emotional trauma and traumatic stress

Male Survivor
www.malesurvivor.org

Men Can Stop Rape
www.mencanstoprape.org
Helping men who rape

PART IV
Psychopharmacology

CHAPTER 21

Attention-Deficit/ Hyperactivity Disorder Medications

Children and adults with attention-deficit/hyperactivity disorder (ADHD) show symptoms of short attention span, impulsivity, and overactivity. Some individuals may not demonstrate hyperactivity and impulsivity but are predominantly inattentive. This condition is referred to as *attention deficit disorder* (ADD). Pharmacological treatments of both conditions are discussed here.

STIMULANTS

Paradoxically, the symptoms of ADHD are treated with stimulant drugs. Responses to these drugs are often dramatic and can quickly increase attention and task-directed behavior while reducing impulsivity, restlessness, and distractibility.

Methylphenidate (Ritalin and other brand names) and mixed amphetamine salts (Adderall) are the most widely used stimulants because of their relative safety and simplicity of use. Not surprisingly, insomnia is a common side effect while taking stimulant medications. Due to insomnia, treating with the minimum effective dose is essential. Administering the medication no later than 4:00 in the afternoon or lowering the last dose of the day helps. The long-acting versions allow for a morning administration with sustained release of the medication over the course of the day and with a decreased incidence of insomnia.

Other common side effects include appetite suppression, headache, abdominal pain, and lethargy.

Among the concerns with the use of psychostimulant drugs are side effects of agitation, exacerbation of psychotic thought processes, hypertension, and growth suppression. As with any controlled substance, there is a risk of misuse such as selling the medication on the street or the use by people for whom the medication was not intended.

NONSTIMULANTS

The U.S. Food and Drug Administration (FDA) has approved three nonstimulants for the treatment of ADHD: atomoxetine (Strattera), guanfacine (Intuniv), and clonidine (Kapvay).

Atomoxetine is a norepinephrine reuptake inhibitor approved for use in children 6 years and older. Common side effects include decreased appetite and weight loss, fatigue, and dizziness. It is contraindicated for patients with severe cardiovascular disease because of its potential to increase blood pressure and heart rate. Therapeutic responses develop slowly, and it may take up to 6 weeks for full improvement. This medication is preferable for individuals whose anxiety is increased with stimulants. It is also useful for those with comorbid anxiety, active substance use disorders, or tics.

Ongoing monitoring of vital signs and regular screening of liver function should be done when using atomoxetine. Rarely, serious allergic reactions occur. Patients and their families should be educated on the risks and benefits of treatment before starting this medication. Atomoxetine should be used with extreme caution in patients with comorbid depression, because its use has been associated with increased suicidal ideation.

Two centrally acting alpha-2 adrenergic agonists, clonidine (Kapvay XR) and guanfacine (Intuniv XR), have traditionally been used to treat hypertension. The FDA-approved forms for ADHD are extended release and are used in children ages 6 to 17 years. Both should be increased slowly and should not be discontinued abruptly. These drugs can be used alone or in conjunction with other ADHD medications.

Of the two drugs, clonidine causes more side effects: somnolence, fatigue, insomnia, nightmares, irritability, constipation, respiratory symptoms, dry mouth, and ear pain.

Guanfacine's most common side effects include sleepiness, low blood pressure, nausea, stomach pain, and dizziness. The drug's effectiveness with teenagers is questionable, and it probably works best in preteens.

See Table 21.1 for a summary of the FDA-approved medications used to treat ADHD.

MANAGING AGGRESSIVE BEHAVIORS IN ATTENTION-DEFICIT/ HYPERACTIVITY DISORDER

To control aggressive behaviors, pharmacological agents including stimulants, mood stabilizers, alpha-adrenergic agonists, and antipsychotics are used. Stimulants have a dose-dependent effect. Low doses stimulate aggressive behaviors, whereas moderate to high doses suppress aggression. Mood stabilizers such as lithium and anticonvulsants reduce aggressive behavior and are recommended for impulsivity, explosive temper, and mood lability.

Because of the side effects of fatigue and somnolence, clonidine and guanfacine are helpful in reducing agitation and rage and in increasing frustration tolerance. Antipsychotic medications have reduced violent behavior, hyperactivity, and social unresponsiveness. However, due to the risk of tardive dyskinesia associated with long-term use, antipsychotic medications are only recommended for severe aggressive behavior.

Table 21.1 **FDA Approved Drugs for Attention-Deficit/Hyperactivity Disorder**

Generic Name	Trade Name	Indications	Duration	Schedule
Stimulants				
Amphetamine	Adzenys XR-ODT	Ages 6 years and older	12 hours	Once a day
	Dyanavel XR	Ages 6 years and older	12 hours	Once a day
	Evekeo	Ages 3 years and older	4-6 hours	Two or three times a day
Dexmethylphenidate	Focalin	Ages 6 years and older	4-5 hours	Two times a day
	Focalin XR	Ages 6 years and older	8-12 hours	Once a day
Dextroamphetamine	Dexedrine	Ages 3-16 years	4-6 hours	Two or three times a day
Lisdexamfetamine dimesylate	Vyvanse	Ages 6 years and older	10-12 hours	Once a day
Methamphetamine	Desoxyn	Ages 6 years and older	6-8 hours	One or two times a day
	Aptensio XR	For 6 years and older	12 hours	Once daily
Methylphenidate	Concerta	Ages 6-65 years	10-12 hours	Once a day
	Cotempla XR-ODT	Ages 6-17 years	12 hours	Once a day

	Daytrana (transdermal patch)	Ages 6-17 years	10-12 hours (up to 3 hours after removal)	Once a day
	Metadate ER	Ages 6-15 years	6-8 hours	One or two times a day
	Metadate CD	Ages 6-15 years	6-8 hours	Once a day
	Methylin ER	Ages 6 years and older	6-8 hours	Once a day
	QuilliChew ER	Ages 6 years and older	12 hours	Once a day
	Quillivant XR	Ages 6-12 years	12 hours	Once a day
	Ritalin	Ages 6-12 years	6-8 hours	One or two times a day
	Ritalin LA	Ages 6-12 years	7-9 hours	Once a day
	Ritalin SR	Ages 6-12 years	6-8 hours	One or two times a day
Mixed amphetamine salts	Adderall	Ages 3 years and older	4-6 hours	Two times a day
	Adderall–XR	Ages 6 years and older	10-12 hours	One or two times a day
Nonstimulants				
Atomoxetine	Strattera	Ages 6-65 years	24 hours	One or two times a day
Clonidine	Kapvay XR	Ages 6-17 years	12 hours	Two times a day
Guanfacine	Intuniv XR	Ages 6-17 years	24 hours	Once a day

Data from Food and Drug Administration. (2017). FDA online label repository. Retrieved from https://labels.fda.gov/

CHAPTER 22

Antipsychotic Medications

Antipsychotic medications, those used to treat psychotic disorders such as schizophrenia and bipolar mania, first became available in the 1950s. Previously available medications provided sedation but did not reduce psychosis. Patients with schizophrenia usually spent months or years in state or private hospitals, resulting in great emotional and financial costs to patients, families, and society. Antipsychotic drugs at last provided symptom control and allowed most patients to live and be treated in the community.

Antipsychotic agents typically take 2 to 6 weeks to achieve the desired effects. Antipsychotics are not addictive. However, they should be discontinued gradually to minimize a discontinuation syndrome that can include dizziness, nausea, tremors, insomnia, electric shock–like pains, and anxiety. Antipsychotics are unlikely to be lethal in overdose situations. Liquid, fast-dissolving forms, and orally inhaled preparations are available that make it difficult for a person to cheek or palm the medication (hide it in the cheek or palm and later dispose of it).

Two types of drugs are used to treat disorders with psychotic symptoms:

1. First-generation antipsychotics are traditional dopamine (D_2 receptor) antagonists. They are also known as typical antipsychotics.
2. Second-generation antipsychotics include serotonin (5-HT_{2A} receptor) and dopamine (D_2 receptor) antagonists such as clozapine (Clozaril). Some drugs in this group are antagonist in areas of high dopamine activity but agonists in areas of low dopamine activity, such as aripiprazole (Abilify). The second-generation antipsychotics are also known as atypical antipsychotics.

FIRST-GENERATION ANTIPSYCHOTICS

The first-generation antipsychotics (FGAs) primarily affect positive symptoms (i.e., hallucinations, delusions, and disorganized thoughts), but have little effect on negative symptoms (e.g., lack of emotion, avolition, alogia, anhedonia, and asociality).

FGAs are used less because of their minimal effect on negative symptoms and the higher level of side effects. However, because they are effective in treating positive symptoms and are relatively inexpensive, for patients untroubled by their side effects, FGAs remain an appropriate choice.

Drug-Induced Movement Disorders

FGAs are dopamine (D_2) antagonists in both limbic and motor centers. Blockage of D_2 receptors in motor areas can cause drug-induced movement disorders (DIMDs). These movement disorders are collectively known as extrapyramidal symptoms (EPSs). The acute EPSs include the following:

- Acute dystonia*:* Sudden, sustained contraction of one or several muscle groups, usually of the head and neck. Acute dystonias can be frightening and painful, but unless they involve muscles affecting the airway, they are not dangerous. They cause significant anxiety and should be treated promptly.
- Akathisia*:* An inner restlessness or an inability to stay still or remain in one place. Akathisia can be severe and distressing to patients and may be mistaken for agitation. This agitation may result in being given more of the drug that caused the akathisia, which makes the side effect worse.
- Parkinsonism: Temporary symptoms that look like Parkinson's disease: tremor, reduced accessory movements (e.g., arms swinging when walking), gait impairment, reduced facial expressiveness (mask facies), and slowing of motor behavior (bradykinesia).

These EPSs can be extremely distressing. They impact medication adherence, reduce quality of life, impair social relationships, and interfere with daily activities such as driving a car. Reducing dosages can minimize movement problems. Using antipsychotics that are less likely to cause

Table 22.1 **Medications Used for Drug-Induced Movement Disorders**

Generic (Brand) Name	Indications
Anticholinergic	
Benztropine (Cogentin) Trihexyphenidyl (Artane)	Dystonias, parkinsonism, akathisia
Dopaminergic	
Amantadine (Symmetrel)	Parkinsonism
Antihistamine	
Diphenhydramine (Benadryl)	Dystonias, parkinsonism
Beta-Adrenergic Antagonist	
Propranolol (Inderal)	Akathisia
Alpha-Adrenergic Antagonist	
Clonidine (Catapres)	Akathisia
Antianxiety Agents	
Clonazepam (Klonopin)	Akathisia, dystonia
Lorazepam (Ativan)	Akathisia, dystonia

these side effects can reduce their incidence. It is important to note that these motor problems often diminish over time.

EPSs can be treated with the addition of other drugs. Anticholinergic drugs are useful, but carry their own side effects including dry mouth, constipation, urinary hesitancy, tachycardia, thickening of secretions, and dry skin. Misuse of anticholinergic drugs is also a problem because they can cause an enjoyable altered sensorium. Other classifications of drugs used for dystonias, akathisia, and parkinsonism are listed in Table 22.1.

Tardive dyskinesia is a delayed and persistent drug-induced movement disorder consisting of involuntary rhythmic movements. Tardive dyskinesia develops in about 10% of patients after chronic exposure to dopamine receptor blockers, which leads to hyperactive dopamine signaling. Tardive dyskinesia often persists even after discontinuing the medication. Early symptoms begin in the mouth and facial muscles and may eventually progress to include the fingers, toes, neck, trunk, or pelvis. More common in women, tardive dyskinesia varies from mild to severe. It can be disfiguring or incapacitating.

The National Institute of Mental Health (NIMH) developed the Abnormal Involuntary Movement Scale (AIMS, Fig. 22.1) to identify and track involuntary movements.

ABNORMAL INVOLUNTARY MOVEMENT SCALE (AIMS)

Public Health Service
Alcohol, Drug Abuse, and Mental Health Administration
National Institute of Mental Health

Name: ____________
Date: ____________
Prescribing Practitioner: ____________

Code: 0 = None
1 = Minimal, may be extreme normal
2 = Mild
3 = Moderate
4 = Severe

Instructions: Complete Examination Procedure before making ratings.

Movement ratings: Rate highest severity observed. Rate movements that occur upon activation one *less* than those observed spontaneously. Circle movement as well as code number that applies.		Rater Date	Rater Date	Rater Date	Rater Date
Facial and Oral Movements	**1. Muscles of facial expression** (e.g., movements of forehead, eyebrows, periorbital area, cheeks, including frowning, blinking, smiling, grimacing)	0 1 2 3 4	0 1 2 3 4	0 1 2 3 4	0 1 2 3 4
	2. Lips and perioral area (e.g., puckering, pouting, smacking)	0 1 2 3 4	0 1 2 3 4	0 1 2 3 4	0 1 2 3 4
	3. Jaw (e.g., biting, clenching, chewing, mouth opening, lateral movement)	0 1 2 3 4	0 1 2 3 4	0 1 2 3 4	0 1 2 3 4
	4. Tongue: Rate only increases in movement both in and out of mouth — *not* inability to sustain movement. Darting in and out of mouth.	0 1 2 3 4	0 1 2 3 4	0 1 2 3 4	0 1 2 3 4
Extremity Movements	**5. Upper (arms, wrists, hands, fingers):** Include choreic movements (i.e., rapid, objectively purposeless, irregular, spontaneous) and athetoid movements (i.e., slow, irregular, complex, serpentine). *Do not include tremor* (i.e., repetitive, regular, rhythmic).	0 1 2 3 4	0 1 2 3 4	0 1 2 3 4	0 1 2 3 4
	6. Lower (legs, knees, ankles, toes) (e.g., lateral knee movement, foot tapping, heel dropping, foot squirming, inversion and eversion of foot)	0 1 2 3 4	0 1 2 3 4	0 1 2 3 4	0 1 2 3 4
Trunk Movements	**7. Neck, shoulder, hips** (e.g., rocking, twisting, squirming, pelvic gyrations)	0 1 2 3 4	0 1 2 3 4	0 1 2 3 4	0 1 2 3 4
Global Judgments	**8. Severity of abnormal movements overall**	0 1 2 3 4	0 1 2 3 4	0 1 2 3 4	0 1 2 3 4
	9. Incapacitation due to abnormal movements	0 1 2 3 4	0 1 2 3 4	0 1 2 3 4	0 1 2 3 4
	10. Patient's awareness of abnormal movements: Rate only patient's report. No awareness 0 Aware, no distress 1 Aware, mild distress 2 Aware, moderate distress 3 Aware, severe distress 4	0 1 2 3 4	0 1 2 3 4	0 1 2 3 4	0 1 2 3 4
Dental Status	**11. Current problems with teeth and/or dentures**	No Yes	No Yes	No Yes	No Yes
	12. Are dentures usually worn?	No Yes	No Yes	No Yes	No Yes
	13. Edentia	No Yes	No Yes	No Yes	No Yes
	14. Do movements disappear in sleep?	No Yes	No Yes	No Yes	No Yes

Fig. 22.1 Abnormal Involuntary Movement Scale (AIMS) Instructions: Rate highest severity observed. Rate movements that occur upon activation one *less* than those observed spontaneously. Circle movement as well as code number that applies. Scoring: 0 = Absent, 1 = Minimal, 2 = Mild, 3 = Moderate, 4 = Severe

Continued

Using the AIMS is an essential nursing role in treating this population. This scale is typically administered every 3 to 6 months or as indicated. A positive AIMS examination is a score of 2 in two or more movements or a score of 3 or 4 in a single movement.

The U.S. Food and Drug Administration ([FDA], 2017) has approved valbenazine (Ingrezza) for the treatment

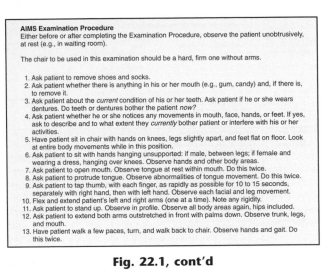

AIMS Examination Procedure
Either before or after completing the Examination Procedure, observe the patient unobtrusively, at rest (e.g., in waiting room).

The chair to be used in this examination should be a hard, firm one without arms.

1. Ask patient to remove shoes and socks.
2. Ask patient whether there is anything in his or her mouth (e.g., gum, candy) and, if there is, to remove it.
3. Ask patient about the *current* condition of his or her teeth. Ask patient if he or she wears dentures. Do teeth or dentures bother the patient *now?*
4. Ask patient whether he or she notices any movements in mouth, face, hands, or feet. If yes, ask to describe and to what extent they *currently* bother patient or interfere with his or her activities.
5. Have patient sit in chair with hands on knees, legs slightly apart, and feet flat on floor. Look at entire body movements while in this position.
6. Ask patient to sit with hands hanging unsupported: if male, between legs; if female and wearing a dress, hanging over knees. Observe hands and other body areas.
7. Ask patient to open mouth. Observe tongue at rest within mouth. Do this twice.
8. Ask patient to protrude tongue. Observe abnormalities of tongue movement. Do this twice.
9. Ask patient to tap thumb, with each finger, as rapidly as possible for 10 to 15 seconds, separately with right hand, then with left hand. Observe each facial and leg movement.
10. Flex and extend patient's left and right arms (one at a time). Note any rigidity.
11. Ask patient to stand up. Observe in profile. Observe all body areas again, hips included.
12. Ask patient to extend both arms outstretched in front with palms down. Observe trunk, legs, and mouth.
13. Have patient walk a few paces, turn, and walk back to chair. Observe hands and gait. Do this twice.

Fig. 22.1, cont'd

of tardive dyskinesia in adults. Valbenazine is a selective vesicular monoamine transporter inhibitor that reduces the severity of abnormal involuntary movements in tardive dyskinesia. Adverse effects include sleepiness and QT prolongation, which can result in sudden death. It is contraindicated with congenital long QT syndrome or with abnormal heartbeats associated with a prolonged QT interval. It should be used with caution for people who drive or operate heavy machinery or do other dangerous activities until it is known how the drug affects them.

Prior to antipsychotic therapy, patients should be screened for undiagnosed movement disorders such as Parkinson's disease. Symptoms of an underlying disease can be mistaken as drug side effects and go untreated.

Anticholinergic Side Effects

The FGAs cause anticholinergic side effects by blocking muscarinic cholinergic receptors. Anticholinergic side effects include urinary retention, dilated pupils, constipation, reduced visual accommodation (blurred near vision), tachycardia, dry mucous membranes, reduced peristalsis (rarely, leading to paralytic ileus and risk of bowel obstruction), and cognitive impairment. Taking multiple medications with anticholinergic side effects increases the risk of anticholinergic toxicity, covered later in this chapter. In general, FGAs have either strong EPS potential or strong anticholinergic potential. That is, when one side effect is prominent, the other is not.

Other First-Generation Antipsychotic Side Effects

FGAs cause sedation, which gradually improves. Orthostatic (postural) hypotension increases the risk of falls when standing suddenly. Lowered seizure threshold increases the risk of seizures. Visual changes such as photosensitivity and cataracts are associated with chlorpromazine (Thorazine) and thioridazine (Mellaril). An increased release of prolactin (hyperprolactinemia) can result in sexual dysfunction (impotence, anorgasmia, impaired ejaculation), galactorrhea (fluid from the breasts), amenorrhea, and gynecomastia (incease in male breast tissue). Weight gain of more than 50 pounds per year often results in psychological distress and an increased risk of cardiovascular disorders and diabetes.

Dangerous side effects are uncommon. Serious responses include anticholinergic toxicity, neuroleptic malignant syndrome, and prolongation of the QT interval. FGAs increase mortality in older adults with dementia. FDA-approved FGAs, formulations, and specific side effects are listed in Table 22.2.

SECOND-GENERATION ANTIPSYCHOTICS

Like FGAs, the second-generation antipsychotics (SGAs) can cause sedation, sexual dysfunction, and seizures. As with FGAs, the SGAs also increase mortality in older adults with dementia. However, most SGAs are less likely to cause significant EPS, especially tardive dyskinesia. Although they have the same potential side effects as the FGAs, SGA side effects are usually fewer, milder, and better tolerated. Some dangerous SGA side effects include anticholinergic toxicity, neuroleptic malignant syndrome, and prolongation of the QT interval.

When the first SGA, clozapine (Clozaril), was approved in 1989, it produced dramatic improvement in patients whose disorder had been resistant to FGAs. Most striking is that they helped to improve negative symptoms. Unfortunately, clozapine causes agranulocytosis in 0.5% to 1% of

Table 22.2 **U.S. Food and Drug Administration–Approved First-Generation Antipsychotics**

Generic (Trade) Name	Route	Specific Side Effects
Chlorpromazine (Thorazine)	Tablet, oral solution, SAIM	NMS, akathisia, EPS, tardive dyskinesia, sedation, weight gain, hypotension, constipation, hyperprolactinemia, photosensitivity
Fluphenazine (Prolixin)	Tablet, oral concentrate, oral elixir, SAIM, LAIM	Sedation, weight gain, hyperprolactinemia, NMS, EPS, akathisia, tardive dyskinesia, dystonia
Haloperidol (Haldol)	Tablet, oral concentrate, SAIM, LAIM	NMS, akathisia, EPS, tardive dyskinesia, dystonia, sedation, hypotension, constipation, hyperprolactinemia
Loxapine (Loxitane)	Capsule	NMS, akathisia, EPS, tardive dyskinesia, sedation, hypotension, constipation, hyperprolactinemia, dystonia
Loxapine (Adusave)	Inhalation powder	Altered taste, sedation. Contraindicated with asthma, and chronic obstructive pulmonary disease.
Molindone (Moban)	Tablet	NMS, akathisia, EPS, tardive dyskinesia, sedation, constipation, hyperprolactinemia, dystonia
Perphenazine (Trilafon)	Tablet	NMS, akathisia, EPS, tardive dyskinesia, sedation, weight gain, hypotension, constipation, hyperprolactinemia, dystonia
Prochlorperazine (Compazine)	Tablet, suppository, SAIM	Hypotension, hyperprolactinemia, NMS, EPS, akathisia, tardive dyskinesia, dystonia
Thioridazine (Mellaril)	Tablet	NMS, akathisia, EPS, tardive dyskinesia, pigmentary retinopathy, sedation, weight gain, hypotension, constipation, hyperprolactinemia, dystonia
Thiothixene (Navane)	Capsule	NMS, akathisia, EPS, tardive dyskinesia, sedation, hypotension, constipation, hyperprolactinemia, dystonia
Trifluoperazine (Stelazine)	Tablet	NMS, akathisia, EPS, tardive dyskinesia, sedation, hypotension, constipation, hyperprolactinemia, dystonia

EPS, Extrapyramidal symptoms; *NMS,* neuroleptic malignant syndrome; *SAIM,* short-acting intramuscular injection; *LAIM,* long-acting intramuscular injection.

those who take it. Other dangerous side effects are myocarditis and life-threatening bowel emergencies. Because of these problems, clozapine use has declined in the United States, and many clinicians reserve its use as a last resort. However, it is the only drug with FDA approval for the treatment of suicidality in schizophrenia.

Metabolic Syndrome

All SGAs carry a risk of metabolic syndrome, which includes weight gain (especially in the abdominal area), dyslipidemia, increased blood glucose, and insulin resistance. This metabolic syndrome is a significant concern and increases the risk of diabetes, certain cancers, hypertension, and cardiovascular disease, making its prevention an important role for nurses.

Some SGAs also have antidepressant properties and are FDA approved for adjunctive use in the treatment of major depressive disorder. As with all antidepressants, they carry a theoretical risk of increased suicidality, particularly in adolescents.

A subset of the SGAs is sometimes referred to as third-generation antipsychotics. These drugs are aripiprazole (Abilify), brexpiprazole (Rexulti), and cariprazine (Vraylar). They are dopamine system stabilizers that reduce dopamine activity in some brain regions while increasing it in other brain regions. Aripiprazole and brexpiprazole act as D_2 partial agonists (meaning they attach to the D_2 receptor without fully activating it, reducing the effective level of dopamine activity). Cariprazine is a partial agonist more on D_3 than D_2 receptors, which may help improve cognitive symptoms.

FDA-approved SGAs, formulations, and specific side effects are listed in Table 22.3.

Table 22.4 summarizes side effects of antipsychotic medication and the nursing care that is associated with these side effects.

Dangerous Antipsychotic Side Effects

Rare but serious and potentially fatal side effects of antipsychotic drugs include anticholinergic toxicity, neuroleptic malignant syndrome, agranulocytosis, prolongation of the QT interval, and liver impairment. Nurses who work in

Text continued on page 355

Table 22.3 **FDA–Approved Second- and Third-Generation Antipsychotics**

Generic (Trade) Name	Route	Specific Side Effects
Aripiprazole (Abilify)	Tablet, SAIM	Dizziness, insomnia, akathisia, activation, nausea, vomiting, sedation
Aripiprazole (Abilify Discmelt)	Orally disintegrating tablet	
Aripiprazole (Abilify Maintena)	LAIM	
Asenapine (Saphris)	Sublingual tablet	Risk of diabetes and dyslipidemia, EPS, hyperprolactinemia, sedation weight gain, akathisia, NMS, tardive dyskinesia, oral hypoesthesia (tongue numbing)
Brexpiprazole (Rexulti)	Tablet	Headache, EPS, dyspepsia
Cariprazine Vraylar)	Capsule	EPS, insomnia, nausea, sedation
Clozapine (Clozaril)	Tablet	Risk of diabetes and dyslipidemia, increased salivation, sweating, agranulocytosis, sedation, weigh gain, constipation, hypotension, seizures
Clozapine (FazaClo)	Orally disintegrating tablet	
Iloperidone (Fanapt)	Tablet	Risk of diabetes and dyslipidemia, EPS, hyperprolactinemia, sedation, weight gain, akathisia, NMS, tardive dyskinesia
Lurasidone (Latuda)	Tablet	Risk of diabetes and dyslipidemia, EPS, hyperprolactinemia, sedation, weight gain, akathisia, NMS, tardive dyskinesia

Olanzapine (Zyprexa)	Tablet, SAIM	Risk of diabetes and dyslipidemia, sedation, weight gain, hyperprolactinemia, constipation, hypotension, seizures
Olanzapine (Zyprexa Relprevv)		
Olanzapine (Zyprexa Zydis)	Orally disintegrating tablet	
Paliperidone (Invega)	Tablet	Risk of diabetes and dyslipidemia, EPS, hyperprolactinemia, sedation, weight gain, tachycardia, headache
Paliperidone (Invega Sustenna, Invega Trinza)	LAIM	
Quetiapine (Seroquel, Seroquel XR)	Tablet	Risk of diabetes and dyslipidemia, dizziness, sedation, weight gain, constipation, hypotension
Risperidone (Risperdal)	Table, oral solution	Risk of diabetes and dyslipidemia, EPS, hyperprolactinemia, sedation, weight gain, akathisia, NMS, tardive dyskinesia
Risperidone (Risperdal Consta)	LAIM	
Risperidone (Risperdal M-Tab)	Orally disintegrating tablet	
Ziprasidone (Geodon)	Capsule, SAIM	Activating, sedation, hypotension, akathisia

EPS, Extrapyramidal symptoms; *NMS,* neuroleptic malignant syndrome; *SAIM,* short-acting intramuscular injection; *LAIM,* long-acting intramuscular injection.

Table 22.4 **Side Effects of Antipsychotic Medication and Associated Nursing Care**

Side Effect	Nursing Care
Extrapyramidal Symptoms (EPS)	
Acute Dystonia	
Acute painful contractions of tongue, face, neck, and back (usually tongue and jaw first) Spasm of the muscles causing backward arching of the head, neck (torticollis), and spine Eyes roll back (oculogyric crisis) Laryngeal dystonia: could threaten airway (rare)	Monitor and ensure open airway. Administer antiparkinsonian agent (IM for faster response). Relief usually occurs in 5–15 minutes. Consider diphenhydramine hydrochloride (Benadryl) 25–50 mg intramuscularly or intravenously. Prevent further dystonias with antiparkinsonian agent. Reassure patient that dystonias are not dangerous except for rare airway complications. Stay with the patient to provide comfort and support.
Akathisia	
Motor restlessness (e.g., pacing, unable to stand still or stay in one location, rocking while seated or shifting from one foot to other while standing)	Consult prescriber regarding possible medication change. Give antiparkinsonian agent, beta-blocker, or lorazepam (Ativan). Propranolol (Inderal), lorazepam (Ativan), or diazepam (Valium) may be used. Relaxation exercises may be helpful. In severe cases, may cause great distress and contribute to suicidality.
Parkinsonism	
Masklike face, stiff and stooped posture, shuffling gait, drooling, tremor, "pill-rolling" finger movements, dysphagia or reduction in spontaneous swallowing	Administer antiparkinsonian agent such as trihexyphenidyl (Artane) or benztropine (Cogentin). If intolerable, consult prescriber regarding dose reduction or medication change. Provide towel or handkerchief to wipe excess saliva. Teach how to reduce fall risk.

Tardive Dyskinesia	
Face: protruding or writhing tongue; blowing, smacking, licking; facial distortion Limbs: Chorea: rapid, purposeless, and irregular movements Athetoid: slow, complex, and serpentine movements Trunk: neck and shoulder movements, hip jerks and rocking, or twisting pelvic thrusts	20% of patients taking these drugs for >2 years may develop tardive dyskinesia. Screening at least every 3 months. Purposeful muscle contraction overrides and masks involuntary tardive movements. Reconsideration medication choice. Provide support. Teach patient ways to conceal involuntary movements such as holding one hand with the other. Valbenazine (Ingrezza) reduces the severity of abnormal involuntary movements.
Hypotension and Orthostatic (Postural) Hypotension Upon standing, systolic rises, diastolic decreases, and pulse increases	Monitor lying or sitting and standing blood pressure and pulse. Hold dose and consult prescriber if systolic pressure is <80 mm Hg when standing. Advise patient to arise slowly to prevent dizziness and to hold on to railings or furniture while rising to reduce falls. If lying down, patient should first move slowly to sitting position and pause until dizziness passes before standing. Effect usually subsides in 1–2 weeks. Ensure adequate hydration.
Anticholinergic	
Dry mouth	Encourage ice chips or frequent sips of water. Sugarless candy or gum stimulates salivation. Xylitol-containing moisture supplements or other saliva substitutes can be helpful.

Continued

Table 22.4 **Side Effects of Antipsychotic Medication and Associated Nursing Care—cont'd**

Side Effect	Nursing Care
Urinary retention and hesitancy	Check for distended bladder. Try running water and a warm moist towel on abdomen. Catheterization may be necessary.
Constipation	Ensure adequate fluid and fiber intake. Promote physical activity. Consider stool softeners, laxatives, or dietary laxatives (e.g., prune juice).
Blurred vision	May improve in 1–2 weeks. Use reading or magnifying glasses. If intolerable, consult prescriber regarding medication change.
Dry eyes	Use artificial tears; minimize wind exposure. Humidifier may help at home.
Sexual dysfunction	Alternative medication may be considered. Suggest artificial lubricants for vaginal dryness.
Metabolic Syndrome	
Weight gain, dyslipidemia (abnormal lipid levels), increased insulin resistance Lead to increased risk of cardiovascular disease, diabetes, and other medical conditions	Minimize weight gain through proper nutrition and physical activity: Help the patient to identify low-calorie snacks. Engage the patient in regular physical activity. Help the patient to identify and pursue physical activities such as walking or cycling. Teach the importance of regular medical evaluation and care to identify symptoms of this syndrome.

Data from Burchum, J., & Rosenthal, L. (2016). *Lehne's pharmacology for nursing care* (9th ed.). St. Louis, MO: Elsevier.

psychiatric settings primary care, and emergency services need to be aware of and monitor for the early signs and symptoms of these side effects. Patients and their families should be taught how to recognize and respond to dangerous side effects.

Anticholinergic toxicity is a potentially life-threatening condition caused by antipsychotics or other medications with anticholinergic effects, including many antiparkinsonian drugs. Older adults and those taking multiple anticholinergic drugs are at greatest risk. Symptoms include autonomic nervous system instability and delirium with altered mental status. Mental status changes can include hallucinations and may be mistaken for a worsening of the patient's psychosis. People whose psychosis is inexplicably worsening should be evaluated for anticholinergic toxicity.

Neuroleptic malignant syndrome (NMS) occurs in about 0.2% to 1% of patients who have taken FGAs. This side effect is less likely with SGAs. Its symptoms are reduced consciousness, increased muscle tone (generalized muscular rigidity), and autonomic dysfunction. A fever in excess of 103 degrees Fahrenheit (39 degrees Celsius) is the most telling symptom. Caused by excessive dopamine receptor blockade, NMS is an emergency that is fatal in up to 10% of cases. It usually occurs early in therapy but has also occurred 20 years into treatment. Early detection, discontinuation of the antipsychotic, management of fluid balance, temperature reduction, and monitoring for complications such as deep vein thrombosis and rhabdomyolysis (protein in the blood from muscle breakdown, which can cause organ failure) are essential.

Agranulocytosis, though most associated with clozapine (Clozaril), is possible with most other antipsychotics. Neutropenia can also develop and can be fatal. Monitoring for neutropenia is done as part of the complete blood count through an absolute neutrophil count (ANC). Symptoms of agranulocytosis include signs of infection (e.g., fever, chills, sore throats) or increased susceptibility to infection.

Prolongation of the QT interval may contribute to sudden death of unknown origin that occasionally occurs in relation to antipsychotic therapy. This prolongation increases the risk of ventricular tachyarrhythmias, which may lead to syncope, cardiac arrest, or sudden death. The FGAs chlorpromazine (Thorazine), haloperidol (Haldol), and thioridazine (Mellaril) may cause this cardiac emergency.

SGAs iloperidone (Fanapt), quetiapine (Seroquel), and ziprasidone (Geodon) can also prolong the QT interval. All patients should be evaluated for existing QT prolongation with an electrocardiogram before beginning antipsychotic therapy.

Liver impairment may also occur, particularly with FGAs. SGAs also lead to serum enzyme elevations but rarely with injury or jaundice. Liver impairment usually occurs in the first weeks of therapy. Signs of liver problems include yellowish skin and eyes, abdominal pain, ascites, vomiting, swelling in the lower extremities, dark urine, pale or tar-colored stool, and easy bruising. The patient may complain of itchy skin, chronic fatigue, nausea, and a loss of appetite. This makes monitoring of liver function values essential.

Table 22.5 summarizes dangerous side effects of antipsychotics and the appropriate nursing care to respond to these side effects.

INJECTABLE ANTIPSYCHOTICS

Some antipsychotics are available in short-acting injectable form, used primarily for treatment of agitation, emergencies such as aggressiveness, or when a patient refuses court-mandated oral antipsychotics. However, side effects can be intensified and less easily managed when medication is administered directly into the system intramuscularly.

Some antipsychotics are available in long-acting injectable formulations that only need to be administered every 2 to 6 weeks and, in one case, every 3 months. Some require special administration protocols (Table 22.6). When less frequent medication administration is necessary, adherence is improved and conflict about taking medications is reduced. The downsides are a lack of dosing flexibility and that patients may feel like they have less control or feel coerced.

Table 22.5 **Dangerous Side Effects of Antipsychotics and Associated Nursing Care**

Side Effect	Nursing Care
Anticholinergic Toxicity *Potentially life-threatening medical emergency* Reduced or absent peristalsis (can lead to bowel obstruction); urinary retention; mydriasis (pupillary dilation); hyperpyrexia without diaphoresis (hot dry skin); delirium with tachycardia, unstable vital signs, agitation, disorientation, hallucinations, reduced responsiveness; worsening of psychotic symptoms; seizure; repetitive motor movements	Hold all medications. Consult prescriber immediately. Implement emergency cooling measures as ordered (cooling blanket, alcohol, or ice bath). Urinary catheterization as needed. Administer a benzodiazepine or other sedation as ordered. Physostigmine, an antidote to reverse the toxicity of anticholinergic effects, may be ordered. Evaluate for anticholinergic toxicity any time psychosis appears to be worsening.
Neuroleptic Malignant Syndrome (NMS) *Rare but dangerous; acute, life-threatening medical emergency* *Early detection increases patient's chance of survival* Hyperpyrexia (fever) over 103°F is most diagnostic symptom. Severe muscle rigidity, dysphasia, flexor-extensor posturing, reduced or absent speech and movement, decreased responsiveness. Autonomic dysfunction: hypertension, tachycardia, diaphoresis, incontinence. Delirium, stupor, coma.	Hold all antipsychotics. Transfer to a critical care unit (if in community, 911 transport to emergency department; notify emergency department of referral and reason). Bromocriptine (Parlodel) and dantrolene (Dantrium) can relieve muscle rigidity and reduce the heat (fever) generated by muscle contractions. Cool body to reduce fever (cooling blankets; alcohol, cool water, or ice bath as ordered). Maintain hydration with oral or intravenous fluids; correct electrolyte imbalance. Treat dysrhythmias. Small doses of heparin may decrease possibility of pulmonary emboli.

Continued

Table 22.5 **Dangerous Side Effects of Antipsychotics and Associated Nursing Care—cont'd**

Side Effect	Nursing Care
Agranulocytosis *Potentially fatal blood dyscrasia* Symptoms include reduced neutrophil counts and increased frequency and severity of infections. Any symptoms suggesting infection (e.g., sore throat, fever, malaise, body aches) should be carefully evaluated.	Monitor for neutropenia weekly for 6 months, then twice monthly for 6 more months, then monthly. If neutropenia develops, hold drug and consult prescriber. Moderate neutropenia (absolute neutrophil count [ANC] 500–999 μL) and severe neutropenia (ANC <500 μL) should result in treatment interruption. In some cases clozapine may be reinstituted once the ANC returns to normal. Reverse isolation may be initiated temporarily. Teach patient to observe for signs of infection and to report these promptly to prescriber.
Prolongation of the QT Interval *Medical emergency, potentially fatal* Prolongation increases the risk of ventricular tachyarrhythmias, which may lead to syncope, cardiac arrest, or sudden death. Tachycardia, irregular pulse, fainting. Seizures may occur because of erratic heartbeats resulting in brain oxygen deprivation.	Evaluate everyone for existing QT prolongation before beginning antipsychotic therapy with electrocardiograms. Monitor pulse for tachycardia and irregularities. Fainting and seizures in a person taking antipsychotics should be considered signs of impending cardiac arrest. Life-saving emergency intervention should be considered.

Table 22.6 **Long-Acting Injectable Antipsychotics**

Generic (Trade) Name	Frequency	Nursing Considerations
Aripiprazole** (Abilify Maintena)	Every 4 weeks	Deltoid or gluteal site. Shake vigorously just before administering.
Aripiprazole** (Aristada)	Every 6 weeks; highest strength every 8 weeks	Deltoid for lowest strength or gluteal site. Shake vigorously just before administering.
Fluphenazine decanoate* (generic only)	Every 2–3 weeks	Viscous, deltoid, or gluteal site. Z-track method.
Haloperidol decanoate* (Haldol Decanoate)	Every 4 weeks	Viscous, deltoid, or gluteal site. Z-track method.
Olanzapine pamoate** (Zyprexa Relprevv)	Every 2–4 weeks	Must monitor patient for excess sedation for 3 hours after each injection. Gluteal site only. Shake vigorously just before administering.
Paliperidone palmitate** (Invega Sustenna)	Every 4 weeks	When initiating, the first two injections must be given deltoid. Deltoid or gluteal site afterward. Shake vigorously just before administering.
Paliperidone palmitate** (Invega Trinza)	Every 3 months	Deltoid or gluteal site. Shake vigorously just before administering.
Risperidone microspheres** (Risperdal Consta)	Every 2 weeks	Deltoid or gluteal site. Shake vigorously just before administering.

*First-generation

**Second-generation

Data from manufacturer's product insert and Burchum, J., & Rosenthal, L. (2016). *Lehne's pharmacology for nursing care* (9th ed.). St. Louis, MO: Elsevier.

CHAPTER 23

Mood Stabilizers

Mood stabilizers are a class of drugs used to treat symptoms associated with bipolar disorder. The original intent of the term mood stabilizer was to indicate that these drugs were effective in the treatment of both mania and depression. This is not precisely true. Although most of the medications in this category are effective in treating mania, not all of them do as well in treating depression.

Table 23.1 summarizes medications used for the treatment of bipolar disorder.

LITHIUM

In 1970 lithium was given U.S. Food and Drug Administration (FDA) approval for the treatment of acute mania, and in 1974 for maintenance therapy in bipolar disorder. For several decades, lithium was the only drug approved for both acute and maintenance treatment. Lithium is a soft natural silvery metal, and most of the lithium in the United States is derived from dry lake beds in South America. Lithium is sold as Eskalith, Eskalith CR, and Lithobid.

Lithium is particularly effective in reducing the following:

- Elation
- Flight of ideas
- Irritability
- Manipulation
- Anxiety

To a lesser extent, lithium controls the following:

- Insomnia
- Psychomotor agitation
- Threatening or assaultive behavior
- Distractibility
- Paranoia
- Hypersexuality

Table 23.1 **FDA Approved Drugs for Bipolar Disorder**

Generic (Trade) Name	Bipolar Depression	Acute Mania	Bipolar Maintenance
Mood Stabilizers			
Lithium (Eskalith, Eskalith CR, Lithobid)	—	FDA approved	FDA approved
Anticonvulsant Mood Stabilizers			
Carbamazepine (Equetro)	—	FDA approved	—
Divalproex sodium delayed release (Depakote), divalproex sodium extended release (Depakote ER)	—	FDA approved	—
Lamotrigine (Lamictal)	—	—	FDA approved
Valproic acid delayed release (Stavzor)	—	FDA approved	—
First-Generation Antipsychotics			
Chlorpromazine (Thorazine)	—	FDA approved	—
Loxapine (Adasuve) orally inhaled	—	FDA approved for bipolar I acute agitation	—
Second-Generation Antipsychotics			
Aripiprazole (Abilify)	—	FDA approved	FDA approved
Asenapine (Saphris)	—	FDA approved	—
Cariprazine (Vraylar)	—	FDA approved	—
Lurasidone (Latuda)	FDA approved	—	—
Olanzapine (Zyprexa)	—	FDA approved	FDA approved

Continued

Table 23.1 **FDA Approved Drugs for Bipolar Disorder—cont'd**

Generic (Trade) Name	Bipolar Depression	Acute Mania	Bipolar Maintenance
Quetiapine (Seroquel, Seroquel XR)	FDA approved	FDA approved	FDA approved
Risperidone (Risperdal, Risperdal Consta)	— —	FDA approved —	— FDA approved
Ziprasidone (Geodon)	—	FDA approved	FDA approved
Combination Second-Generation Antipsychotic and Antidepressant			
Olanzapine (Zyprexa) + fluoxetine (Prozac) = Symbyax	FDA approved	—	—

From U.S. Food and Drug Administration. (2016). FDA online label repository. Retrieved from http://labels.fda.gov/

Lithium's antimanic effect usually takes 7 to 14 days to achieve. Therefore during the initial stages of treatment, another medication such as a second-generation antipsychotic may be given to help decrease psychomotor activity, aggressive behaviors, and prevent exhaustion.

A narrow range exists between the therapeutic dose and toxic dose of lithium. Blood lithium levels should be checked every 3 to 7 days for the first few weeks; once the patient is stable, they can then be checked every 1 to 3 months. Initially, levels should be from 0.8 to 1.2 mEq/L when the patient is in acute mania. Maintenance blood levels of lithium range from 0.6 to 1.2 mEq/L. To prevent serious toxicity, lithium levels should not exceed 1.5 mEq/L. Lithium side effects and signs of lithium toxicity are listed in Table 23.2.

Before administering lithium, complete a baseline assessment of renal function and thyroid status, including levels of thyroxine and thyroid-stimulating hormone. Perform other clinical and laboratory assessments, including an

Table 23.2 **Lithium Side Effects and Signs of Lithium Toxicity**

Plasma Level	Signs	Interventions
Expected Side Effects		
<1.5 mEq/L	Nausea, vomiting, diarrhea, thirst, polyuria (producing too much urine), lethargy, sedation, and fine hand tremor. Renal toxicity may occur with long-term use. Goiter and hypothyroidism.	Symptoms often subside during treatment. Doses should be kept low. Kidney function and thyroid levels should be assessed before treatment and then on an annual basis.
Early Signs of Toxicity		
1.5–2.0 mEq/L	Gastrointestinal upset, coarse hand tremor, confusion, hyperirritability of muscles, electroencephalographic changes, sedation, incoordination.	Medication should be withheld, blood lithium levels measured, and dosage reevaluated.
Advanced Signs of Toxicity		
2.0–2.5 mEq/L	Ataxia, giddiness, serious electroencephalographic changes, blurred vision, clonic movements, large output of dilute urine, seizures, stupor, severe hypotension, coma. Death is usually secondary to pulmonary complications.	Hospitalization is indicated. The drug is stopped, and excretion is hastened. Whole bowel irrigation may be done to prevent further absorption of lithium.
Severe Toxicity		
>2.5 mEq/L	Convulsions, oliguria (producing no or small amounts of urine); death can occur.	In addition to the previously listed interventions, hemodialysis may be used in severe cases.

Data from Sadock, B.J., Sadock, V.A., & Ruiz, P. (2015). *Kaplan and Sadock's synopsis of psychiatry.* Philadelphia, PA: Wolters Kluwer.

electrocardiogram as needed, depending on the individual's physical condition.

Lithium therapy is generally contraindicated in patients with cardiovascular disease, brain damage, renal disease, thyroid disease, or myasthenia gravis. Whenever possible, lithium is not given to women who are pregnant because it may harm the fetus. Lithium use is also contraindicated in mothers who are breast-feeding and in children younger than 12 years.

A fine hand tremor, polyuria, and mild thirst may occur during initial therapy for the acute manic phase and may persist throughout treatment. Transient and mild nausea and general discomfort may also appear during the first few days of lithium administration. Because lithium is a salt, patients should be advised to maintain balanced hydration by drinking an adequate amount of water and consuming a normal level of dietary salt. Dehydration from exercise, heat, vomiting, or diarrhea may result in toxic levels of lithium in the bloodstream. Patient and family teaching is provided in Box 23.1.

ANTICONVULSANTS

Anticonvulsant drugs were developed to treat convulsions associated with epilepsy. They are now commonly used to treat bipolar depression, acute mania, and bipolar maintenance. They generally share several characteristics. They are:

- Superior for continuously cycling patients
- Effective at diminishing impulsive and aggressive behavior in some nonpsychotic patients
- Beneficial in controlling mania (within 2 weeks) and depression (within 3 weeks or longer)
- More effective when there is no family history of bipolar disorder

Divalproex and Valproic Acid

Divalproex sodium (Depakote), divalproex sodium extended release (Depakote ER), and valproic acid delayed release (Stavzor) are FDA approved for the treatment of acute mania. This group of drugs is one of the most widely prescribed mood stabilizers in psychiatry. They work quickly, and most people tolerate them well. Once a sufficient serum level of the drug has been reached (about a

Box 23.1 Patient and Family Teaching: Lithium Therapy

The patient and the patient's family should receive the following information, be encouraged to ask questions, and be given the material in written form as well.

- Lithium is a mood stabilizer and helps prevent relapse. It is important to continue taking the drug even after the current episode subsides.
- Lithium is not addictive.
- Monitor lithium blood levels until a therapeutic level is reached. More frequent testing of blood levels will initially be needed, then once every several months after that.
- It is important to maintain a consistent fluid intake (1500–3000 mL/day or six 12-oz glasses of fluid).
- Aim for consistency in sodium intake. High sodium intake leads to lower levels of lithium and less therapeutic effect. Low sodium intake leads to higher lithium levels, which could produce toxicity.
- Stop taking lithium when experiencing excessive diarrhea, vomiting, or sweating. All of these symptoms can lead to dehydration and increase blood lithium to toxic levels. Inform your care provider if you have any of these problems.
- Lithium levels may be increased while taking ACE inhibitors, angiotensin receptor blockers, thiazide diuretics, and nonsteroidal anti-inflammatory drugs. Let your prescriber know if you are taking any of these medications.
- Talk to your prescriber about having thyroid, parathyroid, and renal function checked periodically due to potential side effects.
- Do not take over-the-counter medicines without checking with your prescriber. Even nonsteroidal anti-inflammatory drugs (e.g., ibuprofen, naproxen) may influence lithium levels.
- Take lithium with meals to prevent stomach irritation.
- In the first week you may gain up to 5 pounds of water weight. Additional weight gain may occur, particularly in women. Discuss how much weight gain is acceptable with your prescriber.
- Groups are available to provide support for people with bipolar disorder and their families. A local self-help group is [give name and telephone number].

week), two-thirds of patients usually respond within 1 to 4 days.

Common side effects include gastrointestinal irritation, nausea, diarrhea, vomiting, weakness, sedation, tremor, weight gain, and hair loss. Significant adverse reactions include sometimes fatal hepatotoxicity, usually in the first 6 months of treatment. Patients should have baseline liver studies before taking these drugs and regularly thereafter. Pancreatitis, including fatal hemorrhagic cases, may result from these drugs.

Women who plan to become pregnant or are pregnant should not take divalproex sodium or valproic acid because of a 5% risk of neural tube defects, especially during the first trimester. Also, decreased cognitive ability is associated with children who are exposed in utero. There have been rare, spontaneous reports of polycystic ovary disease associated with these drugs.

Carbamazepine

Carbamazepine (Equetro) extended release is an alternative to lithium, valproate, or a second-generation antipsychotic in treating acute mania. It seems to work better in patients with rapid cycling and in severely paranoid, angry patients experiencing manias rather than in euphoric, overactive, overfriendly patients experiencing mania. It is also believed to be more effective in dysphoric (i.e., uneasy, dissatisfied) patients experiencing manias.

Liver enzymes should be monitored at least weekly for the first 8 weeks of treatment, because the drug can increase levels of liver enzymes that can speed its own metabolism. In some instances, this can cause bone marrow suppression and liver inflammation. Complete blood counts should also be drawn periodically, because carbamazepine is known to cause leukopenia and aplastic anemia.

Serious and even fatal dermatological reactions—Stevens-Johnson syndrome and toxic epidermal necrolysis—have been reported. Both conditions result in erythema and death of the epidermis and mucous membranes, resulting in serious exfoliation and possible sepsis. Involvement of the mucous membranes can result in gastrointestinal hemorrhage, respiratory failure, ocular abnormalities, and genitourinary complications. These reactions occur in up to 6 per 10,000 new users of Western European descent. The risk in some Asian countries is 10 times higher because of an inherited variation of the HLA-B gene. At-risk people should be screened for this gene before beginning treatment with carbamazepine.

Lamotrigine

Lamotrigine (Lamictal) is an FDA-approved maintenance therapy medication. Patients usually tolerate lamotrigine well. It is more effective in lengthening the time between depressive episodes. The most common side effects are dizziness, ataxia, somnolence, headache, diplopia, blurred vision, and nausea.

About 8% of patients treated with lamotrigine will develop a benign rash in the first 4 months of treatment. If a rash occurs, the medication should be discontinued because of the potential for developing the potentially life-threatening Stevens-Johnson syndrome or toxic epidermal necrosis. Instruct patients to seek immediate medical attention if a rash appears.

SECOND-GENERATION ANTIPSYCHOTICS

Many of the second-generation antipsychotics are FDA approved for acute mania. In addition to showing sedative properties during the early phase of treatment thereby decreasing insomnia, anxiety, and agitation, the second-generation antipsychotics seem to have mood-stabilizing properties.

Second-generation antipsychotics may bring about serious side effects. These side effects stem from a tendency toward weight gain that may lead to insulin resistance, diabetes, dyslipidemia, and cardiovascular impairment. See Chapter 22 for a more complete discussion of antipsychotic medications and their side effects.

Benzodiazepines

Some benzodiazepines (e.g., clonazepam [Klonopin] and lorazepam [Ativan]) have been found to facilitate other antimanic treatments. These drugs are used for a limited time in treatment-resistant mania.

BIPOLAR DEPRESSION

Treatment of bipolar depression with a common antidepressant alone may increase the risk of bringing on a manic episode. This risk is significantly reduced when the antidepressant is combined with a mood stabilizer.

Specific medications are indicated for bipolar depression. The second-generation antipsychotics lurasidone (Latuda) and quetiapine (Seroquel) have FDA approval for the treatment of bipolar depression. Symbyax is another drug with approval for this type of depression. It is made up of the second-generation olanzapine (Zyprexa) and the selective serotonin reuptake inhibitor fluoxetine (Prozac).

CHAPTER 24

Antidepressants

At the cellular level major depressive disorders are caused by problems with neurotransmitters. It follows that medications that alter brain chemistry are an important component in their treatment. Antidepressant therapy is an effective strategy for most cases of major depressive disorder, particularly in severe cases. A combination of psychotherapy and antidepressant therapy is superior to either psychotherapy or pharmacological treatment alone.

ANTIDEPRESSANT DRUGS

Antidepressant drugs can positively impact poor self-concept, social withdrawal, vegetative signs of depression, and activity level. Target symptoms include the following:

- Sleep disturbance (decreased or increased)
- Appetite disturbance (decreased or increased)
- Fatigue
- Limited or absent sex drive
- Psychomotor retardation or agitation
- Diurnal variations in mood (often worse in the morning)
- Impaired concentration or memory
- Anhedonia (inability to experience pleasure)
- Feelings of guilt and self-loathing

A drawback of antidepressant drugs is that improvement in mood may take 1 to 3 weeks or longer. If a patient is acutely suicidal, a somatic treatment such as electroconvulsive therapy (discussed in Chapter 29) may be a reliable and effective alternative.

The goal of antidepressant therapy is the complete remission of symptoms. Often, the first antidepressant prescribed is not the one that will ultimately bring about remission. Aggressive treatment helps in finding the proper treatment. An adequate trial for the treatment of depression is 3 months. Individuals experiencing their first depressive episode are maintained on antidepressants for 6 to

9 months after symptoms of depression remit. Some people may have multiple episodes of depression or may have a chronic form and benefit from indefinite antidepressant therapy.

Antidepressants may precipitate a manic episode in a patient with bipolar disorder. Patients with bipolar disorder often receive a mood-stabilizing drug along with an antidepressant, which usually prevents a manic episode.

CHOOSING AN ANTIDEPRESSANT

All antidepressants work to increase the availability of one or more of the neurotransmitters—serotonin, norepinephrine, and dopamine. All antidepressants demonstrate similar efficacy in pharmaceutical trials. Each of the antidepressants has different adverse effects, costs, safety issues, and maintenance considerations. Selection of the appropriate antidepressant is based on the following considerations:

- Symptom profile of the patient
- Side effect profile (e.g., sexual dysfunction, weight gain)
- Ease of administration
- History of past response
- Safety and medical considerations

Increasingly, prescribers (e.g., psychiatric–mental health registered nurse practitioners and psychiatrists) are using drug–gene testing to help determine which drug to use. The human body uses P450 enzymes to process medications. The particular enzyme with the most variation among people is CYP2D6, which processes many antidepressants. CYP450 tests can offer clues about how an individual may respond to a new drug.

Among the information provided by drug–gene testing is the quality of drug metabolism. People fall into one of four categories:

1. Poor metabolizers are missing an enzyme, resulting in slow processing of certain drugs. This can cause the medication to build up and increase the likelihood of side effects. The medication may still be used, but at lower doses.
2. Intermediate metabolizers have reduced enzyme function, resulting in suboptimal processing of certain drugs, which can increase side effects and drug interactions.
3. Normal metabolizers (commonly referred to as extensive metabolizers) are more likely to benefit from treatment

and experience fewer side effects than those who do not process the medication as well.

4. Ultrarapid metabolizers process medications too quickly before they have a chance to work properly. Individuals in this category will require higher-than-usual doses of medications.

DISCONTINUING AN ANTIDEPRESSANT

An underrecognized problem may occur with abrupt discontinuation of antidepressant medications. This withdrawal reaction, known as discontinuation syndrome, occurs at a high rate—about 20%—in patients after taking medication for at least 6 weeks. Symptoms include flu-like aching, insomnia, nausea, imbalance, sensory disturbances, and hyperarousal. These symptoms tend to last 1 or 2 weeks, or are eliminated quickly if the drug is restarted.

The syndrome is more common with longer duration of treatment and a shorter half-life of the drug. All approved antidepressant drugs carry the potential of this problem. Nurses should assess for the syndrome and provide education to prevent it, such as slow tapering off of the antidepressant.

ANTIDEPRESSANT CLASSIFICATION

This chapter reviews several classifications of antidepressants from the most commonly prescribed groups to the least. Table 24.1 provides an overview of antidepressants used in the United States and discussed in this chapter.

Selective Serotonin Reuptake Inhibitors

The selective serotonin reuptake inhibitors (SSRIs) selectively block the neuronal uptake of serotonin (e.g., 5-HT, 5-HT_1 receptors). This blockage increases the availability of serotonin in the synaptic cleft. Some SSRIs tend to be more activating while others tend to be more sedating; the choice of drug depends, in part, on the patient's symptoms.

The first SSRI to be introduced was fluoxetine (Prozac) in 1987. This drug proved to be extremely popular and effective. Within 2 years, pharmacies were filling 65,000 fluoxetine prescriptions per month in the United States alone.

Table 24.1 **U.S. Food and Drug Administration–Approved Drugs for Major Depressive Disorder**

Generic (Trade) Name	Side Effects	Warnings
Selective Serotonin Reuptake Inhibitors (SSRIs)		
Citalopram (Celexa) Escitalopram (Lexapro) Fluoxetine (Prozac, Prozac Weekly) Paroxetine (Paxil, Paxil CR, Pexeva) Sertraline (Zoloft)	Agitation, insomnia, headache, nausea and vomiting, sexual dysfunction, hyponatremia	Discontinuation syndrome—dizziness, insomnia, nervousness, irritability, nausea, and agitation—may occur with abrupt withdrawal (depending on half-life); taper slowly.
Serotonin Norepinephrine Reuptake Inhibitors (SNRIs)		
Desvenlafaxine (Pristiq, Khedezla)	Nausea, headache, dizziness, insomnia, diarrhea, dry mouth, sweating, constipation	Neonates with in utero exposure may require respiratory support and tube feeding.
Duloxetine (Cymbalta)	Nausea, dry mouth, insomnia, somnolence, constipation, reduced appetite, fatigue, sweating, blurred vision	May reduce pain associated with depression and is approved for fibromyalgia, pain of diabetic peripheral neuropathy, and chronic musculoskeletal pain.
Levomilnacipran (Fetzima)	Nausea, orthostatic hypotension, constipation, sweating, increased heart rate, palpitations, difficulty urinating, decreased appetite, sexual dysfunction	May increase the effects of anticoagulants.

Venlafaxine (Effexor, Effexor XR)	Hypertension, nausea, insomnia, dry mouth, sedation, sweating, agitation, headache, sexual dysfunction	Monitor blood pressure, especially at higher doses and with a history of hypertension. Discontinuation syndrome.
Serotonin Antagonists and Reuptake Inhibitors (SARIs)		
Nefazodone (generic only)	Sedation, hepatotoxicity, dizziness, hypotension, paresthesias	Life-threatening liver failure is possible but rare; priapism of the penis or clitoris is a rare but serious side effect.
Trazodone (generic only) Trazodone ER (Oleptro)	Severe sedation, hypotension, nausea	Priapism has been reported.
Vilazodone (Viibryd)	Diarrhea, nausea, vomiting, dry mouth, dizziness, insomnia	Palpitations, ventricular premature beats, serotonin syndrome.
Vortioxetine (Trintellix)	Constipation, nausea, vomiting	Hyponatremia, rare induction of manic states, serotonin syndrome
Norepinephrine Dopamine Reuptake Inhibitor (NDRI)		
Bupropion (Wellbutrin, Aplenzin, Forfivo XL, Zyban for smoking cessation)	Agitation, insomnia, headache, nausea and vomiting. Sexual dysfunction is rare.	High doses increase seizure risk, especially in people who are predisposed to them.
Noradrenergic and Specific Serotonergic Antidepressant (NaSSA)		
Mirtazapine (Remeron)	Weight gain/appetite stimulation, sedation, dizziness, headache; sexual dysfunction is rare	Drug-induced somnolence exaggerated by alcohol, benzodiazepines, and other central nervous system depressants.

Continued

Table 24.1 **U.S. Food and Drug Administration–Approved Drugs for Major Depressive Disorder—cont'd**

Generic (Trade) Name	Side Effects	Warnings
Tricyclic Antidepressants (TCAs)		
Amitriptyline (generic only) Amoxapine (generic only) Desipramine (Norpramin) Doxepin (Sinequan) Imipramine (Tofranil) Maprotiline (generic only) Nortriptyline (Aventyl, Pamelor) Protriptyline (Vivactil) Trimipramine (Surmontil)	Dry mouth, constipation, urinary retention, blurred vision, hypotension, cardiac toxicity, sedation	Lethal in overdose; use cautiously in the elderly and with cardiac disorders, elevated intraocular pressure, urinary retention, hyperthyroidism, seizure disorders, and liver or kidney dysfunction.
Monoamine Oxidase Inhibitors (MAOIs)		
Isocarboxazid (Marplan) Phenelzine (Nardil) Selegiline (Eldepryl, EMSAM - Transdermal System Patch) Tranylcypromine (Parnate)	Insomnia, nausea, agitation, and confusion; hypertensive crisis	Contraindicated in people taking SSRIs, used cautiously in people taking TCAs; tyramine-rich food could bring about a hypertensive crisis. Many other strong drug and dietary interactions.

From U.S. Food and Drug Administration. (2017). FDA online label repository. Retrieved from www.labels.fda.gov

Indications

SSRIs are commonly the first-line treatment in depression. In addition to their use in treating depressive disorders, the SSRIs are prescribed for anxiety disorders. Generalized anxiety disorder, panic disorder, social anxiety disorder, and obsessive–compulsive disorder are all treated with U.S. Food and Drug Administration (FDA) approved SSRIs. Fluoxetine (Prozac) has FDA approval for bulimia nervosa. Fluoxetine, sertraline (Zoloft), and controlled-release paroxetine (Paxil CR) have FDA approval for the treatment of premenstrual dysphoric disorder. Another paroxetine, Brisdelle, is used to treat moderate to severe vasomotor symptoms (e.g., hot flashes, night sweats) associated with menopause.

Common Adverse Reactions

Agents that selectively enhance synaptic serotonin within the central nervous system (CNS) may induce agitation, anxiety, sleep disturbance, tremor, sexual dysfunction (primarily anorgasmia), or tension headache. Autonomic reactions (e.g., dry mouth, sweating, weight change, mild nausea, and loose bowel movements) may also be experienced with the SSRIs.

Potential Toxic Effects

A rare and life-threatening event associated with SSRIs, and by any of the antidepressants that increase serotonin, is serotonin syndrome. This syndrome is related to overactivation of the central serotonin receptors caused by either too high a dose or interaction with other drugs. Many symptoms are possible: abdominal pain, diarrhea, sweating, fever, tachycardia, elevated blood pressure, altered mental state (delirium), myoclonus (muscle spasms), increased motor activity, irritability, hostility, and mood change. Severe manifestations can induce hyperpyrexia (excessively high fever), cardiovascular shock, or death.

The risk of this syndrome seems to be greatest when an SSRI is administered in combination with a second serotonin-enhancing agent, such as a monoamine oxidase inhibitor (MAOI). A patient should discontinue all SSRIs for 2 to 5 weeks before starting an MAOI. Box 24.1 lists the signs of serotonin syndrome and provides emergency treatment guidelines.

Box 24.1 Signs of Serotonin Syndrome and Treatment Guidelines

Signs

- Hyperactivity or restlessness
- Tachycardia → cardiovascular shock
- Fever → hyperpyrexia
- Elevated blood pressure
- Altered mental states (delirium)
- Irrationality, mood swings, hostility
- Seizures → status epilepticus
- Myoclonus, incoordination, tonic rigidity
- Abdominal pain, diarrhea, bloating
- Apnea → death

Interventions

- Discontinue offending agent(s)
- Initiate symptomatic treatment:
  - Serotonin-receptor blockade with cyproheptadine, methysergide, propranolol
  - Cooling blankets
  - Dantrolene, diazepam for muscle rigidity or rigors
  - Anticonvulsants
  - Artificial ventilation
  - Induction of paralysis

Serotonin Norepinephrine Reuptake Inhibitors

Serotonin norepinephrine reuptake inhibitors (SNRIs) increase both serotonin and norepinephrine. Venlafaxine (Effexor) acts more like a serotonergic agent at lower therapeutic doses and promotes norepinephrine reuptake blockade at higher doses, leading to the dual SNRI action. Hypertension may be induced in about 5% of patients and is a dose-dependent effect based on norepinephrine reuptake blockade. Doses greater than 150 mg a day can increase diastolic blood pressure by approximately 7 to 10 mm Hg. In addition to treating depression, venlafaxine has FDA approval for treating generalized anxiety disorder, panic disorder, and social anxiety disorder.

Desvenlafaxine (Pristiq) is the primary active metabolite of venlafaxine. When people take venlafaxine, most benefit comes from venlafaxine being metabolized into desvenlafaxine. Therefore the mechanism of action and side effects of the two antidepressants are similar. Nausea is a prominent side effect of this drug.

Duloxetine (Cymbalta) is an SNRI that has FDA approval for both depression and generalized anxiety disorder. It is also approved for treating diabetic peripheral neuropathy, fibromyalgia, and chronic musculoskeletal pain.

Levomilnacipran (Fetzima) is an SNRI with a greater effect on norepinephrine reuptake than the other SNRIs. Increasing norepinephrine may be responsible for increases in heart rate and blood pressure in some patients.

Serotonin Antagonist and Reuptake Inhibitors

Nefazodone, formerly sold under the name Serzone, is a novel drug indicated only for depression. It is a serotonin antagonist and reuptake inhibitor (SARI) that works by blocking serotonin receptors and weakly inhibiting the reuptake of norepinephrine and serotonin. The most common side effects are sedation, headache, fatigue, dry mouth, nausea, constipation, dizziness, and blurred vision. Weight gain and sexual dysfunction are minimal. This drug should be used with caution to prevent life-threatening liver failure and should never be given to people with preexisting liver problems. Early detection of drug-induced hepatic injury and immediate withdrawal of the drug increases the likelihood for recovery.

Trazodone, formerly sold under the name Desyrel, is a weak antidepressant often prescribed for the treatment of insomnia, because sedation is one of its common side effects. A trademarked version, Oleptro, has FDA approval as an extended-release drug indicated for the use of major depressive disorder in adults. Its antidepressant effects are related to its action as a 5-HT reuptake inhibitor and 5-HT2A/2C antagonist.

Common side effects of trazodone are sedation, dizziness, and orthostatic hypotension. Potent alpha-1 antagonists with little anticholinergic effects, such as trazodone, can lead to priapism. Priapism is a painful prolonged penile or clitoral erection.

Vilazodone (Viibryd) enhances the release of serotonin by inhibiting the serotonin transporter (similar to SSRIs) and by stimulating serotonin (5-HT1A) receptors through partial agonism (similar to the antianxiety medication buspirone [BuSpar]). Weight gain is not associated with this drug and sexual side effects are limited. Patients should take this antidepressant with food for better bioavailability and avoid nighttime doses to prevent insomnia. Common side effects include diarrhea, nausea, insomnia, and vomiting. Vilazodone should be used with caution in people taking medications that affect coagulation since it can increase the risk of bleeding. The decision to use vilazodone in pregnant or nursing women should take into account the potential risks to the fetus or baby versus the benefit to the mother.

Vortioxetine (Trintellix) has a similar side effect and contraindication profile to vilazodone. Nausea is the most common reason identified for discontinuing vortioxetine treatment. Constipation and vomiting have also been reported.

Norepinephrine Dopamine Reuptake Inhibitor

Bupropion (Wellbutrin) is an antidepressant also used for smoking cessation (Zyban). It acts as a norepinephrine and dopamine reuptake inhibitor (NDRI). With no serotonergic activities, it carries a lower risk of sexual dysfunction than most other antidepressants. Side effects include insomnia, tremor, anorexia, and weight loss. It is contraindicated in patients with a seizure disorder, in patients with a current or prior diagnosis of bulimia or anorexia nervosa, and in patients undergoing abrupt discontinuation of alcohol or sedatives (including benzodiazepines) because of the potential for seizures.

Norepinephrine and Specific Serotonin Antidepressant

The class of drugs known as the norepinephrine and specific serotonin antidepressant (NaSSA) is represented by only one drug, mirtazapine (Remeron). Mirtazapine increases norepinephrine and serotonin transmission by antagonizing (blocking) presynaptic alpha-2 adrenergic receptors. This drug provides both antianxiety and antidepressant effects with minimal sexual dysfunction, fewer gastrointestinal symptoms, and improved sleep. Common side effects are sedation, appetite stimulation, and weight gain. This drug should be used with caution in patients with renal and hepatic insufficiency.

Tricyclic Antidepressants

The tricyclic antidepressants (TCAs) inhibit the reuptake of norepinephrine and serotonin by the presynaptic neurons in the CNS, increasing the amount of time norepinephrine and serotonin are available to the postsynaptic receptors. This increase in norepinephrine and serotonin in the brain is believed to be responsible for mood elevations. They also block the actions of acetylcholine, and some TCAs also affect histamine.

The first TCAs were imipramine (Tofranil) and amitriptyline formerly sold as Elavil). These tricyclic antidepressants were introduced in the early 1960s.

Patients must take therapeutic doses of TCAs for 10 to 14 days or longer before they begin to work. Full effects may not be seen for 4 to 8 weeks. Positive effects on some symptoms of depression, such as insomnia and anorexia, may be noted earlier

Indications

The TCAs are all indicated for the treatment of depression. Side effect profiles are taken into account when choosing a particular TCA. A stimulating TCA, such as desipramine (Norpramin) or protriptyline (Vivactil), may be best for a patient who is lethargic and fatigued. If a more sedating effect is needed for agitation or restlessness, drugs such as amitriptyline and doxepin (Sinequan) may be more appropriate choices. Regardless of which TCA is given, the initial dose should always be low and be increased gradually.

Common Adverse Reactions

The chemical structure of the TCAs closely resembles that of antipsychotic medications, and the anticholinergic actions are similar (e.g., dry mouth, blurred vision, tachycardia, constipation, urinary retention, and esophageal reflux). These side effects are more common and more severe in patients taking antidepressants. They usually are not serious and are often transitory, but urinary retention and severe constipation require immediate medical attention. Weight gain is also a common complaint among people taking TCAs.

The alpha-adrenergic blockade of the TCAs can produce orthostatic hypotension and tachycardia. Hypotension can lead to dizziness and increase the risk of falls. For this reason older adults on TCAs must be monitored carefully for dizziness and fall risk.

The sedative effects of the TCAs are attributed to the blockade of histamine receptors. Administering the total daily dose of TCA at night is beneficial for two reasons. First, most TCAs have sedative effects and thereby aid sleep. Second, the minor side effects occur while the individual is sleeping, which increases compliance with drug therapy.

Potential Toxic Effects

The most serious effects of the TCAs are cardiovascular: dysrhythmias, tachycardia, myocardial infarction, and heart block. Because the cardiac side effects are so serious, TCA use is considered a risk in older adults and patients with cardiac disease. Patients should have a thorough cardiac workup before beginning TCA therapy.

One of the most troubling aspects of TCAs are their potential for poisoning through overdose. Choosing this classification of antidepressant should be accomplished by carefully weighing out the risks versus the benefits.

Adverse Drug Interactions

A few of the more common medications usually *not* given while TCAs are being used are MAOIs, phenothiazines, barbiturates, disulfiram (Antabuse), oral contraceptives (or other estrogen preparations), anticoagulants, some antihypertensives (clonidine, guanethidine, reserpine), benzodiazepines, and alcohol. A patient who is taking any of these medications along with a TCA should have medical clearance, because some of the reactions can be fatal.

Contraindications

People who have recently had a myocardial infarction (or other cardiovascular problems), those with narrow-angle glaucoma or a history of seizures, and women who are pregnant should not be treated with TCAs except with extreme caution and careful monitoring.

Monoamine Oxidase Inhibitors

The enzyme monoamine oxidase is responsible for inactivating, or breaking down, monoamine neurotransmitters in the brain such as norepinephrine, serotonin, dopamine, and tyramine. When a person takes an MAOI, fewer amines get inactivated, resulting in an increase of the mood-elevating neurotransmitters.

Monoamine oxidase is also responsible for breaking down tyramine, an amino acid that helps regulate blood pressure. Tyramine occurs naturally in the body and is found in certain foods. The inability to break down tyramine normally can result in a serious problem. Certain foods are quite rich in tyramine. Individuals who take MAOIs and eat these foods are at risk for a hypertensive crisis, which is discussed below under potential toxic effects. People taking these drugs must reduce or eliminate their intake of foods that contain high amounts of tyramine. Table 24.2 identifies unsafe and safe foods for people taking MAOIs.

Indications

MAOIs are particularly effective for people with unconventional depression (characterized by mood reactivity, oversleeping, and overeating), as well as panic disorder, social phobia, generalized anxiety disorder, obsessive–compulsive disorder, posttraumatic stress disorder, and bulimia. MAOIs with FDA approval are phenelzine (Nardil), tranylcypromine (Parnate), and isocarboxazid (Marplan). A transdermal patch, selegiline (EMSAM), does not require strict dietary restrictions at its lowest dose.

Common Adverse Reactions

Some common and troublesome long-term side effects of the MAOIs are orthostatic hypotension, weight gain, edema, change in cardiac rate and rhythm, constipation, urinary hesitancy, sexual dysfunction, vertigo, overactivity, muscle twitching, insomnia, weakness, and fatigue. Hypomania and mania may be activated with MAOIs.

Potential Toxic Effects

The most serious reaction to the MAOIs is an increase in blood pressure with the possible development of intracranial hemorrhage, hyperpyrexia, convulsions, coma, and death. Therefore routine monitoring of blood pressure, especially during the first 6 weeks of treatment, is necessary.

Because many drugs, foods, and beverages can increase blood pressure in patients taking MAOIs, hypertensive

Table 24.2 **Safe and Unsafe Foods With Monoamine Oxidase Inhibitors**

Category	Unsafe Foods (High Tyramine Content)	Safe Foods (Little or No Tyramine)
Vegetables	Avocados, especially if overripe; fermented bean curd; fermented soybean; soybean paste	Most vegetables
Fruits	Figs, especially if overripe; bananas, in large amounts	Most fruits
Meats	Meats that are fermented, smoked, or otherwise aged; spoiled meats; liver, unless very fresh	Meats that are known to be fresh (exercise caution in restaurants; meats may not be fresh)
Sausages	Fermented varieties; bologna, pepperoni, salami, others	Non-fermented varieties
Fish	Dried or cured fish; fish that is fermented, smoked, or otherwise aged; spoiled fish	Fish that is known to be fresh; vacuum-packed fish, if eaten promptly or refrigerated only briefly after opening
Milk, milk products	Practically all cheeses	Milk, yogurt, cottage cheese, cream cheese
Foods with yeast	Yeast extract (e.g., Marmite, Bovril)	Baked goods that contain yeast
Beer, wine	Some imported beers, Chianti wines	Major domestic brands of beer; most wines
Other foods	Protein dietary supplements; soups (may contain protein extract); shrimp paste; soy sauce	

Foods That Contain Other Nontyramine Vasopressors

Food	Comments
Chocolate	Contains phenylethylamine, a pressor agent; large amounts can cause a reaction.
Fava beans	Contain dopamine, a pressor agent; reactions are most likely with overripe beans.
Ginseng	Headache, tremulousness, and mania-like reactions have occurred.
Caffeine	Caffeine is a weak pressor agent; large amounts may cause a reaction.

From Burchum, J.R., & Rosenthal, L.D. (2016). *Lehne's pharmacology for nursing care* (9th ed.). St. Louis, MO: Elsevier.

Table 24.3 **Adverse Reactions to and Toxic Effects of Monoamine Oxidase Inhibitors**

Adverse Reactions	Comments
Hypotension Sedation, weakness, fatigue Insomnia Changes in cardiac rhythm Muscle cramps Anorgasmia or sexual impotence Urinary hesitancy or constipation Weight gain	Hypotension is an expected side effect. Orthostatic blood pressures should be taken—first lying down, then sitting or standing after 1–2 minutes. This may be a dangerous side effect, especially in older adults who may fall and sustain injuries as a result of dizziness from the blood pressure drop.
Toxic Effects	**Comments**
Hypertensive crisis: Severe headache Tachycardia, palpitations Hypertension Nausea and vomiting	Patient should go to local emergency department immediately—blood pressure should be checked. One of the following may be given to lower blood pressure: 5 mg intravenous phentolamine or sublingual nifedipine to promote vasodilation. Patients may be prescribed a 10-mg nifedipine capsule to carry in case of emergency.

crisis is a constant concern. The hypertensive crisis usually occurs within 15 to 90 minutes of ingestion of the contraindicated substance. Early symptoms include irritability, anxiety, flushing, sweating, and a severe headache. The patient then becomes anxious and restless and develops a fever. Eventually the fever becomes severe, seizures ensue, and coma or death are possible.

When a hypertensive crisis is suspected, immediate medical attention is crucial. If ingestion is recent, gastric lavage and charcoal may be helpful. Pyrexia is treated with hypothermic blankets or ice packs. Fluid therapy is essential, particularly with hyperthermia. A short-acting antihypertensive agent such as nitroprusside, nitroglycerine, or phentolamine may be used. Intravenous benzodiazepines are useful for agitation and seizure control.

Table 24.3 identifies common side effects and toxic effects of the MAOIs.

Contraindications

The use of MAOIs may be contraindicated with the following:

- Cerebrovascular disease
- Hypertension and congestive heart failure
- Liver disease
- Consumption of foods containing tyramine, tryptophan, and dopamine
- Use of certain medications
- Recurrent or severe headaches
- Surgery in the previous 10 to 14 days
- Age younger than 16 years

ANTIDEPRESSANT USE IN SPECIAL POPULATIONS

Use of Antidepressants by Pregnant Women

The risk of depression in pregnant women may be as high as 20% (Olivier et al., 2015). There is evidence that depression has a negative effect on birth outcomes. Preeclampsia, diabetes, and hypertension have all been associated with maternal depression. Low birth weight, preterm birth, and small size for gestational age have been noted effects in infants born to depressed mothers. Antidepressants cross the placenta. The benefits of treatment of severe depression, particularly with suicidal ideation, must outweigh the risks.

Black Box Warning for Children and Adolescents

Although antidepressant medications undoubtedly help children and adolescents with depression, there has been some concern that they may actually induce suicidal behavior in young people. In 2004 the FDA issued a public warning about an increased risk of suicidal thoughts or behavior in children and adolescents treated with SSRIs. A 2007 metaanalysis (Bridge et al.) reviewed 2200 children treated with SSRIs. No completed suicides occurred. However, 4% of these children experienced suicidal thinking or behavior, including suicide attempts at twice the rate of the control group.

In response to this study, the FDA adopted a black box label warning, the most serious type of warning in prescription drug labeling. The label states that antidepressants may increase the risk of suicidal thinking and behavior in some children and adolescents with major depressive disorder. Young people taking SSRIs should be closely monitored for worsening depression, emergence of suicidal thinking or behavior, or unusual changes in behavior such as agitation. This close monitoring is recommended during the first 4 weeks of treatment and during dose changes.

Use of Antidepressants by Older Adults

Polypharmacy and the normal metabolic processes of aging contribute to concerns about prescribing antidepressants for older adults. SSRIs are a first-line treatment for older adults, but they have the potential for aggravated side effects. Starting doses are recommended to be half the lowest adult dose, with dose adjustments occurring no more frequently than every 7 days ("start low and go slow").

Despite the conventional wisdom that SSRIs are safest for older adults, some research is beginning to call this practice into question. In a 2011 study (Coupland et al.), researchers reviewed records of nearly 70,000 older adults. All of the adults in the study had diagnoses of depression. Researchers reviewed adverse events in the participants. They found that the greatest risk during the course of a year came from SSRIs, followed by TCAs, and that taking no medication posed the lowest risk in this population.

Cardiotoxicity is possible with TCAs, and hypotension is common with both TCAs and MAOIs. Any medication with a side effect of hypotension or sedation in older adults increases the risk of falls. Older adults should be cautioned against abrupt discontinuation of antidepressants because of the possibility of discontinuation syndrome, which causes anxiety, dysphoria, flu-like symptoms, dizziness, excessive sweating, and insomnia.

CHAPTER 25

Antianxiety Medications

Anxiety disorders are chronic and incurable conditions, but they are treatable in most cases. Psychopharmacology is an important adjunct to use with other therapies, especially cognitive–behavioral therapy (CBT). Several classes of medications have been found to be effective in the treatment of anxiety disorders.

- Selective serotonin reuptake inhibitors (SSRIs) are the first-line treatment for all anxiety disorders, especially panic disorders.
- Serotonin norepinephrine reuptake inhibitors (SNRIs) are becoming increasingly popular for anxiety disorders.
- Antianxiety agents such as benzodiazepines are quite effective but should be used short term; they are not recommended for use by patients with substance use problems.
- Buspirone (BuSpar) can be used for long-term management of generalized anxiety disorder and is ideal for individuals who may have substance use problems.

Table 25.1 summarizes medications approved by the U.S. Food and Drug Administration (FDA) for the treatment of anxiety disorders.

ANTIDEPRESSANTS

SSRIs are considered the first line of defense in most anxiety and obsessive–compulsive–related disorders. These SSRIs include paroxetine (Paxil), fluoxetine (Prozac), escitalopram (Lexapro), fluvoxamine (Luvox), and sertraline (Zoloft). Some of these antidepressants exert more of an activating effect than others and may actually increase anxiety initially. Fluoxetine and sertraline tend to be the most activating. Paroxetine seems to have a more calming effect than the other SSRIs. Antidepressants have the secondary benefit of treating comorbid depressive disorders.

Table 25.1 **FDA Approved Drugs for the Treatment of Anxiety Disorders**

Anxiety Disorder	Selective Serotonin Reuptake Inhibitors	Serotonin Norepinephrine Reuptake Inhibitors	Benzodiazepines	Other
Generalized anxiety disorder	Escitalopram (Lexapro) Paroxetine (Paxil)	Venlafaxine (Effexor) Duloxetine[a] (Cymbalta)	Alprazolam (Xanax) Chlordiazepoxide (Librium) Clorazepate (Tranxene) Diazepam (Valium) Lorazepam (Ativan) Oxazepam (Serax)	Buspirone (BuSpar)
Panic disorder	Fluoxetine (Prozac) Paroxetine (Paxil) Sertraline (Zoloft)	Venlafaxine (Effexor)	Alprazolam (Xanax) Clonazepam (Klonopin)	
Social anxiety disorder	Paroxetine (Paxil) Sertraline (Zoloft)	Venlafaxine (Effexor)		
Obsessive–compulsive disorder	Fluoxetine[a] (Prozac) Fluvoxamine[b] (Luvox) Paroxetine (Paxil) Sertraline[c] (Zoloft)			Clomipramine[d] [x](Anafranil)

[a]Approved for children and adolescents age 7 to 17 years.
[b]Approved for children and adolescents age 8 to 17 years.
[c]Approved for children and adolescents age 6 years and up.
[d]Approved for children and adolescents age 10 years and up.
From U.S. Food and Drug Administration. (2017). FDA online label repository. Retrieved from www.labels.fda.gov

Venlafaxine (Effexor) is an SNRI that is quite successful in the treatment of several anxiety disorders. Another SNRI, duloxetine (Cymbalta), is effective in the treatment of generalized anxiety disorder.

Monoamine oxidase inhibitors (MAOIs) are reserved for treatment-resistant conditions. A life-threatening hypertensive crisis could occur if the patient does not follow dietary restrictions of avoiding tyramine-containing foods. Patients must be given specific dietary instructions. The risk of hypertensive crisis also makes the use of MAOIs contraindicated in patients with comorbid substance use disorders. See Chapter 24 for more information about the MAOIs and other antidepressant medications.

ANTIANXIETY DRUGS

Antianxiety drugs are often used to treat the somatic and psychological symptoms of anxiety disorders. Benzodiazepines are most commonly used because they have a quick onset of action. When moderate or severe anxiety is reduced, patients are better able to participate in treatment of their underlying problems. Despite the fitting name of this classification of drugs for treating anxiety disorder, they are actually second-line treatment options. As U.S. Drug Enforcement Administration schedule IV controlled substances, there is potential for misuse and physical habituation. Ideally, these drugs should be used for short periods until other medications or treatments reduce symptoms.

An important nursing intervention is to monitor for side effects of benzodiazepines, including sedation, ataxia, and decreased cognitive function. Paradoxical reactions—reactions that are the exact opposite of intended responses—sometimes occur. Symptoms such as anxiety, agitation, talkativeness, and loss of impulse control may occur when using this classification of medications. Benzodiazepines are not recommended for patients with a substance use disorder and should not be given to women during pregnancy or breast-feeding. They are not recommended for older adult patients because of the risk of delirium, falls, and fractures.

These medications require tapering if used long term to avoid withdrawal effects. Tapering can last weeks to months depending on the circumstance, namely the dose and half-life of the drug and duration of therapy. Since these drugs are depressants, rebound hyperactivity occurs with sudden removal of the substance. Hence, autonomic hyperactivity, tremor, insomnia, psychomotor agitation, anxiety, and grand mal seizures can occur. Benzodiazepine withdrawal is unusual in that symptoms tend to wax and wane from day to day and week to week.

Buspirone (BuSpar) is an alternative antianxiety medication that does not cause dependence and is not a controlled substance. It takes 2 to 4 weeks for it to reach full effects. Buspirone may be used for long-term treatment and should be taken regularly.

OTHER CLASSES OF MEDICATIONS

Other classes of medications sometimes used to treat anxiety disorders include beta-blockers, antihistamines, anticonvulsants, and antipsychotics. These agents are often added if the first course of treatment is ineffective. Beta-blockers block the receptors that, when stimulated, cause the heart to beat faster and have been used to treat social anxiety disorder. Medications such as propranolol (Inderal) reduce physical manifestations of anxiety such as slowing the heart rate and reducing blushing.

Anticonvulsants have shown some benefit in the management of generalized anxiety disorder and social anxiety disorder. Gabapentin (Neurontin) and pregabalin (Lyrica), for example, have been studied and are commonly prescribed.

Antihistamines can be a safe, nonaddictive alternative to reducing anxiety levels. They may be helpful in treating patients with concurrent substance use problems. Hydroxyzine (Vistaril) is an effective short-term (up to 4 months) antianxiety agent. A commonly used antihistamine, diphenhydramine (Benadryl), can be used to treat sleep loss associated with anxiety based on its significant sedative properties.

The antihistamines are also anticholinergics, that is, they block the binding of acetylcholine to neural receptors. Anticholinergic side effects, including dry mouth, constipation, and cognitive effects, should be monitored. These drugs should be avoided or used with caution in older adults since the body's production of acetylcholine diminishes with age. A large-scale study by Risacher and colleagues (2016) demonstrated brain atrophy, dysfunction, and clinical decline in older adults who use anticholinergic drugs and recommend against their use in this population.

Antipsychotic medications are effective in treating more severe symptoms of anxiety disorders. The risks of metabolic side effects, as well as the consequences of the dopamine blockade, significantly reduce the use of antipsychotics for anxiety disorders. The FDA has not approved any antipsychotics for these disorders.

HERBAL THERAPY AND INTEGRATIVE APPROACHES

Herbal therapy and dietary supplements are commonly used, but they are not subject to the same rigorous testing as prescription medications. Also, herbs and dietary supplements may not be uniformly prepared or dosed, and there is no guarantee of bioequivalence of the active compound among preparations. Problems that can occur with the use of psychotropic herbs include toxic side effects and herb–drug interactions. Nurses and other health care providers should improve their knowledge of these products so that discussions with their patients provide informed and reliable information.

One example is kava (or kava-kava), which is derived from the roots of *Piper methysticum,* a South American plant is used as a sedative with antianxiety effects. Before seeking professional care, people with anxiety disorders may try kava in the belief that herbs are safer than medications. Kava supplements have been found to exert a small effect on reducing anxiety

However, in 2010 the FDA issued a warning regarding a correlation between kava's use and a risk of liver damage. Kava is known to dramatically inhibit a liver enzyme (P450) necessary for the metabolism of many medications. This inhibition could result in liver failure, especially when taken along with alcohol or other medications such as central nervous system depressants (antianxiety agents fall into this category). Long-term use of high doses of kava has also been associated with dry, scaly skin or yellowing of the skin.

Valerian is a perennial flowering plant that is used for conditions related to anxiety and psychological stress, but it is most commonly used for insomnia and anxiety. Although it has proven effective for insomnia, there is insufficient scientific evidence to rate its safety. Unlike kava, valerian is considered safe for most people when used in medicinal

Table 25.2 **Essential Oils Used in Mental Health–Related Concerns**

Essential Oil	Use
Roman chamomile	Relieving anxiety
Clary sage	Relaxing and relieving anxiety
Lavender	Calming and decreasing anxiety
Mandarin	Calming
Neroli	Relieving and decreasing anxiety
Rose	Relieving and decreasing anxiety
Vetiver	Calming

From National Association of Holistic Aromatherapy. (2016). *Most commonly used essential oils.* Retrieved from www.naha.org/explore-aromatherapy/about-aromatherapy/most-commonly-used-essential-oils

amounts on a short-term basis. Some side effects of valerian are headaches, excitability, uneasiness, and even insomnia.

German chamomile is an herb whose flowers are used to make a supplement that has been used for generalized anxiety disorder. There have been reports of allergic reactions, including rare cases of anaphylaxis, in response to chamomile products. Allergies to other ragweed plants seem to predispose people to such reactions.

Essential oils that are either inhaled or massaged into the skin. may also reduce anxiety and stress. Table 25.2 provides an overview of anxiety- and stress-relieving oils.

ANXIETY TREATMENT USE IN SPECIAL POPULATIONS

Anxiety Treatment in Children

A few drugs are approved specifically for anxiety and obsessive–compulsive disorders in children and adolescents. The FDA approved the SNRI duloxetine (Cymbalta) in 2014 for children aged 7 to 17 years for generalized anxiety disorder. The FDA has approved four medications for use in children with obsessive–compulsive disorder. They are clomipramine (Anafranil), fluoxetine (Prozac), fluvoxamine (Luvox), and sertraline (Zoloft).

However, medications approved for other age groups are still prescribed off label without specific FDA approval. SSRIs are being used for generalized anxiety disorder, panic disorder, and social anxiety disorder with good results.

They are also often used for children with obsessive–compulsive and related disorders.

Anxiety Treatment in Older Adults

Anxiety disorders are just as common in older adults as in younger people. The most common anxiety disorder in this population is generalized anxiety disorder. The treatment adage of "start low and go slow" is important due to changes in drug absorption and action in the aging body. Medications such as antidepressants are begun with one-half or one-quarter of the usual starting dose and increased slowly.

CHAPTER 26

Sleep-Promoting Medications

Many patients use medication to address their sleep problems. Nurses frequently provide education about the purpose, benefits, and side effects of sleep-promoting medications. Nurses explain that medications are usually prescribed for no more than 2 weeks, because tolerance and withdrawal may result. In many settings, the nurse also monitors the effectiveness of the medication.

This chapter focuses on medications used to promote sleep. Table 26.1 provides an overview of pharmacological treatment of insomnia with U.S. Food and Drug Administration (FDA) approval. Over-the-counter and herbal and dietary sleep aids are briefly discussed. Other classifications of drugs are used off-label without specific FDA approval to promote sleep. These drugs include antidepressants, anticonvulsants, and antihistamines. Second-generation antipsychotics improve sleep in people using them for other problems such as schizophrenia.

BENZODIAZEPINES

Benzodiazepines potentiate, or promote, the activity of gamma-aminobutyric acid (GABA) by binding to a specific site on the GABA receptor complex. This binding results in an increased frequency of chloride channel opening causing membrane hyperpolarization, which reduces the cellular excitation. If cellular excitation is decreased, the result is a calming effect.

All benzodiazepines can cause sedation at higher therapeutic doses. There are five benzodiazepines approved by the FDA for treatment of insomnia with a predominantly hypnotic (sleep-inducing) effect: estazolam (ProSom), flurazepam (Dalmane), quazepam (Doral), temazepam (Restoril), and triazolam (Halcion).

Table 26.1 **FDA Approved Drugs for Insomnia**

Generic (Trade) Name	Onset of Action (min)	Duration of Action	Use in Insomnia		Habit Forming?
			DFA	DMS	
Benzodiazepines					
Estazolam (ProSom)	15–60	Intermediate	✔	✔	Yes, all drugs in this class are schedule IV.
Flurazepam (Dalmane)[a]	30–60	Long	✔	✔	
Quazepam (Doral)[a]	20–45	Long	✔	✔	
Temazepam (Restoril)	45–60	Intermediate	–	✔	
Triazolam(Halcion)	15–30	Short	✔	–	
Nonbenzodiazepine Receptor Agonists					
Eszopiclone (Lunesta)	60	Intermediate	✔	✔	Yes, all drugs in this class are schedule IV.
Zaleplon (Sonata)	15–30	Ultra short	✔	–	
Zolpidem immediate release (Ambien)	30	Short	✔	–	
Immediate release (Intermezzo)[b]	30	Short	–	✔	
Extended release (Ambien CR)	30	Intermediate	✔	✔	
Melatonin Receptor Agonist					
Ramelteon (Rozerem)	30	Short	✔	–	No
Orexin Receptor Antagonist					
Suvorexant (Belsomra)	30	Intermediate	✔	✔	Yes, schedule IV.
Tricyclic Antidepressant					
Doxepin (Silenor)	>60	Intermediate	–	✔	No

DFA, Difficulty falling asleep; *DMS*, difficulty maintaining sleep.
[a]This drug is generally not recommended due to its long duration of action.
[b]A sublingual taken in the middle of the night when there are at least 4 hours left to sleep.
From U.S Food and Drug Administration. (2015). Drug label repository/. Retrieved from https://labels.fda.gov/.

Nurses must caution patients taking benzodiazepines about engaging in activities that could be dangerous if reflexes and attention are impaired, including activities, such as working in construction or driving a car. In older adults, the use of benzodiazepines may contribute to falls and bone fractures since ataxia is a common side effect secondary to the abundance of GABA receptors in the cerebellum.

This class of drugs may be misused and are categorized as schedule IV drugs by the U.S. Drug Enforcement Administration (DEA). Craving, tolerance, and withdrawal can develop even when taken for their intended indication. See Chapter 12 for more discussion of sedative-, hypnotic-, and anxiolytic-related substance use disorders.

When used alone these drugs rarely inhibit the brain to the degree of respiratory depression, coma, and death. However, when combined with other central nervous system (CNS) depressants, such as alcohol, opiates, or tricyclic antidepressants, the inhibitory actions of the benzodiazepines can lead to life-threatening CNS depression.

NONBENZODIAZEPINE RECEPTOR AGONISTS

The Z-hypnotics include eszopiclone (Lunesta), zaleplon (Sonata), and zolpidem (Ambien). Zolpidem comes in two additional types. Intermezzo is an immediate release drug and is used to help people fall back to sleep if they wake in the middle of the night. Ambien CR has two separate layers, one that dissolves quickly and promotes falling asleep, and the other dissolves more slowly to help in continuing sleep.

They have sedative effects without the antianxiety, anticonvulsant, or muscle relaxant effects of benzodiazepines. They are selective for $GABA_A$ receptors containing alpha-1 subunits. The drugs' affinity to alpha-1 subunits confers the potential for amnestic and ataxic side effects.

It is important to inform patients taking this classification of drugs about their quick onset of action and to take them only when they are ready to go to sleep. These drugs have short half-lives. Eszopiclone has the longest duration of action (an average of 7 to 8 hours of sleep) while the other two are shorter. Eszopiclone also has a unique side effect of an unpleasant bitter taste upon awakening.

Tolerance and dependence are less frequent than with benzodiazepines. Still, the Z-hypnotics are categorized as schedule IV by the DEA. There have been reports of sleep-walking, -eating, and even-driving with the Z-hypnotics. These CNS adverse effects have been reported with other hypnotics as well. Doses for immediate-release zolpidem are lower for women and older adults.

MELATONIN RECEPTOR AGONIST

Melatonin is a hormone that is only excreted at night as part of the normal circadian rhythm. Ramelteon (Rozerem) is a melatonin (MT) receptor agonist and acts much the same way as natural melatonin. It has a high selectivity and potency at the MT1 receptor site—which regulates sleepiness—and at the MT2 receptor site—which regulates circadian rhythms.

This medication is not classified as a scheduled substance since it lacks potential for misuse. Side effects include headache and dizziness. Long-term use of ramelteon above therapeutic doses can lead to increased prolactin and associated side effects (e.g., sexual dysfunction).

OREXIN RECEPTOR AGONIST

Orexin is a neurotransmitter produced in the hypothalamus that promotes normal wakefulness. Suvorexant (Belsomra) is an orexin receptor antagonist approved for its properties of selectively blocking the binding of orexin to suppress wakefulness.

Suvorexant may result in daytime impairment, making activities such as driving dangerous. When taken with other CNS depressants, this drug will increase the intensity of sleepiness. Sleep paralysis, hypnagogic (immediately before sleep) and hypnopompic (immediately before waking) hallucinations and cataplexy (loss of muscle tone) have been reported as side effects of suvorexant. Abnormal thinking, behavioral changes, worsening of depression, and increased suicidal ideation have also occurred while taking this drug.

TRICYCLIC ANTIDEPRESSANT

Doxepin (Silenor) is the low-dose formulation of an old tricyclic antidepressant. Doxepin has FDA approval for the treatment of insomnia characterized by difficulty in maintaining sleep. The mechanism of action for its sedative effect is most likely from a strong histamine-1 receptor blockade.

Patients with severe urinary retention or on monoamine oxidase inhibitors (MAOIs) should avoid this medication. The use of other CNS depressants and sedating antihistamines should also be avoided. Doxepin has mainly been studied in the older adult population where it showed an improvement in total sleep duration with no significant decrease in time of sleep onset.

OVER-THE-COUNTER SLEEP AIDS

People use a variety of over-the-counter sleep aids to get a good night's sleep. Many of these drugs contain diphenhydramine (Benadryl), an antihistamine commonly used for allergy symptoms. One of its side effects is drowsiness, making this a popular option as a sleep aid. They can cause unwanted sleepiness in the morning, difficulty urinating, and confusion and delirium. Some of the over-the-counter products that contain diphenhydramine include the following:

- Exedrin PM
- Nytol
- Tylenol PM
- ZzzQuil

Another active sleep-promoting antihistamine ingredient is doxylamine, which is found in Unisom. Common side effects include dry mouth, ataxia, urinary retention, drowsiness, and memory problems. Severe consequences of taking this drug include hallucinations, psychosis, and an increased sensitivity to external stimuli.

Antihistamines are also anticholinergics, that is, they block the binding of acetylcholine to neural receptors. Anticholinergic side effects, including dry mouth, constipation, and cognitive effects, should be monitored. These drugs should be avoided or used with caution in older adults since the body's production of acetylcholine diminishes with age. Older adults taking anticholinergic drugs demonstrate brain atrophy, dysfunction, and clinical decline (Risacher et al., 2016). Therefore, their use is strongly discouraged in this population.

These over-the-counter drugs work best when used for mild and infrequent insomnia. Despite the "non–habit forming" label, there is reason for concern. Most over-the-counter sleep aids result in habituation and should not be used longer than 2 weeks.

HERBAL AND DIETARY SUPPLEMENTS FOR INSOMNIA

Valerian is a plant native to Asia and Europe. It is used as a dietary supplement for insomnia, anxiety, and other conditions such as depression and menopause symptoms. The evidence for its efficacy in treating insomnia is insufficient. It is generally considered safe for short periods. No information is available about the long-term safety of valerian or its safety in children younger than 3 years, pregnant women, or nursing mothers. Mild side effects could include morning fatigue, headaches, dizziness, and upset stomach.

Melatonin is a hormone occurring naturally in the body that plays a role in sleep. The production and release of melatonin is dependent on the time of day with levels increasing in the evening and decreasing in the morning. Its production is blocked at night because of the absence of light. Dietary supplements containing melatonin have been found to help with sleep disorders, such as jet lag, dysfunction with the body's internal clocks, and night shift work sleep problems.

German chamomile, nicknamed "sleep tea," is a traditional herbal remedy for insomnia. Its use for a variety of conditions including diarrhea, skin conditions, and mouth sores dates back to ancient Greece, Egypt, and Rome (National Institute for Complementary and Integrative Health Care, 2016).

The flowering tops of the plant are used for teas, extracts, and topical ointments. Sedative effects may be due to the flavonoid apigenin that binds to benzodiazepine receptors in the brain. However, no empirical studies support chamomile's medical use other than being a relaxing drink before bedtime. Rare serious allergic reactions, including anaphylaxis, which may be related to other plant allergies such as ragweed, have been reported. Drug interactions with warfarin, cyclosporine, and other medications may occur.

CHAPTER 27

Substance Use Disorder Medications

Pharmacological treatment for substance use disorders is generally aimed at helping people during acute intoxication and overdose, to withdraw from the substance, and then to abstain from the substance. The overall term for using medication along with counseling and behavioral therapies to treat substance use disorders is referred to as medication-assisted treatment (MAT). Medication is used to normalize brain chemistry, reduce the euphoric effects of alcohol and substances, address physiological cravings, and assist with the body's return to normal functioning.

ALCOHOL

Alcohol Overdose

An alcohol overdose occurs after drinking more than the body can safely process. Blood alcohol levels can continue to rise even when a person is no longer drinking because of continued absorption from the stomach and intestines Symptoms of alcohol poisoning are listed in Box 27.1

It is dangerous to assume that a person will be able to sleep it off because they may not wake up. Medical care includes managing breathing problems with an artificial airway if necessary, monitoring cardiac status, administering fluids to increase hydration and blood glucose, and flushing the stomach to clear the body of alcohol. Heated blankets may be used to manage hypothermia.

Alcohol Withdrawal

The types of symptoms of alcohol withdrawal occur because alcohol is a central nervous system depressant. Two neurotransmitters are involved:

Box 27.1 Signs of Alcohol Poisoning

- Vomiting
- Dulled responses, such as no gag reflex (can result in choking and asphyxiation)
- Slow respirations (fewer than 8 breaths per minute)
- Irregular breathing (10 seconds or more between breaths)
- Hypothermia (low body temperature)
- Bluish, pale, clammy skin
- Mental confusion, stupor, coma, or inability to wake up
- Seizures

1. Alcohol affects gamma-aminobutyric acid (GABA), a major inhibitory (calming) neurotransmitter in the brain. GABA receptors contain alcohol-specific binding sites that become less sensitive with chronic exposure to ethanol. Reduction or cessation of alcohol from chronically elevated concentrations results in decreased inhibitory tone.
2. Glutamate is a major excitatory (stimulating) amino acid. Chronic alcohol use results in adaption by increasing the number of glutamate receptors in an attempt to maintain a normal state of arousal. Reduction or cessation of alcohol results in unregulated excess excitation.

Mild alcohol withdrawal usually occurs within 24 hours of the last drink and is characterized by tremulousness (the "shakes"), increased blood pressure and pulse, insomnia, anxiety, panic, twitching, sweating, and stomach upset. Moderate alcohol withdrawal usually occurs 24 to 36 hours after the cessation of alcohol intake. Its manifestations include intense anxiety, tremors, insomnia, seizures, hallucinations, hypertension, and racing pulse. Benzodiazepines such as chlordiazepoxide (Librium), diazepam (Valium), or lorazepam (Ativan) are useful in reducing mild to moderate symptoms of alcohol withdrawal.

Psychotic and perceptual symptoms may begin in 8 to 10 hours. If a patient is undergoing withdrawal to the point of psychosis, it should be considered a medical emergency because of the risks of unconsciousness, seizures, and delirium. Benzodiazepines such as lorazepam or chlordiazepoxide can be given either orally or intramuscularly and tapered over the next 5 to 7 days.

Withdrawal seizures may occur within 12 to 24 hours after alcohol cessation. These seizures are generalized and tonic-clonic. Additional seizures may occur within hours of the first seizure. Diazepam given intravenously is a common treatment for withdrawal seizures.

Alcohol withdrawal delirium, also known as *delirium tremens (DTs),* is a medical emergency that can result in death in 20% of untreated patients, usually as a result of medical problems such as pneumonia, renal disease, hepatic insufficiency, or heart failure (Sadock et al., 2015). Alcohol withdrawal delirium may happen anytime in the first 72 hours. Autonomic hyperactivity may result in tachycardia, diaphoresis, fever, anxiety, insomnia, and hypertension. Delusions and visual and tactile hallucinations are common in alcohol withdrawal delirium.

Delusions and hallucinations may result in unpredictable behaviors as patients try to protect themselves from what they believe are genuine dangers. All patients are at risk for this condition after cessation of heavy drinking for 3 days and are a danger to themselves and others. However, it is rare to see this syndrome in individuals in good physical health. Serious physical illness such as hepatitis or pancreatitis increases the likelihood of alcohol withdrawal delirium.

Prevention of alcohol withdrawal delirium is the goal. Oral diazepam may be useful in the symptomatic relief of acute agitation, tremor, impending or acute delirium tremens, and hallucinosis. Chlordiazepoxide is also used to relieve symptoms. However, once delirium appears, intravenous therapy with benzodiazepines is required.

Temporary mechanical restraint may be necessary for patients experiencing delirium tremens to protect both the patient and caretakers. Dehydration, often exacerbated by diaphoresis and fever, can be corrected with oral or intravenous fluids.

Alcohol-Induced Persisting Amnestic Disorder

People with long-term heavy use of alcohol may experience short-term memory disturbances. One memory-reducing problem is Wernicke's (alcoholic) encephalopathy, an acute and reversible condition. A more severe form of this problem is Korsakoff's syndrome, a chronic condition with a low recovery rate (about 20%). The two conditions are a result of a thiamine deficiency, which may be caused by poor nutrition or by malabsorption of nutrients.

Along with memory disturbances, symptoms of Wernicke's encephalopathy are an altered gait, vestibular (balance) dysfunction, and ocular abnormalities. Sluggish reaction to light and unequal pupil size are also symptoms. Wernicke's encephalopathy responds rapidly to large doses of intravenous thiamine two to three times daily for 1 or 2 weeks. Treatment of Korsakoff syndrome is also thiamine for 3 to 12 months. While patients with Korsakoff's syndrome may never fully recover, cognitive improvement may occur with thiamine and nutritional support.

Alcohol Relapse Prevention

There are three primary medications used to prevent relapse and to help people recovering from alcohol use disorder resist the temptations to drink. The most widely used medications in the treatment of alcohol use disorder are disulfiram (Antabuse), naltrexone (ReVia, Vivitrol), and acamprosate (Campral).

Disulfiram

Disulfiram (Antabuse) was the first drug approved by the U.S. Food and Drug Administration (FDA) for alcohol misuse. People taking disulfiram become extremely sick if they drink alcohol. Normally, metabolism of ethanol goes from oxidation by alcohol dehydrogenase to the formation of acetaldehyde, which is further metabolized to acetyl-coenzyme A by aldehyde dehydrogenase. Disulfiram is an aldehyde dehydrogenase inhibitor. Inhibition of this enzyme results in an accumulation of acetaldehyde in the blood.

Disulfiram motivates individuals to avoid alcohol out of a fear of experiencing intense and unpleasant symptoms, similar to a severe hangover. These symptoms include nausea, throbbing headache, vomiting, hypertension, flushing, sweating, thirst, dyspnea, tachycardia, chest pain, vertigo, and blurred vision. The reaction happens rapidly and may last up to 2 hours. Elimination of the drug from the body takes 1 to 2 weeks.

Severe reactions may occur with greater amounts of alcohol. These reactions are respiratory depression, cardiovascular collapse, arrhythmias, myocardial infarction, acute congestive heart failure, unconsciousness, convulsions, and death.

In the absence of alcohol, disulfiram is well tolerated. Common side effects include fatigue, dermatitis, impotence, optic neuritis, and cognitive changes. It may exacerbate psychosis. Disulfiram is associated with a low rate of serum aminotransferase elevations and may cause severe and even fatal liver injury. Because of this rare complication, this drug is given at lower doses and is used less widely than alternative medications.

Disulfiram is contraindicated in patients with myocardial disease or coronary occlusion, psychoses, or pregnancy and in those with high levels of impulsivity and suicidality. Patients who are taking metronidazole, paraldehyde, and alcohol-containing products such as cough syrups or using aftershave should not be given disulfiram.

Naltrexone

Naltrexone is used once abstinence has been achieved. It is an opiate antagonist widely used for both alcohol and opioid use disorder. Naltrexone competitively binds to opioid receptors. Naltrexone reduces the pleasure associated with drinking and reduces the cravings to use and abuse. This drug is available in an oral form (ReVia) and a long-acting injectable form (Vivitrol).

This medication is well tolerated by most people recovering from alcohol use disorder, and most people will not experience serious side effects after the first few days. Common side effects include nausea, headache, dizziness, nervousness, fatigue, insomnia, vomiting, anxiety, and somnolence. Hepatitis and liver dysfunction have been associated with the use of naltrexone.

Patients should be opioid free for 7 to 10 days before initiating this therapy. No opiates, even codeine-containing cough syrups, can be taken along with naltrexone. Most patients will use naltrexone for the first few months of sobriety, during which time the cravings to use are strongest.

A contraindication for naltrexone use is current opioid analgesic use. Intramuscular injection should not be used with patients whose body mass precludes the use of a 2-inch needle. Subcutaneous injections may cause a severe injection-site reaction.

Acamprosate

Acamprosate (Campral) works like naltrexone to reduce the intensity of experienced cravings in people who have quit drinking. Its mechanism of action is to counteract the imbalance between the excitatory glutamatergic and inhibitory GABA activity. This stabilization allows the brain to recover slowly while reducing some of the discomforts of withdrawal symptoms.

Along with reducing alcohol cravings, acamprosate also seems to help people to sleep better during recovery. Improved sleep is significant in alcohol use disorder, because insomnia is a major contributor to relapse.

Common side effects are usually mild and transient. They include headache, diarrhea, flatulence, abdominal pain, paresthesias, and skin reactions. Acamprosate may be discontinued abruptly without symptoms and is not addictive. Acamprosate is contraindicated with renal impairment.

Table 27.1 identifies medications used in the treatment of alcohol withdrawal and relapse prevention.

CANNABIS

Abstinence and support are the main principles of treatment for cannabis use disorder. Hospitalization or outpatient care may be required. Individual, family, and group therapies can provide support. Antianxiety medication may be useful for short-term relief of withdrawal symptoms. Patients with underlying anxiety and depression may respond to antidepressant therapy.

OPIOIDS

Opioid Overdose

Overdose is common among people who misuse illicit substances such as heroin or pain medications such as oxycodone, hydrocodone, and morphine. An opioid overdose is a medical emergency. Signs of opioid overdose are listed in Box 27.2.

Any patient with signs of opioid overdose, or when this is suspected, should be administered naloxone. It is a safe drug that produces no clinical effects in non-opioid users or non-opioid intoxicated individuals. Treatment for an opioid overdose begins with aspirating secretions, inserting an airway, using mechanical ventilation, and providing oxygen. In the absence of medical equipment, rescue breathing should be performed.

Table 27.1 **Common Medications Used for Alcohol Use Disorder**

Generic (Trade) Name	Uses	Notes
Benzodiazepines: Lorazepam (Ativan), Chlordiazepoxide (Librium), Diazepam (Valium)	Withdrawal	Sedation, decreased anxiety and blood pressure Assess for seizures that could lead to delirium tremens (DTs); if not treated this can lead to coma and ultimately death.
Anticonvulsants: Carbamazepine (Tegretol), Phenobarbital (Luminal)	Withdrawal	Older treatments that are still used. Other treatments have proven more effective and safer. Assess for seizures that could lead to delirium tremens if not treated; coma and ultimately death may result.
Clonidine *(Catapres)*	Mild to moderate withdrawal	Alpha-agonist antihypertensive agent. Give every 4–6 hours as needed. Side effects include dizziness, hypotension, fatigue, and headache.
Disulfiram (Antabuse)	Maintenance, relapse prevention, aversion therapy	Physical effects when alcohol is used include intense nausea and vomiting, headache, sweating, flushed skin, respiratory difficulties, and confusion. Avoid all alcohol and substances as cough syrup and mouthwash that contain alcohol.

Continued

Table 27.1 **Common Medications Used for Alcohol Use Disorder—cont'd**

Generic (Trade) Name	Uses	Notes
Naltrexone (ReVia, Vivitrol)	Withdrawal, relapse prevention, decreases pleasurable feelings and cravings	Oral or long-acting (once a month) injectable form. Nausea usually goes away after first month; headache and sedation may occur. Pain at injection site; patient needs to be opiate-free 10 days before initiation of medication.
Acamprosate calcium (Campral)	Relapse prevention	Begin after abstinence from alcohol. Tablets are taken three times a day. Side effects include diarrhea, gastrointestinal upset, appetite loss, dizziness, anxiety, and difficulty sleeping. Contraindicated in patients with renal impairment.

From Substance Abuse and Mental Health Services Administration and National Institute on Alcohol Abuse and Alcoholism. (2015). *Medication for the treatment of alcohol use disorder: A brief guide. HHS Publication No. (SMA) 15-4907*. Rockville, MD: Author.

Box 27.2 **Signs of Opioid Overdose**

- Extreme sleepiness
- Unresponsive to verbal stimuli or sternal rub
- Fingernails or lips turning blue/purple
- Constricted pinpoint pupils
- Slow pulse and/or low blood pressure
- Slow to shallow breathing in a patient that cannot be awakened
- Respiratory death rattle—exhalation with a distinct, labored sound from the throat

Table 27.2 **Methods of Naloxone Delivery**

Brand Name	Delivery Method	Notes
Narcan	Subcutaneous, intramuscular, intravenous	Most rapid onset of action is intravenous administration
Narcan Nasal Spray	Intranasal	Pre-filled device that requires no assembly Delivers a single dose into one nostril Two doses per package
Evzio Auto Injector	Intramuscular or subcutaneous	Hand-held automatic injection into outer thigh Device provides verbal instruction on how to deliver the medication

Naloxone, a specific opioid antagonist, can be given by intranasal spray, intramuscularly, subcutaneously, or intravenously. The most rapid onset of action is by intravenous administration, which is recommended in emergency situations. The smallest effective dose that maintains spontaneous normal respiratory drive should be used. Too much naloxone may produce withdrawal symptoms. Duration of action for naloxone is short compared with many opioids (20 to 90 minutes), so repeated administration may be required.

Naloxone usually results in a rapid response of increased respirations and pupillary dilation within 3 to 5 minutes. Methods of naloxone delivery are listed in Table 27.2.

Patients should be monitored for recurrence of opioid toxicity for at least 4 hours after naloxone use. Overdoses on long-acting opioids should be monitored for a longer period of time.

Opioid Withdrawal and Relapse Prevention

The principles of opioid detoxification/withdrawal are to:

1. Substitute a longer-acting, pharmacologically equivalent of the misused drug.
2. Stabilize the patient on the substituted drug.
3. Gradually withdraw the substituted drug.

The following drugs are opioid agonists, partial agonists, and antagonists. Agonists and partial agonists are used for detoxification and maintenance purposes. Antagonists are used to accelerate detoxification and then to prevent relapse.

Methadone

Methadone (Dolophine, Methadose) is a synthetic narcotic opioid used to decrease the painful symptoms of opiate withdrawal and also for maintenance of abstinence. A full opioid agonist, methadone tricks the brain into thinking it is still getting the drug by activating opioid receptors. It blocks the euphoric effects of other opiate drugs such as heroin, morphine, and codeine, as well as semisynthetic opioids like oxycodone and hydrocodone.

Methadone is a U.S. Drug Enforcement Administration (DEA) schedule II drug with high abuse potential. It can only be dispensed through an opioid treatment program certified by a government substance use agency. Methadone, too, will eventually need to be withdrawn to prevent dependence. In pregnant users, a low dose of methadone may be the safest course. Neonatal withdrawal is usually mild and can be managed with paregoric.

Some serious side effects may result from methadone. Patients should be instructed to seek medical care if they experience difficulty breathing. Feeling lightheaded, faint, chest pain, and a pounding heartbeat may be symptoms of QT prolongation, a serious cardiac arrhythmia. Hives, rash, or swelling of the face, lips, tongue, or throat could also be serious symptoms. Hallucinations or confusion should also be reported to a care provider.

Buprenorphine

Buprenorphine reduces or eliminates withdrawal symptoms and drug craving without dangerous side effects of heroin and other opioids. It is used to help people reduce or quit their use of heroin or other opiates such as pain relievers like morphine. Buprenorphine both blocks and activates opiate receptors and is known as a partial opioid agonist.

A DEA schedule III drug, buprenorphine can be prescribed by providers who have completed special education. Some buprenorphine products also contain naloxone. The naloxone in the combined formulation causes a withdrawal reaction if it is intravenously injected, thereby deterring misuse.

Side effects of buprenorphine include nausea, vomiting, constipation, muscle aches and cramps, insomnia, irritability, and fever. This drug is used only after abstaining from opioids for 12 to 24 hours and in the early stages of opioid withdrawal. It can bring on acute withdrawal for patients who are not in the early stages of withdrawal and who have other opioids in their bloodstream. Because buprenorphine is a long-acting drug, once patients have been stabilized, they can sometimes switch to alternate-day dosing instead of dosing every day.

Naltrexone

Naltrexone is an opioid antagonist indicated for the prevention of relapse to opioid dependence opioid detoxification is completed. Naltrexone is available as ReVia, a tablet form of the drug. A long-acting injectable version, Vivitrol, is given once a month. If a person using naltrexone relapses and uses the misused drug, naltrexone blocks the euphoric and sedative effects.

Common adverse reactions with ReVia include difficulty sleeping, anxiety, nervousness, abdominal pain/cramps, nausea and/or vomiting, low energy, joint and muscle pain, and headache. The most common adverse reactions with Vivitrol are hepatic enzyme abnormalities, injection site pain, nasopharyngitis, insomnia, and toothache. Naltrexone is contraindicated in acute hepatitis or liver failure. Hepatitis and clinically significant liver dysfunction has occurred in patients taking naltrexone. Patients should be warned of the risk of hepatic injury.

Table 27.3 identifies medications used in the treatment of opioid use disorder.

HALLUCINOGENS

Patients who have ingested phencyclidine (PCP) cannot be talked down and may require restraint and a calming medication such as a benzodiazepine. Mechanical cooling may be necessary for severe hyperthermia.

INHALANTS

Inhalant intoxication usually does not require any treatment. However, serious and potentially fatal responses such as coma, cardiac arrhythmias, or bronchospasm do

Table 27.3 **FDA Approved Medications for Opioid Use Disorder**

Medication and Action	Form	Use
Methadone (opioid agonist)		Withdrawal and maintenance treatment
• Dolophine	Tablet	
• Methadose	Tablet, oral concentrate	
Buprenorphine (partial opioid agonist)		Withdrawal and maintenance treatment
• Subutex (buprenorphine)	Sublingual tablet	
• Bunavail (buprenorphine and naloxone)	Buccal film	
• Suboxone (buprenorphine and naloxone)	Sublingual tablet	
• Zubsolv (buprenorphine and naloxone)	Sublingual tablet	
• Probuphine (buprenorphine)	Implanted rods	
Naltrexone (opioid antagonist)		Relapse prevention
• ReVia	Tablet	
• Vivitrol	Long-acting injectable	

happen. A psychotic response can be induced by inhalant intoxication. This self-limiting (a few hours to a few weeks) problem may require careful use of haloperidol (Haldol) to manage severe agitation.

SEDATIVES, HYPNOTICS, AND BENZODIAZEPINES

Like alcohol, repeated sedative, hypnotic, and benzodiazepine use results in repeated dampening of the central nervous system. This dampening results in the body's daily attempt to return to homeostasis. In the absence of the substance, rebound hyperactivity is manifested. Hence symptoms such as autonomic hyperactivity, tremor, insomnia, psychomotor agitation, anxiety, and grand mal seizures occur. The degree and timing of the withdrawal syndrome depend on the specific substance. Half-life is an important predictor of withdrawal time.

Gradual reduction of these substances will prevent seizures and other withdrawal symptoms. Benzodiazepine withdrawal can be aided by using a long-acting barbiturate such as phenobarbital.

AMPHETAMINES

Depending on the amphetamine used, specific drugs may be used short term to treat withdrawal symptoms. Antipsychotics may be prescribed for a few days. If there is no psychosis, diazepam (Valium) is useful in treating agitation and hyperactivity. Once the patient has been withdrawn from the amphetamine, depression can be treated with antidepressants such as bupropion (Wellbutrin).

NICOTINE

Withdrawal from and treatment for nicotine use disorders is facilitated by nicotine replacement therapies. This highly successful nicotine replacement is available in the form of gum, lozenges, nasal sprays, inhalers, and patches. Non-nicotine therapy options include the antidepressant bupropion (Zyban), which reduces the cravings for nicotine. Clonidine (Catapres) decreases sympathetic activity and reduces withdrawal symptoms. Varenicline (Chantix) provides some nicotine effects to ease withdrawal symptoms and blocks the effects of nicotine from cigarettes if smoking is resumed.

CHAPTER 28

Neurocognitive Medications

Several medications have been approved by the U.S. Food and Drug Administration (FDA) for the treatment of Alzheimer's disease. These medications are widely used and have demonstrated statistically significant effects compared with placebos. However, they produce only a marginal improvement in cognition and functioning, and the benefits of these medications diminish after 1 to 2 years. Considering the potential side effects, which double in people older than 85 years, their use should be carefully weighed against the potential benefits.

CHOLINESTERASE INHIBITORS

Because a deficiency of acetylcholine has been linked to Alzheimer's disease, medications aimed at preventing its breakdown have been developed. Drugs in this classification work by preventing an enzyme called acetylcholinesterase or, more simply, cholinesterase from breaking down acetylcholine in the brain. As a result, an increased concentration of acetylcholine leads to temporary improvement of some symptoms. Symptom improvement may diminish as the disease process advances and fewer cholinergic neurons remain functionally intact. Despite slight variations in the type of action of the cholinesterase inhibitors, there is no evidence of any differences between them with regard to effectiveness.

The FDA approved the first cholinesterase inhibitor, tacrine (Cognex), in 1993 for the treatment of mild to moderate symptoms of Alzheimer's disease. Unfortunately, tacrine was associated with a high frequency of side effects, including gastrointestinal effects, elevated liver transaminase levels, and liver toxicity. It was withdrawn from the market by the FDA in 2012.

Donepezil

The most commonly prescribed cholinesterase inhibitor, donepezil (Aricept), was approved by the FDA in 1996. Indications for donepezil include mild, moderate, and severe Alzheimer's disease. It appears to improve cognitive functions without the potentially serious liver toxicity attributed to tacrine.

Some individuals may experience nausea and diarrhea while taking the drug. These side effects are dose-related, so a decreased dose helps minimize them. Other side effects include muscle cramps, fatigue, and weight loss. Donepezil should be taken in the evening, just before going to sleep. It can be taken with or without food. It is available both as a tablet and an orally disintegrating tablet.

Rivastigmine

Oral rivastigmine (Exelon) was approved for use in 2000 for mild to moderate dementia of both Alzheimer's disease and Parkinson's disease. The transdermal patch delivery system is approved for severe dementia.

The most common side effects of rivastigmine are nausea, vomiting, loss of appetite, and weight loss. In most cases, these side effects are temporary. Patients should always take rivastigmine with food to reduce gastrointestinal side effects. The most common causes of discontinuation of therapy during clinical trials were nausea, vomiting, anorexia, and dizziness.

Another side effect of rivastigmine is skin-related. Disseminated allergic dermatitis, an acute, symmetrical, and generalized eczema, is extremely itchy and sleep disturbing. Its appearance should lead to discontinuation of this medication.

Rivastigmine is available in a capsule, an oral solution, or a patch. The transdermal patch has FDA approval for mild, moderate, and severe Alzheimer's symptoms. It is applied once a day and has no food requirement because the drug enters the body through the bloodstream. It is useful for people who have trouble swallowing pills. In addition to the common adverse reactions previously discussed, the patch may cause application site erythema. Patients and families should be cautioned to always remove the old patch before applying the new one to prevent serious side effects.

Galantamine

Galantamine (Razadyne [formerly marketed as Reminyl]) gained FDA approval in 2001. It is prescribed in the mild to moderate stages of dementia. In addition to inhibiting cholinesterase, galantamine also stimulates nicotinic receptors to release more acetylcholine. As with the other cholinesterase inhibitors, its therapeutic effect decreases as the disease progresses.

The most common side effects of galantamine include nausea, vomiting, diarrhea, dizziness, headache, decreased appetite, and decreased weight. The most common causes of discontinuation of this drug in clinical trials were nausea, vomiting, decreased appetite, and dizziness. Bradycardia and syncope have been associated with this class of drugs. They should be used with caution when patients are taking nonsteroidal anti-inflammatory drugs (NSAIDs).

Serious skin reactions (i.e., Stevens-Johnson syndrome and acute generalized exanthematous pustulosis) have been reported in patients receiving galantamine. It should be discontinued at the first appearance of a skin rash, unless the rash is clearly not drug-related.

Galantamine is available as a tablet or oral solution. It is also available in an extended-release capsule.

N-METHYL-D-ASPARTATE RECEPTOR ANTAGONIST

Memantine (Namenda) was approved for use with Alzheimer's disease in 2003. It is approved for treatment of moderate to severe dementia, but not mild dementia. This medication is typically added after trying the cholinesterase inhibitors.

Memantine regulates the activity of glutamate, a neurotransmitter that plays a role in information processing, storage, and retrieval. Persistent activation of *N*-methyl-D-aspartate (NMDA) receptors by glutamate has been hypothesized to contribute to the Alzheimer's disease symptoms. Memantine binds to these NMDA receptors and protects against excessive neuronal stimulation by glutamate.

Memantine can be taken with or without food. Capsules can be swallowed intact or opened and sprinkled on applesauce. After using memantine twice a day, patients may be switched to long-acting memantine XR for once-a-day dosing.

Common side effects include headache, diarrhea, and dizziness. In clinical trials, the most common cause of discontinuation was dizziness.

Drugs approved by the FDA for treatment of Alzheimer's disease are described in Table 28.1.

MEDICATIONS FOR BEHAVIORAL SYMPTOMS OF ALZHEIMER'S DISEASE

Other medications are often useful in managing the behavioral symptoms of individuals with dementia, but these need to be used with extreme caution. The rule of thumb for older adults is "start low and go slow." Another is to use the smallest dose for the shortest duration possible and discontinue if they are not effective. In addition, because people with dementia are at high risk of developing delirium, always add medications with caution.

Most people with neurocognitive disorders will experience behavioral symptoms that reduce their quality of life, are distressing to them and their caregivers, and may lead to placement in a residential care facility. Some of the troubling behaviors are psychotic symptoms (hallucinations, paranoia), severe mood swings (depression is common), wandering, anxiety, agitation, and verbal or physical aggression (combativeness). Not only are these behaviors distressing, but they may also lead to injuries from falls, infections, and incontinence.

Psychotropic medications may be prescribed. Drug classifications that are used off-label without specific FDA approval include antidepressants, antipsychotics, antianxiety agents, and anticonvulsants. Of these, antipsychotics have been used most often. Unfortunately, these medications are associated with a risk of mortality, mostly from cardiovascular and infectious causes. Antipsychotics should be avoided or used only when benefits outweigh risks and for the shortest duration possible.

Table 28.1 **FDA Approved Drugs for Alzheimer's Disease**

Generic (Trade)	Action	Indications	Side Effects
Cholinesterase Inhibitors			
Donepezil (Aricept)	Prevents the breakdown of acetylcholine by inhibiting its hydrolysis by cholinesterase	Mild, moderate, and severe stages	Nausea, diarrhea, cramps, fatigue, and weight loss
Rivastigmine (Exelon, Exelon Patch)	Prevents the breakdown of acetylcholine by inhibiting its hydrolysis by cholinesterase	Oral: mild to moderate stages Patch: mild, moderate, and severe stages	Nausea, vomiting, loss of appetite, and weight loss Application site erythema with patch
Galantamine (Razadyne, Razadyne ER)	Prevents the breakdown of acetylcholine by inhibiting its hydrolysis by cholinesterase Stimulates nicotinic receptors to release more acetylcholine	Mild to moderate stages	Nausea, vomiting, diarrhea, dizziness, headache, decreased appetite, and decreased weight
***N*-Methyl-D-Aspartate (NMDA) Receptor Antagonist**			
Memantine (Namenda, Namenda XR)	Regulates glutamate activity by blocking NMDA receptors, decreasing excitatory neurotoxicity caused by overstimulation of NMDA receptors by glutamate	Moderate to severe stages	Headaches, diarrhea, and dizziness
NMDA Receptor Antagonist/Cholinesterase Inhibitor			
Memantine/donepezil (Namzaric)	See memantine and donepezil	Moderate to severe stages	See side effects listed under memantine and donepezil

From U.S. Food and Drug Administration. (2017). FDA online label repository. Retrieved from www.labels.fda.gov

PART V
Nonpharmacological Approaches

CHAPTER 29

Psychotherapeutic Models

Nurses who are prepared at the basic level are qualified to provide counseling, support, and education to their patients. Registered nurses and nursing students promote the stabilization of symptoms and the reinforcement of healthy behaviors and interactions in the context of a therapeutic relationship.

Psychiatric–mental health advanced practice registered nurses are prepared to provide a more complex form of counseling known as psychotherapy. Psychotherapy, informally referred to as "talk therapy," is a term for a variety of treatment techniques that help individuals identify and change self-defeating feelings, thoughts, and behavior.

Most of the therapies in this chapter require advanced education for their actual application and for third party reimbursement. Yet it is important for nurses working and training in a psychiatric setting to be familiar with the types of therapies available. Among the benefits of becoming familiar with these therapies is the ability to do the following:

1. Use basic concepts of the models as interventions, such as recognizing negative thought patterns as used in cognitive–behavioral therapy (CBT) or taking part in token economies when working with children and adolescents as used in behavioral therapy.

2. Understand the therapy being recommended to or being provided for your patient, and being able to discuss the proposed therapy or the work currently being done.

This chapter offers snapshots of some of the most common psychotherapies. Most of these therapies are provided for individuals, families, and groups. They include the following:

- Cognitive-behavioral therapy
- Dialectical behavioral therapy
- Eye movement and desensitization and reprocessing therapy
- Interpersonal therapy
- Behavioral therapy
  - Modeling
  - Operant conditioning
  - Systematic desensitization
  - Aversion
  - Biofeedback
- Milieu therapy
- Group therapy

COGNITIVE–BEHAVIORAL THERAPY

Cognitive-behavioral therapy (CBT) is an active, time-limited, and structured approach. This evidence-based therapy is used to treat a variety of psychiatric disorders such as depression, anxiety, phobias, and pain. It is based on the underlying theoretical principle that feelings and behaviors are largely determined by the way people think about the world and their place in it (Beck, 1979). Their cognitions (verbal or pictorial events in their streams of consciousness) are based on attitudes or assumptions developed from previous experiences. These cognitions may be fairly accurate or distorted.

People have schemas, or unique assumptions, about themselves, others, and the world in general. For example, if a man has the schema, "The only person I can trust is myself," he will have expectations that everyone else has questionable motives, is dishonest, and will eventually hurt him. Other negative schemas include incompetence, abandonment, evilness, and vulnerability. People are typically not aware of such cognitive biases.

Rapid, unthinking responses based on schemas are known as automatic thoughts. These responses are particularly intense and common in psychiatric disorders such as depression and anxiety. Often automatic thoughts, or cognitive distortions, are irrational and lead to false assumptions and misinterpretations. For example, if a woman interprets all experiences in terms of whether she is competent and adequate, her thinking may be dominated by the cognitive distortion, "Unless I do everything perfectly, I'm a failure." Consequently, that person reacts to situations in terms of adequacy, even when these situations are unrelated to whether she is personally competent. Table 29.1 describes common cognitive distortions.

Therapeutic techniques are designed to identify, reality test, and correct distorted conceptualizations and the dysfunctional beliefs underlying them. Patients are taught to challenge their own negative thinking and substitute it with positive, rational thoughts. They learn to recognize when thinking is based on distortions and misconceptions.

Homework assignments play an important role in CBT. A particularly useful technique is a four-column thought diary to record the precipitating event or situation, the resulting automatic thought, and the preceding feelings and behaviors. Finally, a challenge to the negative thoughts based on rational evidence and thinking is listed in the last column. Box 29.1 illustrates an entry in a thought diary.

DIALECTICAL BEHAVIOR THERAPY

Dialectical behavior therapy (DBT) is an evidence-based therapy developed to treat chronically suicidal persons with borderline personality disorder (Linehan, 1993). Data on the use of DBT with individuals experiencing comorbid personality disorders (such as obsessive–compulsive personality disorder) and other psychiatric disorders (such as major depression, generalized anxiety, substance abuse, and eating disorders) have been confirmed.

DBT combines cognitive and behavioral techniques with mindfulness, which emphasizes being aware of thoughts and actively shaping them. The goals of DBT are to increase the patient's ability to manage distress, improve interpersonal effectiveness skills, and enhance the therapist's effectiveness in working with this population. Treatment focuses on behavioral targets, beginning with identification of and interventions for suicidal behaviors and then progressing to a focus on interrupting destructive behaviors. Finally, DBT addresses quality-of-life behaviors across a hierarchy of care.

Table 29.1 **Common Cognitive Distortions**

Distortion	Definition	Example
All-or-nothing thinking	Thinking in black and white, reducing complex outcomes into absolutes	Although Valentina earned the second-highest score in the state's cheerleading competition, she consistently referred to herself as "a loser."
Overgeneralization	Using a bad outcome (or a few bad outcomes) as evidence that nothing will ever go right again	Andrew had a minor traffic accident. He is reluctant to drive and says, "I shouldn't be allowed on the road."
Labeling	A form of generalization in which a characteristic or event becomes definitive and results in an overly harsh label for self or others	"Because I failed the advanced statistics examination, I am a failure. I might as well give up. I may as well quit and look for an easier major."
Mental filter	Focusing on a negative detail or bad event and allowing it to taint everything else	Anne's boss evaluated her work as exemplary and gave her a few suggestions for improvement. She obsessed about the suggestions and ignored the rest.
Disqualifying the positive	Maintaining a negative view by rejecting information that supports a positive view as being irrelevant, inaccurate, or accidental	"I've just been offered the job I thought I always wanted. There must have been no other applicants."
Jumping to conclusions	Making a negative interpretation despite the fact that there is little or no supporting evidence	"My fiance, Juan, didn't call me for 3 hours, which just proves he doesn't love me anymore."

a. Mind-reading	Inferring negative thoughts, responses, and motives of others	Isabel is giving a presentation and a man in the audience is sleeping. She panics, "I must be boring."
b. Fortune-telling error	Anticipating that things will turn out badly as an established fact	"I'll ask her out, but I know she won't have a good time."
Magnification or minimization	Exaggerating the importance of something (such as a personal failure or the success of others) or reducing the importance of something (such as a personal success or the failure of others)	"I'm alone on a Saturday night because no one likes me. When other people are alone, it's because they want to be."
Catastrophizing	An extreme form of magnification in which the very worst is assumed to be a probable outcome	"If I don't make a good impression on the boss at the company picnic, she will fire me."
Emotional reasoning	Drawing a conclusion based on an emotional state	"I'm nervous about the examination. I must not be prepared. If I were, I wouldn't be afraid."
"Should" and "must" statements	Rigid self-directives that presume an unrealistic amount of control over external events	Renee believes that a patient with diabetes has high blood sugar today because she is not a very good nurse and that her patients should always get better.
Personalization	Assuming responsibility for an external event or situation that was likely outside personal control	"I'm sorry your party wasn't more fun. It's probably because I was there."

Modified from Beck, A. T. (1979). *Cognitive therapy and the emotional disorders*. New York: International Universities Press.

Box 29.1 **Thought Diary Entry**

Event	Automatic Thought	Feeling 0 (low) – 10 (high)	Alternate Thoughts
I went to my favorite restaurant. The waitress, Rebecca, who I know well, barely acknowledged me.	Rebecca doesn't like me anymore. I must have said something stupid. I wonder who else doesn't like me here.	Hurt (6)	Rebecca doesn't feel well. She may be upset about something going on in her life. The restaurant was crowded; she may have felt overwhelmed.

EYE MOVEMENT DESENSITIZATION AND REPROCESSING THERAPY

Eye movement densensitization and reprocessing therapy (EMDR) therapy is an innovative evidence-based approach used by professionals to treat traumatized children and adults. EMDR therapy processes traumatic memories though a specific eight-phase protocol. The clinician asks the patient to think about the traumatic event. At the same time the patient attends to other stimulation, such as eye movements, audio tones, or tapping. The combination of thinking and other stimuli brings about neurological and physiological changes that help people process and integrate traumatic memories.

INTERPERSONAL THERAPY

Interpersonal therapy is an effective short-term therapy. The number of sessions is generally between 12 and 16. The assumption with this therapy is that psychiatric disorders are influenced by interpersonal interactions and the social context. The goal of interpersonal therapy is to reduce or eliminate psychiatric symptoms by improving interpersonal functioning and satisfaction with social relationships.

Interpersonal therapy has proven successful in the treatment of depression, particularly related to grief and loss, interpersonal conflict, role transitions, and deficits related to interpersonal skills. Treatment is based on the notion that disturbances in important interpersonal relationships (or a deficit in one's capacity to form those relationships) can play a role in initiating or maintaining clinical depression. In interpersonal psychotherapy, the therapist identifies the nature of the problem to be resolved and then selects strategies consistent with that problem area.

BEHAVIORAL THERAPY

Behavioral therapy is based on the assumption that changes in maladaptive behavior can occur without insight into the underlying cause. This approach works best when it is directed at specific problems and the goals are well defined. Behavioral therapy is effective in treating people with phobias, alcoholism, schizophrenia, and many other conditions. Five types of behavior therapy are modeling, operant conditioning, systematic desensitization, aversion therapy, and biofeedback.

Modeling

In modeling, the therapist provides a role model for specific identified behaviors, and the patient learns through imitation. The therapist may do the modeling, provide another person to model the behaviors, or present a video for the purpose. For example, clinicians can help patients reduce their phobias about nonpoisonous snakes. They do this by having them first view close-up filmed encounters between people and snakes that resulted in successful outcomes. Afterward they view live encounters between people and snakes that also have successful outcomes.

In a similar fashion, some behavior therapists demonstrate patterns of behavior that might be more effective than those usually engaged in and then have the patients practice these new behaviors. For example, a student who does not know how to ask a professor for an extension on a term paper would watch the therapist portray a potentially effective way of making the request. The clinician would then help the student practice the new skill in a similar role-playing situation.

Operant Conditioning

Operant conditioning is the basis for behavior modification and uses positive reinforcement to increase desired behaviors. For example, when desired goals are achieved or behaviors are performed, patients might be rewarded with tokens. These tokens can be exchanged for food, small luxuries, or privileges. This reward system is known as a token economy.

Operant conditioning has been useful in improving the verbal behaviors of mute, autistic, and developmentally disabled children. In patients with severe and persistent mental illness, behavior modification has helped increase levels of self-care, social behavior, group participation, and more. You may find this a useful technique as you proceed through your clinical rotations.

A familiar case in point of positive reinforcement is a mother who takes her preschooler to the grocery store, and the child starts acting out, demanding candy, nagging, crying, and yelling. Box 29.2 lists three ways the child's behavior can be reinforced.

Box 29.2 **Behavioral Reinforcement Approaches**

Action	Result
1. The mother gives the child the candy.	The child continues to use this behavior. This is positive reinforcement of negative behavior.
2. The mother scolds the child.	Acting out may continue, because the child gets what he really wants—attention. This positively rewards negative behavior.
3. The mother ignores the acting out but gives attention to the child when he is acting appropriately.	The child gets a positive reward for appropriate behavior.

Systematic Desensitization

Systematic desensitization is another form of behavior modification therapy that involves the development of behavior tasks customized to the patient's specific fears; these tasks are presented to the patient while he or she uses learned relaxation techniques. The process involves four steps:

1. The patient's fear is broken down into its components by exploring the particular stimulus cues to which the patient reacts. For example, certain situations may precipitate a phobic reaction, whereas others do not. Crowds at parties may be problematic, whereas similar numbers of people in other settings do not cause the same distress.
2. The patient is exposed to the fear little by little. For example, a patient who has a fear of flying is introduced to short periods of visual presentations of flying—first with still pictures, then with videos, and finally in a busy airport. The situations are confronted while the patient is in a relaxed state. Gradually, over a period of time, exposure is increased until anxiety about or fear of the object or situation has ceased.
3. The patient is instructed in how to design a hierarchy of fears. For a fear of flying, a patient might develop a set of statements representing the stages of a flight, order the statements from the most fearful to the least fearful, and use relaxation techniques to reach a state of relaxation while progressing through the list.
4. The patient practices these techniques every day.

Aversion Therapy

Aversion therapy is used to treat behaviors such as alcoholism, paraphilic disorders, shoplifting, violent and aggressive behavior, and self-mutilation. Aversion therapy is the pairing of a negative stimulus with a specific target behavior, thereby suppressing the behavior. This treatment may be used when other, less drastic, measures have failed to produce the desired effects.

Simple examples of extinguishing undesirable behavior through aversion therapy include painting foul-tasting substances on the fingernails of nail biters or the thumbs of thumb suckers. Other examples of aversive stimuli are chemicals that induce nausea and vomiting, unpleasant odors, unpleasant verbal stimuli (e.g., descriptions of disturbing scenes), costs or fines in a token economy, and denial of positive reinforcement (e.g., isolation).

Before initiating any aversive protocol, the therapist, treatment team, or society must answer the following questions:

- Is this therapy in the best interest of the patient?
- Does its use violate the patient's rights?
- Is it in the best interest of society?

If the therapist believes aversion therapy as the most appropriate treatment, ongoing supervision, support, and evaluation of those administering it must occur.

Biofeedback

Through the use of sensitive instrumentation, biofeedback provides immediate and exact information regarding muscle activity, brain waves, skin temperature, heart rate, blood pressure, and other bodily functions. Indicators of the particular internal physiological process are detected and amplified by a sensitive recording device. An individual can achieve greater voluntary control over phenomena once considered to be exclusively involuntary if he or she knows instantaneously, through an auditory or visual signal, whether a somatic activity is increasing or decreasing.

The use of biofeedback was once reserved for clinicians with specialized training. Now, with increasingly sophisticated technology, most people can use some form of biofeedback themselves. Exercise trackers and smart watches provide users with the ability to track sleep patterns and heart rates. One high-tech gadget is a clip-on device that tracks respiration changes that indicate tension. A companion application (app) suggests relaxation techniques such as meditation. A hand-held device that measures skin conductance (sweat) that indicates stress also comes with an app that teaches calming techniques.

MILIEU THERAPY

Milieu (mil'yo͞o) is a word of French origin (mi "middle" + lieu "place") and refers to surroundings and physical environment. In a therapeutic context, it refers to the overall environment and interactions within that environment. It is an all-inclusive term that recognizes the people (patients and staff), the setting, the structure, and the emotional climate as important to healing. Regardless of whether the setting involves treatment of psychotic children, adult patients in a psychiatric hospital, substance users in a residential treatment center, or psychiatric patients in a day treatment program, a well-managed milieu offers patients a sense of security and promotes healing. Structured aspects of the milieu include activities, rules, reality orientation practices, and environment.

GROUP THERAPY

Group therapy is an evidence-based practice that allows multiple patients to be treated at the same time. Members benefit from the knowledge, insights, and life experience of both the leader and participants. A therapeutic group is a safe setting to learn new ways of relating to other people and to practice new communication skills. Groups can also promote feelings of belonging and a sense of cohesiveness (e.g., "We're in this together.").

Group work is characterized by both content and process. Group content is the actual words that are used in the setting. Group process is the term used to describe everything else that goes on in a group. It refers to the way group members interact with one another such as being supportive, interruptive, or silent.

Registered nurses provide group therapy for the purpose of education, tasks, and support. Nurse leaders set the foundation for open communication and mutual respect. The degree to which the leader controls the direction of the group depends on the group's needs. Autocratic leaders do not encourage much interaction and exert control over the group. This leadership style works best for time-limited tasks such as community meetings. Democratic leaders promote group interaction while maintaining the role of leader. This style works well in most groups in the psychiatric setting. Laissez-faire leaders allow the group to control its direction. This works well in creative groups such as art or horticulture groups.

Yalom and Leszcz (2005) identify core principles that make a group therapeutic. These curative (healing) factors are powerful aspects of group work success. Table 29.2 summarizes these curative factors.

Table 29.2 **Curative Factors in Group Therapy**

Curative Factor	Description
Interpersonal learning	Members gain insight into themselves based on the feedback from others during later group phases.
Catharsis	Through experiencing and expressing feelings, therapeutic discharge of emotions is shared.
Instillation of hope	The leader shares optimism about successes of group treatment, and members share their improvements.
Universality	Members realize that they are not alone with their problems, feelings, or thoughts.
Imparting of information	Participants receive formal teaching by the leader or advice from peers.
Altruism	Members gain or profit from giving support to others, leading to improved self-value.
Corrective experience of primary family	Members repeat patterns of behavior in the group that they learned in their families; with feedback from the leader and peers, they learn about their own behavior.
Socializing techniques	Members learn new social skills based on others' feedback and modeling.
Imitative behavior	Members may copy behavior from the leader or peers and can adopt healthier habits.
Group cohesiveness	Group member feels connected to the other members, the leader, and the group as a whole; members can accept positive feedback and constructive criticism.
Existential resolution	Members examine aspects of life (e.g., loneliness, mortality, responsibility) that affect everyone in constructing meaning.

From Yalom, I. D., & Leszcz, M. (2005). *The theory and practice of group psychotherapy* (5th ed.). New York, NY: Basic Books.

CHAPTER 30

Brain Stimulation Therapies

Although medication is the foundation of somatic (physical) treatment for psychiatric disorders and psychiatric symptoms, other treatments are available. Brain stimulation therapy has been in use since 1938 when electroshock therapy was used to treat almost every known psychiatric condition. Since then brain stimulation therapies have become more sophisticated and are even considered high technology. These therapies all involve activating or inhibiting the brain directly with electricity. The following brain stimulation therapies are discussed in this chapter:

- Electroconvulsive therapy (ECT)
- Repetitive transcranial magnetic stimulation (rTMS)
- Magnetic seizure therapy (MST)
- Vagus nerve stimulation (VNS)
- Deep brain stimulation (DBS)

ELECTROCONVULSIVE THERAPY

Despite being a highly effective somatic treatment for psychiatric disorders, ECT has a bad reputation. This may be related, in part, to the past practice of restraining a conscious individual while inducing a full-blown seizure. In fact, before paralytic drugs, more than 30% of ECT patients experienced compression fractures of the spine (Welch, 2016). Given the current sophistication of anesthetic and paralytic agents, ECT is actually not dramatic at all.

Indications

ECT is the most effective acute treatment for major depressive disorder (Welch, 2016). Psychotic illnesses are the second most common indication for ECT. For drug-resistant patients with psychosis, a combination of

ECT and antipsychotic medication has resulted in sustained improvement about 80% of the time. Depression associated with bipolar disorder remits in about 50% of the cases after ECT. It is also useful in treatment-refractory cases of obsessive–compulsive disorder.

Although medication is generally the first line of treatment for ease of use, ECT may be a primary treatment in the following circumstances:

- When the patient is severely malnourished, exhausted, and dehydrated because of lengthy depression (after rehydration)
- When ECT is more safe than medications because of certain medical conditions
- When the patient has delusional depression
- When previous medication trials have failed
- When the patient has schizophrenia with catatonia

Risk Factors

Using ECT requires clinicians to weigh the risk of using this method versus the risk of suicide and diminished quality of life. Several conditions pose risks and require careful workup and management. Because the heart can be stressed at the onset of the seizure and for up to 10 minutes after, careful assessment and management in hypertension, congestive heart failure, cardiac arrhythmias, and other cardiac conditions is warranted (Welch, 2016). ECT also stresses the brain as a result of increased cerebral oxygen, blood flow, and intracranial pressure. Conditions such as brain tumors and subdural hematomas may increase the risk when using ECT.

Procedure

The procedure is explained to the patient, and informed consent is obtained if the patient is being treated voluntarily. For a patient treated involuntarily, permission may be obtained from the next of kin, although in some states such treatment must be court-ordered. The patient is usually given a general anesthetic to induce sleep and a muscle-paralyzing agent to prevent muscle distress and fractures. These medications have revolutionized the comfort and safety of ECT.

Patients should have a pre-ECT workup that includes chest radiography, an electrocardiogram (ECG), a urinalysis, a complete blood count, blood urea nitrogen, and an electrolyte panel. Benzodiazepines should be discontinued before the procedure, because they will interfere with the seizure process.

An electroencephalogram (EEG) monitors brain waves, and an electrocardiogram monitors cardiac responses. Brief seizures (30–60 seconds) are deliberately induced by an electrical current (as brief as 1 second) transmitted through electrodes attached to one or both sides of the head. To ensure that patients experience a seizure over the entire brain, a blood pressure cuff may be inflated on the lower arm or leg before administration of the paralytic agent. In that way, the convulsion can be visualized in the unparalyzed extremity.

The usual course of ECT for a patient with depression is two or three treatments per week to a total of 6 to 12 treatments. Continuation ECT along with medication may help to decrease relapse rates.

Side Effects

Patients wake about 15 minutes after the procedure. The patient is often confused and disoriented for several hours. The nurse and family may need to orient the patient frequently during the course of treatment. Most people experience what is called *retrograde amnesia,* which is a loss of memory of events leading up to and including the treatment itself.

REPETITIVE TRANSCRANIAL MAGNETIC STIMULATION

rTMS is a noninvasive modality used in the treatment of major depressive disorder. The rTMS system is an electromagnetic device that non-invasively delivers a rapidly pulsed magnetic field to the cerebral cortex to activate neurons within a limited volume without inducing a seizure.

Indications

In 2008 the U.S. Food and Drug Administration (FDA) approved the use of rTMS for major depressive disorder. Specifically, this treatment is approved for adult patients who have failed to achieve satisfactory improvement from one prior antidepressant medication at or above the minimal effective dose and duration in the current episode. It may also be a promising treatment for generalized anxiety disorder. Some researchers even suggest that rTMS be used to enhance cognitive function in healthy, non-depressed individuals.

Risk Factors

The only absolute contraindication to rTMS is the presence of metal in the area of stimulation. Cochlear implants, brain stimulators, or medication pumps are examples of metals that could interfere with the procedures.

Procedure

Outpatient treatment with rTMS takes about 30 minutes and is typically ordered for 5 days a week for 4 to 6 weeks. Patients are awake and alert during the procedure. An electromagnet is placed on the patient's scalp, and short, magnetic pulses pass into the prefrontal cortex of the brain. These pulses are similar to those used for magnetic resonance imaging but are more focused. The pulses cause electrical charges to flow and induce neurons to fire or become active. During the procedure, patients feel a slight tapping or knocking in the head, contraction of the scalp, and tightening of the jaws.

Side Effects

After the procedure, patients may experience a headache and lightheadedness. No neurological deficits or memory problems have been noted. Seizures are a rare complication of rTMS. Most of the common side effects of rTMS are mild and include scalp tingling and discomfort at the administration site.

MAGNETIC SEIZURE THERAPY

MST combines certain elements from both ECT and rTMS. Like rTMS, MST uses magnetic pulses instead of electricity to stimulate a precise area of the brain (National Institute of Mental Health, 2016). Like ECT, MST aims to induce a seizure. The seizure is accomplished by using higher-frequency pulses than the ones given in rTMS.

The goal of MST is to achieve the effectiveness of ECT while reducing its cognitive side effects. ECT leads to a much more widespread seizure induction. This widespread effect is probably responsible for cognitive problems after ECT. MST uses a more focal seizure expression with less involvement of hippocampal and deep brain structures.

Indications

Although MST is in the early stages of testing for psychiatric disorders, results are promising. Recent research indicates that MST has been effective in triggering remission in 30% to 40% of individuals treated for major depressive disorder and bipolar disorder. It is also being investigated as a treatment for schizophrenia and obsessive–compulsive disorder.

Procedure

The patient must be anesthetized and given a muscle relaxant to prevent movement during the procedure. The motor activity of the right foot is assessed visually to track the duration of the motor seizure. An EEG is used to track seizure activity in the brain. Up to 600 pulses are delivered. Generally, two or three MST sessions are delivered each week. Some research reports using a total of 24 sessions or continued use until symptoms abate.

Side Effects

Common side effects after MST are headache, dizziness, nausea, vomiting, muscle aches, and fatigue. These side effects can be explained by anesthesia exposure and the induction of a seizure. Studies in both animals and humans have found that MST produces the following:

- Fewer memory side effects
- Shorter seizures
- A shorter recovery time than is experienced with ECT

VAGUS NERVE STIMULATION

The use of VNS originated as a treatment for epilepsy. Clinicians noted that in addition to decreasing seizures, VNS also seemed to improve mood in a population that normally experiences higher rates of depression. The theory behind VNS relates to the action of the vagus nerve, the longest cranial nerve, which extends from the brainstem to organs in the neck, chest, and abdomen. Electrical stimulation of the vagus nerve results in boosting the level of neurotransmitters, thereby improving mood and also enhancing the action of antidepressants.

Indications

Nearly a decade after VNS was approved for use in Europe, the FDA granted approval for its use in the United States for treatment-resistant depression. The efficacy of VNS in treating depression is still being established. Other potential applications of VNS include anxiety, obesity, and pain.

Procedure

The surgery to implant VNS is typically an outpatient procedure. A pacemaker-like device is implanted surgically into the left chest wall. The device is connected to a thin flexible wire that is threaded up and wrapped around the vagus nerve on the left side of the neck. After surgery, an infrared magnetic wand is held against the chest while a personal computer or personal digital assistant is used to program the frequency of pulses. Pulses are usually delivered for 30 seconds, every 5 minutes, 24 hours a day. Antidepressant action usually occurs in several weeks.

Side Effects

The implantation of VNS is a surgical procedure, carrying with it the risks inherent in any surgical procedure (e.g., pain, infection, sensitivity to anesthesia). Side effects of active VNS therapy are related to the proximity of the lead on the vagus nerve, which is close to the laryngeal and pharyngeal branches of the left vagus nerve. Voice alteration occurs in nearly 60% of patients. Other side effects include neck pain, cough, paresthesia, and dyspnea, which tend to decrease with time. The device can be temporarily turned off by placing a special magnet over the implant. This may be especially helpful when engaging in public speaking or heavy exercise.

DEEP BRAIN STIMULATION

DBS is a treatment whereby electrodes are surgically implanted into specific areas of the brain to stimulate those regions identified to be underactive in depression. Electrical pulses are delivered continuously and are believed to "reset" the malfunctioning area of the brain.

Indications

DBS is a long-approved surgical treatment for Parkinson disease. Clinical trials are investigating its use in patients with treatment-resistant depression and obsessive–compulsive disorder. One of the challenges is identifying the optimal neuroanatomical target in the brain.

Procedure

As in VNS, a device is implanted in the chest wall that is designed to provide electrical stimulation. It differs from VNS in that electrodes are implanted directly into the brain to modify brain activity. Before the procedure, the head is shaved and then attached with screws to a frame to prevent the head from moving. The patient is awake during the procedure to provide the surgeon with feedback.

Two holes are dilled into the head under a local anesthetic. A slender tube is threaded to specific areas and electrodes are inserted. In the case of depression, several areas of the brain have been targeted by DBS. In the case of obsessive–compulsive disorder, the electrodes are placed in the ventral capsule and ventral striatum, the areas of the brain believed to be associated with obsessive thoughts and compulsive behavior.

After placement, the patient provides feedback and then is placed under general anesthesia. The electrodes are then attached to wires inside the body that run from the head to the chest. A pair of battery-operated generators is implanted in the chest that continuously delivers electrical pulses.

Adverse Reactions

DBS is also more invasive and as such carries risks associated with any type of brain surgery. For example, the procedure may lead to the following:

- Bleeding in the brain or stroke
- Infection
- Disorientation or confusion
- Unwanted mood changes
- Movement disorders
- Lightheadedness
- Sleep disturbances

Because of its recent introduction, it is likely that not all side effects have been identified.

LIGHT THERAPY

Light therapy has been researched for nearly 20 years and is accepted as a first-line treatment for seasonal affective disorder (SAD). SAD is considered a subtype of major depressive disorder. People with SAD often live in regions in which there are marked seasonal differences in the amount of daylight. For those affected by SAD, light therapy has been found to be as effective in reducing depressive symptoms as medications.

Light therapy's effectiveness is thought to be the influence of light on melatonin. Melatonin is secreted by the pineal gland and is necessary for maintaining and shifting biological rhythms. Patients with SAD may have longer periods of nocturnal melatonin secretion during winter than during summer. Light therapy treatment may improve SAD symptoms by shortening the nocturnal duration of melatonin.

Ideal treatment consists of 30 to 45 minutes of exposure daily to a 10,000-lux light source. Morning exposure is best. However, success has been reported when exposure occurs at other times of the day or in divided doses. Anecdotal reports suggest that increasing the available light by adding additional light sources may also help to elevate mood.

Negative side effects include headache and jitteriness. People with past or current eye problems such as glaucoma, cataracts, or eye damage from diabetes should consult eye specialists before beginning light therapy.

References

Agency for Healthcare Research and Quality. (2012). Improving patient safety systems for patients with limited English proficiency. Retrieved from https://www.ahrq.gov/professionals/systems/hospital/lepguide/lepguide1.html.

Ahmedani, B. K., Simon, G. E., Stewart, C., et al. (2014). Health care contacts in the year before suicide death. *Journal of General Internal Medicine, 29*(6), 870–877. doi:10.1007/s11606-014-2767-3.

Alonso, P., Cuadras, D., Gabriels, L., et al. (2015). Deep brain stimulation for obsessive-compulsive disorder: A meta-analysis of treatment outcome and predictors of response. *PLOS* [online]. Retrieved from http://journals.plos.org/plosone/article?id=10.1371/journal.pone.0133591.

Alzheimer's Association. (2014). Alzheimer's Association Report: 2014 Alzheimer's disease facts and figures. *Alzheimer's and Dementia, 10*, e47–e92.

American Association of Neurological Surgeons. (2017). A pilot study of deep brain stimulation in treatment-resistant schizophrenia. *ScienceDaily*, from www.sciencedaily.com/releases/2017/04/170425153818.htm. (Retrieved 12 September 2017).

American Nurses Association, American Psychiatric Nurses Association, & the International Society of Psychiatric-Mental Health Nurses. (2014). *Psychiatric-mental health nursing: Scope and standards of practice.* Silver Spring, MD: nursesbooks.org.

American Psychiatric Association. (2013). *Diagnostic and statistical manual of mental health disorders* (5th ed.). Washington, DC: Author.

Beck, A. T. (1979). *Cognitive therapy and the emotional disorders*. New York: International Universities Press.

Bridge, J. A., Iyengar, S., Salary, C. B., et al. (2007). Clinical response and risk for reported suicidal ideation and suicide attempts in pediatric antidepressant treatment: A meta-analysis of randomized controlled trials. *JAMA: The Journal of the American Medical Association, 297*, 1683–1696.

Bulechek, G. M., Butcher, H. K., Dochterman, J. M., et al. (2013). *Nursing interventions classification (NIC)* (6th ed.). St. Louis, MO: Mosby.

Caplan, G. (1964). *Principles of preventive psychiatry.* New York, NY: Basic Books.

Center for Behavioral Health Statistics and Quality. (2015). Behavioral health trends in the United States: Results from the 2014 National Survey on Drug Use and Health (HHS Publication No. SMA 15-4927, NSDUH Series H-50). Retrieved from http://www.samhsa.gov/data/.

Centers for Disease Control and Prevention. (2010). Adverse childhood experiences reported by adult—Five states, 2009. *Morbidity and Mortality Weekly Report, 59*(49), 1609–1613.

Centers for Disease Control and Prevention. (2013). Mental health surveillance among children—United States 2005-2011. Retrieved from https://www.cdc.gov/mmwr/preview/mmwrhtml/su6202a1.htm?s_cid=su6202a1_w.

Centers for Disease Control and Prevention. (2016). Suicide facts at a glance: 2015. Retrieved from http://www.cdc.gov/violenceprevention/pdf/suicide-datasheet-a.pdf.

Christensen, D. L., Baio, J., Braun, K. V., et al. (2016). Prevalence and characteristics of autism spectrum disorder among children age 8 years. *Surveillance Summaries, 65*, DOI: http://dx.doi.org/10.15585/mmwr.ss6503a1.

Coupland, C., Dhiman, P., Morriss, R., et al. (2011). Antidepressant use and risk of adverse outcomes in older people: Population based cohort study. *BMJ (Clinical Research Ed.), 343*, d4551.

Ebert, D. H., Finn, C. T., & Smoller, J. W. (2016). Genetics and psychiatry. In T. A. Stern, M. Fava, T. E. Wilens, et al. (Eds.), *Massachusetts General Hospital comprehensive clinical psychiatry* (2nd ed., p. 681). Philadelphia, PA: Saunders.

Gordon, C., & Bereson, E. V. (2016). The doctor-patient relationship. In T. A. Stern, M. Fava, T. E. Wilens, et al. (Eds.), *Massachusetts General Hospital comprehensive clinical psychiatry* (2nd ed., pp. 1–7). Philadelphia, PA: Saunders.

Halter, M. (2018). *Varcarolis' foundations of psychiatric-mental health nursing* (8th ed.). St. Louis, MO: Elsevier.

Harrington, B. C., Jimerson, M., Haxton, C., et al. (2015). Initial evaluation, diagnosis, and treatment of anorexia nervosa and bulimia nervosa. *American Family Physician,*

91(1), 46–52. Retrieved from http://ezproxy.twu.edu:2048/login?url=http://search.ebscohost.com/login.aspx?direct=true&db=ccm&AN=109693701&site=ehost-live&scope=site.

Huang, Y., Kotov, R., de Girolamo, G., et al. (2009). DSM-IV personality disorders in the WHO world mental health surveys. *British Journal of Psychiatry, 195*(1), 46–53. doi:10.1192/bjp.bp.108.058552.

Kaster, T. S., Daskalakis, Z. J., & Blumberger, D. M. (2017). Clinical effectiveness and cognitive impact of electroconvulsive therapy for schizophrenia: A large retrospective study. *Journal of Clinical Psychiatry, 78*(4), e383–e389. doi:10.4088/JCP.16m10686.

Kessler, R. C., Sonnega, A., Bromet, E., et al. (1995). Posttraumatic stress in the national comorbidity survey. *Archives of General Psychiatry, 52*, 1048–1060.

Kilpatrick, D. G., Resnick, H. S., & Friedman, M. J. (2013). Severity of posttraumatic stress symptoms scale. Retrieved from APA_DSM5_Severity-of-Posttraumatic-Stress-Symptoms-Adult%20(7).pdf.

Kübler-Ross, E. (1969). *On death and dying*. New York, NY: Macmillan.

Linehan, M. M. (1993). *Cognitive-behavioral treatment of borderline personality disorder*. New York: NY: Guilford.

McInnis, M. G., Riba, M., & Greden, J. F. (2014). Depressive disorders. In R. E. Hales, S. C. Yudofsky, & L. W. Roberts (Eds.), *Textbook of psychiatry*. Washington, DC: American Psychiatric Publishing.

Moorhead, S., Johnson, M., Maas, M., et al. (2013). *Nursing outcomes classification (NOC)* (5th ed.). St. Louis, MO: Mosby.

National Council of State Boards of Nursing. (2015). *2016 NCLEX-RN detailed test plan—candidate version*. Retrieved from https://www.ncsbn.org/2016_RN_Test_Plan_Candidate.pdf.

National Institute for Complementary and Integrative Care. (2016). Chamomile. Retrieved from https://nccih.nih.gov/health/chamomile/ataglance.htm.

National Institute of Mental Health. (2012). *Older adults: Depression and suicide facts (fact sheet)*. Retrieved from http://www.nimh.nih.gov/health/publications/older-adults-and-depression/older-adults-and-depression_141998.pdf.

National Institute of Mental Health. (2015). Post-traumatic stress disorder among adults. Retrieved from https://

www.nimh.nih.gov/health/statistics/prevalence/post-traumatic-stress-disorder-among-adults.shtml.

National Institute of Mental Health. (2016). Brain stimulation therapies. Retrieved from https://www.nimh.nih.gov/health/topics/brain-stimulation-therapies/brain-stimulation-therapies.shtml#part_152880.

National Institute on Drug Abuse. (2015). Strategic plan 2016–2020. Retrieved from http://www.drugabuse.gov/about-nida/strategic-plan.

National League for Nursing. (2015). Debriefing across the curriculum. Retrieved from http://www.nln.org/docs/default-source/about/nln-vision-series-(position-statements)/nln-vision-debriefing-across-the-curriculum.pdf?sfvrsn=0.

Olivier, J. D. A., Akerud, H., & Promomaa, I. S. (2015). Antenatal depression and antidepressants during pregnancy. *European Journal of Pharmacology*, *753*, 257–262.

Peplau, H. E. (1968). A working definition of anxiety. In S. F. Burd & M. A. Marshall (Eds.), *Some clinical approaches to psychiatric nursing* (pp. 323–327). New York, NY: Macmillan.

Peplau, H. E. (1999). *Interpersonal relations in nursing: A conceptual frame of reference for psychodynamic nursing*. New York, NY: Springer.

Quality and Safety Education for Nurses. (2012). Patient centered care. Retrieved from http://www.qsen.org/definition.php?id=1.

Risacher, S. L., McDonald, B. C., Tallman, E. F., et al. (2016). Association between anticholinergic medication use and cognitition, brain metabolism, and brain atrophy in cognitively normal older adults. *JAMA Neurology*, *73*(6), 721–732. doi:10.1001/jamaneurol.2016.0580.

Rosenvinge, J., & Petterson, G. (2015). Epidemiology of eating disorders part II: An update with a special reference to the DSM-5. *Advances in Eating Disorders*, *3*(2), 198–220. doi:10.1080/21662630.2014.940549.

Sadock, B. J., Sadock, V. A., & Ruiz, P. (2015). *Kaplan and Sadock's synopsis of psychiatry*. Philadelphia, PA: Wolters Kluwer.

Sansone, R., & Sansone, L. A. (2011). Personality disorders: A nation-based perspective on prevalence. *Innovation in Clinical Neuroscience*, *8*(4), 13–18.

Skodol, A. E., Bender, D. S., Morey, L. C., et al. (2011). Personality disorder types proposed for DSM-5. *Journal of Personality Disorders*, *25*(2), 136–169.

Spielman, A., & Glovinsky, P. (2004). A conceptual framework of insomnia for primary care providers: Predisposing, precipitating, and perpetuating factors. *Sleep Medicine Alert*, *9*(1), 1–6.

Substance Abuse and Mental Health Services Administration. (2014). Gambling problems: An introduction for behavioral health services providers. Retrieved from http://www.ncpgambling.org/wp-content/uploads/2014/04/Gambling-Addiction-An-Introduction-for-Behavioral-Health-Providers-SAMHSA-2014.pdf.

Substance Abuse and Mental Health Services Administration. (2015). *Behavioral health trends in the United States: Results from the 2014 National Survey on Drug Use and Health. (HHS Publication No. SMA 15-4927, NSDUH Series H-50)*. Retrieved from http://www.samhsa.gov/data/sites/default/files/NSDUH-FRR1-2014/NSDUH-FRR1-2014.pdf.

U.S. Department of Justice. (2012). An updated definition of rape. Retrieved from https://www.justice.gov/opa/blog/updated-definition-rape.

U.S. Food and Drug Administration. (2017). FDA online label repository. Retrieved from http://labels.fda.gov/.

van Munster, B. C., & de Rooij, S. E. (2014). Delirium: A synthesis of current knowledge. *Clinical Medicine*, *14*(2), 192–195.

Welch, C. A. (2016). Electroconvulsive therapy. In T. A. Stern, M. Fava, T. E. Wilens, et al. (Eds.), *Comprehensive clinical psychiatry* (2nd ed.). St. Louis, MO: Elsevier.

APPENDIX A

Patient-Centered Assessment

A patient-centered assessment such as this can be used to structure admission data. Key findings from an initial assessment provide direction for determining patient problems and planning. Most of the checkboxes included in this assessment tool should be supplemented with more thorough descriptions of abnormal findings. The patient-centered assessment begins with general information, then covers essential information (e.g., substance use and sleep), and progresses to the more detailed mood and cognitive domains.

GENERAL INFORMATION

Name (or initials):
Age:
Sex: ☐ Female ☐ Male
Race:
☐ White ☐ Black or African American ☐ American Indian or Alaska Native
☐ Asian ☐ Native Hawaiian or Other Pacific Islander
Ethnicity:
☐ Non-Hispanic, Latino, or Spanish origin ☐ Hispanic, Latino, or Spanish origin
Language:
☐ English ☐ English as second language ☐ Other:
Height: Weight: Recent weight gain/loss (amount):
Marital status: ☐ Single ☐ Married ☐ Cohabitating ☐ Divorced ☐ Other:
Education: ☐ <High school ☐ High school
☐ Some associates/technical/trade ☐ Associates/technical/trade
☐ Some undergraduate ☐ Undergraduate
☐ Some graduate ☐ Graduate

Employment: □ Currently employed □ Full-time
□ Part-time
Occupation:
Residence: □ Rents □ Owns home □ Other:
Lives with:

PRESENTING PROBLEM, STRENGTHS, GOALS, AND COPING

1. Use a question such as, "Identify the purpose of you being admitted/treated here" to provide a statement in the patient's own words in quotations, the reason for treatment.
2. Ask the patient to identify three strengths.
3. Ask the patient to identify three goals for hospitalization/treatment.
4. Ask the patient to identify coping methods for stress, anxiety, and when angry.

RELEVANT HISTORY

1. Do any family members have psychiatric problems?
2. Do you have a history of emotional, physical, or sexual abuse and/or neglect?
3. Have you ever experienced a traumatic event or traumatic events?

PSYCHIATRIC HISTORY

Treatment Dates	Therapist/Facility	Outcome

History of suicidality (ideation, gesture, attempt, method):
Current suicidality (ideation, gesture, plan, means):
History of violence/homicidality:
Current thoughts of violence/homicidality:

MEDICATION (INCLUDING OVER-THE-COUNTER)

Medication	Dose	Frequency	Dates of Use

ALCOHOL/SUBSTANCE USE

History of alcohol and/or substance use:
Treatment for alcohol and/or substance use:
Current alcohol and/or substance use:

SLEEP PATTERN

Quantity: □ 0 to 2 hours □ 2 to 4 hours □ 4 to 6 hours □ 6 to 8 hours □ 9 + hours
Initiation: □ No problem falling asleep □ Difficulty falling asleep
Maintenance: □ Continuous sleep □ Wakes repeatedly □ Wakes and has difficulty returning to sleep
Quality: □ Refreshing □ Not refreshing

APPEARANCE

Eye contact: □ Direct □ Poor □ Intermittent □ Staring □ Intense
Pupils: □ Normal □ Constricted □ Dilated
Age: □ Appears stated age □ Appears older than stated age
Posture: □ Neutral □ Slouched □ Straight □ Tense
Gait: □ Normal □ Shuffling □ Staggering □ Spastic
Attire: □ Neat □ Unkempt □ Appropriate □ Inappropriate attire
Hygiene: □ Good □ Neglected
Skin: □ Healthy □ Impaired integrity

ATTITUDE

□ Cooperative □ Engaged □ Disengaged □ Defensive □ Elusive □ Poor historian

BEHAVIOR

Psychomotor: □ Normal □ Hyperactive □ Agitated □ Retarded
Movement: □ Akathisia □ Catatonia □ Echopraxia □ Waxy flexibility
□ Verbal tics □ Motor tics □ Fine hand tremor □ Course hand tremor □ Dystonia
□ Tardive dyskinesia (attach AIMs scale from Chapter 22)

MOOD

Mood is assessed by asking the patient, "How do you feel?" and then summarized by the nurse.
□ Euthymic (normal) □ Depressed □ Euphoric (elated) □ Angry
□ Irritable □ Anxious □ Apathetic □ Anhedonic □ Alexithymic (unable to describe mood)

AFFECT

Affect is determined by observations of the nurse.
□ Appropriate to situation □ Inappropriate to situation
□ Congruent with mood □ Incongruent with mood
□ Even □ Intense □ Blunt □ Flat □ Heightened □ Dramatic
□ Constricted □ Fixed □ Immobile □ Labile

SPEECH

Presence: □ Present □ Absent/mute □ Aphasic
Rate: □ Slow □ Hesitant □ Normal □ Rapid □ Pressured
Volume: □ Soft □ Normal □ Loud
Articulation: □ Clear □ Mumbled □ Garbled □ Overemphasis □ Stuttered
Speech patterns: □ Echolalia (repeating others' words) □ Palilalia (repeating own words) □ Neologisms (creating new words)

THOUGHT PROCESSES

□ Poverty of thought □ Normal quantity of thought □ Overabundance of thought
□ Retarded □ Perseveration □ Circumstantiality □ Tangentiality □ Loose associations
□ Flight of ideas □ Logical □ Disorganized □ Blocking

THOUGHT CONTENT

Delusions: □ Paranoid □ Ideas of reference □ Persecutory □ Grandiose □ Erotomanic
□ Somatic □ Jealousy □ Control □ Guilt □ Poverty □ Nihilistic □ Religious
Outside control: □ Thought broadcasting □ Thought withdrawal □ Thought insertion
Intrusive thoughts: □ Obsessions □ Phobias
Preoccupation: □ Suicidality □ Aggression □ Homicidality □ Suspicions □ Fears

PERCEPTIONS

Hallucinations: □ Auditory □ Visual □ Tactile □ Olfactory □ Gustatory
Auditory hallucinations: □ Inside own head □ Outside own head □ Pleasant/positive □ Negative □ Insulting □ Command □ Distractible
Frequency:
Other: □ Illusions □ Depersonalization □ Derealization □ Déjà vu

COGNITION

Alertness: □ Alert □ Clouded □ Drowsy □ Stuporous
Orientation: □ Person □ Time □ Date □ Place □ Situation
Attention and concentration:
Serial sevens (counting backward from 100 by 7s)
□ Able □ Makes mistakes □ Unable
Spelling a five-letter word (such as world) backward
□ Able □ Makes mistakes □ Unable
Memory:
Immediate memory (repeating a set of words)
□ Able □ Makes mistakes □ Unable
Short-term memory (repeating a set of words after an interval)
□ Able □ Makes mistakes □ Unable
Long-term memory (recalling an historical or geographical fact)
□ Able □ Makes mistakes □ Unable
Cognitive/visual functioning:
Complex task (draw the face of a clock)
□ Able □ Makes mistakes □ Unable

INSIGHT

Recognition of psychiatric disorder
□ Insight intact □ Some insight □ Insight absent
Participation in care decisions
□ Actively participates □ Some participation □ No participation □ Resists participation
Understands that symptoms are part of a psychiatric disorder
□ Insight intact □ Some insight □ Insight absent

JUDGMENT

□ Judgment intact □ Judgment fair □ Judgment impaired □ Judgment critically impaired

APPENDIX B

DSM-5 Classification

Before each disorder name, ICD-10-CM codes are provided. Blank lines indicate that the ICD-10-CM code is not applicable. For some disorders, the code can be indicated only according to the subtype or specifier.

After chapter titles and disorder names, page numbers for the corresponding text or criteria are included in parentheses.

Note that for all mental disorders related to another medical condition, indicate the name of the other medical condition in the name of the mental disorder with "due to [the medical condition]." The code and name for the other medical condition should be listed first immediately before the mental disorder related to the medical condition.

NEURODEVELOPMENTAL DISORDERS (31)

Intellectual Disabilities (33)

—.—	Intellectual Disability (Intellectual Developmental Disorder) (33)
	Specify current severity:
F70	Mild
F71	Moderate
F72	Severe
F73	Profound
F88	Global Developmental Delay (41)
F79	Unspecified Intellectual Disability (Intellectual Developmental Disorder) (41)

Communication Disorders (41)

F80.9	Language Disorder (42)
F80.0	Speech Sound Disorder (44)
F80.81	Childhood-Onset Fluency Disorder (Stuttering) (45)
	Note: Later-onset cases are diagnosed as 307.0 (F98.5) Adult-Onset Fluency Disorder.
F80.98	Social (Pragmatic) Communication Disorder (47)
F80.9	Unspecified Communication Disorder (49)

Autism Spectrum Disorder (50)

F84.0	Autism Spectrum Disorder (50)
	Specify if: Associated with a known medical or genetic condition or environmental factor; Associated with another neurodevelopmental, mental or behavioral disorder
	Specify current severity for Criterion A and Criterion B: Requiring very substantial support, Requiring substantial support, Requiring support
	Specify if: With or without accompanying intellectual impairment, With or without accompanying language impairment, With catatonia (use additional code 293.89 [F06.1])

Attention-Deficit/Hyperactivity Disorder (59)

—.—	Attention-Deficit/Hyperactivity Disorder (59)
	Specify whether:
F90.2	Combined presentation
F90.0	Predominantly inattentive presentation
F90.1	Predominantly hyperactive/impulsive presentation
	Specify if: In partial remission
	Specify current severity: Mild, Moderate, Severe
F90.8	Other Specified Attention-Deficit/Hyperactivity Disorder (65)
F90.9	Unspecified Attention-Deficit/Hyperactivity Disorder (66)

Specific Learning Disorder (66)

—.—	Specific Learning Disorder (66)
	Specify if:
F81.0	With impairment in reading (specify if with word reading accuracy, reading rate or fluency, reading comprehension)
F81.81	With impairment in written expression (specify if with spelling accuracy, grammar and punctuation accuracy, clarity or organization of written expression)
F81.2	With impairment in mathematics (specify if with number sense, memorization or arithmetic facts, accurate or fluent calculation, accurate math reasoning)
	Specify current severity: Mild, Moderate, Severe

Motor Disorders (74)

F82	Developmental Coordination Disorder (74)
F98.4	Stereotypic Movement Disorder (77)
	Specify if: With self-injurious behavior, Without self-injurious behavior
	Specify if: Associated with a known medical or genetic condition, neurodevelopmental disorder, or environmental factor
	Specify current severity: Mild, Moderate, Severe

Tic Disorders

F95.2	Tourette's Disorder (81)
F95.1	Persistent (Chronic) Motor or Vocal Tic Disorder (81)
	Specify if: With motor tics only, With vocal tics only
F95.0	Provisional Tic Disorder (81)
F95.8	Other Specified Tic Disorder (85)
F95.9	Unspecified Tic Disorder (85)

Other Neurodevelopment Disorders (86)

F88	Other Specified Neurodevelopmental Disorder (86)
F89	Unspecified Neurodevelopmental Disorder (86)

SCHIZOPHRENIA SPECTRUM AND OTHER PSYCHOTIC DISORDERS (87)

The following specifiers apply to Schizophrenia Spectrum and Other Psychotic Disorders where indicated:

F21	Schizotypal (Personality) Disorder (90)
F22	Delusional Disorder[a,c] (90)
	Specify whether: Erotomanic type, Grandiose type, Jealous type, Persecutory type, Somatic type, Mixed type, Unspecified type
	Specify if: With bizarre content
F23	Brief Psychotic Disorder[b,c] (94)
	Specify if: With marked stressor(s), Without marked stressor(s), With postpartum onset
F20.81	Schizophreniform Disorder[b,c] (96)
	Specify if: With good prognostic features, Without good prognostic features
F20.9	Schizophrenia[a,b,c] (99)
—.—	Schizoaffective Disorder[a,b,c] (105)
	Specify whether:
F25.0	Bipolar type
F25.1	Depressive type
—.—	Substance/Medication-Induced Psychotic Disorder[c] (110)
	Note: See the criteria set and corresponding recording procedures for substance-specific codes and ICD-10-CM coding.
	Specify if: With onset during intoxication, With onset during withdrawal
—.—	Psychotic Disorder Due to Another Medical Condition[c] (115)
	Specify whether:
F06.2	With delusions
F06.0	With hallucinations
F06.1	Catatonia Associated With Another Mental Disorder (Catatonia Specifier) (119)
F06.1	Catatonic Disorder Due to Another Medical Condition (120)
F06.1	Unspecified Catatonia (121)
	Note: Code first 781.99 (R29.818) other symptoms involving nervous and musculoskeletal systems.

Continued

F28	Other Specified Schizophrenia Spectrum and Other Psychotic Disorder (122)
F29	Unspecified Schizophrenia Spectrum and Other Psychotic Disorder (122)

[a]Specify if: The following course specifiers are only to be used after a 1-year duration of the disorder: First episode, currently in acute episode; First episode, currently in partial remission; First episode, currently in full remission; Multiple episodes, currently in acute episode; Multiple episodes, currently in partial remission; Multiple episodes, currently in full remission; Continuous; Unspecified
[b]Specify if: With catatonia (use additional code 293.89 [F06.1])
[c]Specify current severity of delusions, hallucinations, disorganized speech, abnormal psychomotor behavior, negative symptoms, impaired cognition, depression, and mania symptoms

BIPOLAR AND RELATED DISORDERS (123)

The following specifiers apply to Bipolar and Related Disorders where indicated:

—.—	Bipolar I Disorder[a] (123)
—.—	Current or most recent episode manic
F31.11	Mild
F31.12	Moderate
F31.13	Severe
F31.2	With psychotic features
F31.73	In partial remission
F31.74	In full remission
F31.9	Unspecified
F31.0	Current or most recent episode hypomanic
F31.73	In partial remission
F31.74	In full remission
F31.9	Unspecified
—.—	Current or most recent episode depressed
F31.31	Mild
F31.32	Moderate
F31.4	Severe
F31.5	With psychotic features
F31.75	In partial remission
F31.76	In full remission
F31.9	Unspecified
F31.9	Current or most recent episode unspecified
F31.81	Bipolar II Disorder[a] (132)
	Specify current or most recent episode: Hypomanic, Depressed

	Specify course if full criteria for a mood episode are not currently met: In partial remission, In full remission
	Specify severity if full criteria for a mood episode are not currently met: Mild, Moderate, Severe
F34.0	Cyclothymic Disorder (139)
	Specify if: With anxious distress
—.—	Substance/Medication-Induced Bipolar and Related Disorder (142)
	Note: See the criteria set and corresponding recording procedures for substance-specific coded and ICD-10-CM coding.
	Specify if: With onset during intoxication, With onset during withdrawal
—.—	Bipolar and Related Disorder Due to Another Medical Condition (145)
	Specify if:
F06.33	With manic features
F06.33	With manic- or hypomanic-like episode
F06.33	With mixed features
F31.89	Other specified Bipolar and Related Disorder (148)
F31.9	Unspecified Bipolar and Related Disorder (149)

[a]Specify: With anxious distress (specify current severity: mild, moderate, moderate-severe, severe); With mixed features; With rapid cycling; With melancholic features; With atypical features; With mood-congruent psychotic features; With mood-incongruent psychotic features; With catatonia (use additional code 293.89 [F06.1]); With peripartum onset; With seasonal pattern

DEPRESSIVE DISORDERS (155)

The following specifiers apply to Depressive Disorders where indicated:

F34.8]	Disruptive Mood Dysregulation Disorder (156)
—.—	Major Depressive Disorder[a] (160)
—.—	Single episode
F32.0	Mild
F32.1	Moderate
F32.2	Severe
F32.3	With psychotic features
F32.4	In partial remission
F32.5	In full remission
F32.9	Unspecified
—.—	Recurrent episode
F33.0	Mild
F33.1	Moderate

Continued

F33.2	Severe
F33.3	With psychotic features
F33.41	In partial remission
F33.42	In full remission
F33.9	Unspecified
F34.1	Persistent Depressive Disorder (Dysthymia)[a] (168)
	Specify if: In partial remission, In full remission
	Specify if: Early onset, Late onset
	Specify if: With pure dysthymic syndrome; With persistent major depressive episode; With intermittent major depressive episodes, with current episode; With intermittent major depressive episodes, without current episode
	Specify current severity: Mild, Moderate, Severe
N94.3	Premenstrual Dysphoric Disorder (171)
___.___	Substance/Medication-Induced Depressive Disorder (175)
	Note: See the criteria set and corresponding recording procedures for substance-specific codes and ICD-10-CM coding.
	Specify if: With onset during intoxication, With onset during withdrawal
___.___	Depressive Disorder Due to Another Medical Condition (180)
	Specify if:
F06.31	With depressive features
F06.32	With major depressive-like episode
F06.34	With mixed features
F32.8	Other Specified Depressive Disorder (183)
F32.9	Unspecified Depressive Disorder (184)

[a]Specify: With anxious distress (specify current severity: mild, moderate, moderate-severe, severe); With mixed features; With melancholic features; With atypical features; With mood-congruent psychotic features; With mood-incongruent psychotic features; With catatonia (use additional code 293.89 [F06.1]); With peripartum onset; With seasonal pattern

ANXIETY DISORDERS (189)

F93.0	Separation Anxiety Disorder (190)
F94.0	Selective Mutism (195)
___.___	Specific Phobia (197)
	Specify if:
F40.218	Animal
F40.228	Natural environmental
___.___	Blood-injection-injury

F40.230	Fear of blood
F40.231	Fear of injections and transfusions
F40.232	Fear of other medical care
F40.233	Fear of injury
F40.248	Situational
F40.298	Other
F40.10	Social Anxiety Disorder (Social Phobia) (202)
	Specify if: Performance only
F41.0	Panic Disorder (208)
—.—	Panic Attack Specifier (214)
F40.00	Agoraphobia (217)
F41.1	Generalized Anxiety Disorder (222)
—.—	Substance/Medication-Induced Anxiety Disorder (226)
	Note: See the criteria set and corresponding recording procedures for substance-specific codes and ICD-10-CM coding.
	Specify if: With onset during intoxication, With onset during withdrawal, With onset after medication use
F06.4	Anxiety Disorder Due to Another Medical Condition (230)
F41.8	Other Specified Anxiety Disorder (233)
F41.9	Unspecified Anxiety Disorder (233)

OBSESSIVE–COMPULSIVE AND RELATED DISORDERS (235)

The following specifiers apply to Obsessive–Compulsive and Related Disorders where indicated:

F42	Obsessive–Compulsive Disorder[a] (237)
	Specify if: Tic-related
F45.22	Body Dysmorphic Disorder[a] (242)
	Specify if: With muscle dysmorphia
F42	Hoarding Disorder[a] (247)
	Specify if: With excessive acquisition
F63.2	Trichotillomania (Hair-Pulling Disorder) (251)
L98.1	Excoriation (Skin-Picking) Disorder (254)
—.—	Substance/Medication-Induced Obsessive–Compulsive and Related Disorder (257)
	Note: See the criteria set and corresponding recording procedures for substance-specific codes and ICD-10-CM coding.

Continued

	Specify if: With onset during intoxication, With onset during withdrawal, With onset after medication use
F06.8	Obsessive–Compulsive and Related Disorder Due to Another Medical Condition (260)
	Specify if: With obsessive–compulsive disorder-like symptoms, With appearance preoccupations, With hoarding symptoms, With hair-pulling symptoms, With skin-picking symptoms
F42	Other Specified Obsessive–Compulsive and Related Disorder (263)
F42	Unspecified Obsessive–Compulsive and Related Disorder (264)

[a]Specify if: With good or fair insight, With poor insight, With absent insight/delusional beliefs

TRAUMA- AND STRESSOR-RELATED DISORDERS (265)

F94.1	Reactive Attachment Disorder (265)
	Specify if: Persistent
	Specify current severity: Severe
F94.2	Disinhibited Social Engagement Disorder (268)
	Specify if: Persistent
	Specify current severity: Severe
F43.10	Posttraumatic Stress Disorder (includes Posttraumatic Stress Disorder for Children 6 Years and Younger) (271)
	Specify whether: With dissociative symptoms
	Specify if: With delayed expression
F43.0	Acute Stress Disorder (280)
___.___	Adjustment Disorder (286)
	Specify whether:
F43.21	With depressed mood
F43.22	With anxiety
F43.23	With mixed anxiety and depressed mood
F43.24	With disturbance of conduct
F43.25	With mixed disturbance of emotions and conduct
F43.20	Unspecified
F43.8	Other Specified Trauma- and Stressor-Related Disorder (289)
F43.9	Unspecified Trauma- and Stressor- Related Disorder (290)

DISSOCIATIVE DISORDERS (291)

F44.81	Dissociative Identity Disorder (292)
F44.0	Dissociative Amnesia (298)
	Specify if:
F44.1	With dissociative fugue
F48.1	Depersonalization/Derealization Disorder (302)
F44.89	Other Specified Dissociative Disorder (306)
F44.9	Unspecified Dissociative Disorder (307)

SOMATIC SYMPTOM AND RELATED DISORDERS (309)

F45.1	Somatic Symptom Disorder (311)
	Specify if: With predominant pain
	Specify if: Persistent
	Specify current severity: Mild, Moderate, Severe
F45.21	Illness Anxiety Disorder (315)
	Specify whether: Care-seeking type, Care-avoidant type
—.—	Conversion Disorder (Functional Neurological Symptom Disorder) (318)
	Specify symptom type:
F44.4	With weakness or paralysis
F44.4	With abnormal movement
F44.4	With swallowing symptoms
F44.4	With speech symptom
F44.5	With attacks or seizures
F44.6	With anesthesia or sensory loss
F44.6	With special sensory symptom
F44.7	With mixed symptoms
	Specify if: Acute episode, Persistent
	Specify if: With psychological stressor (specify stressor), Without psychological stressor
F54	Psychological Factors Affecting Other Medical Conditions (322)
	Specify current severity: Mild, Moderate, Severe, Extreme
F68.10	Factitious Disorder (includes Factitious Disorder Imposed on Self, Factitious Disorder Imposed on Another) (324)
	Specify: Single episode, Recurrent episodes
F45.8	Other Specified Somatic Symptom and Related Disorder (327)
F45.9	Unspecified Somatic Symptom and Related Disorder (327)

FEEDING AND EATING DISORDERS (329)

The following specifiers apply to Feeding and Eating Disorders where indicated:

—.—	Pica[a] (329)
F98.3	In children
F50.8	In adults
F98.21	Rumination Disorder[a] (332)
F50.8	Avoidant/Restrictive Food Intake Disorder[a] (334)
—.—	Anorexia Nervosa[b,c] (338)
	Specify whether:
F50.01	Restricting type
F50.02	Binge-eating/purging type
F50.2	Bulimia Nervosa[b,c] (345)
F50.8	Binge-Eating Disorder[b,c] (350)
F50.8	Other Specified Feeding or Eating Disorder (353)
F50.9	Unspecified Feeding or Eating Disorder (354)

[a]Specify if: In remission
[b]Specify if: In partial remission, In full remission
[c]Specify current severity: Mild, Moderate, Severe, Extreme

ELIMINATION DISORDERS (355)

F98.0	Enuresis (355)
	Specify whether: Nocturnal only, Diurnal only, Nocturnal and diurnal
F98.1	Encopresis (357)
	Specify whether: With constipation and overflow incontinence, Without constipation and overflow incontinence
—.—	Other Specified Elimination Disorder (359)
N39.498	With urinary symptoms
R15.9	With fecal symptoms
—.—	Unspecified Elimination Disorder (360)
R32	With urinary symptoms
R15.9	With fecal symptoms

SLEEP–WAKE DISORDERS (361)

The following specifiers apply to Sleep–Wake Disorders where indicated:

G47.00	Insomnia Disorder[a] (362)
	Specify if: With nonsleep disorder mental comorbidity, With other medical comorbidity, With other sleep disorder
G47.10	Hypersomnolence Disorder[b,c] (368)
	Specify if: With mental disorder, With medical condition, With another sleep disorder
___.___	Narcolepsy[c] (372)
	Specify whether:
G47.419	Narcolepsy without cataplexy but with hypocretin deficiency
G47.411	Narcolepsy with cataplexy but without hypocretin deficiency
G47.419	Autosomal dominant cerebellar ataxia, deafness, and narcolepsy
G47.419	Autosomal dominant narcolepsy, obesity, and type 2 diabetes
G47.429	Narcolepsy secondary to another medical condition

[a]Specify if: Episodic, Persistent, Recurrent
[b]Specify if: Acute, Subacute, Persistent
[c]Specify current severity: Mild, Moderate, Severe

Breathing-Related Sleep Disorders (378)

G47.33	Obstructive Sleep Apnea Hypopnea[c] (378)
___.___	Central Sleep Apnea (383)
	Specify whether:
G47.31	Idiopathic central sleep apnea
R06.3	Cheyne-Stokes breathing
G47.37	Central sleep apnea comorbid with opioid use
	Note: First code opioid use disorder, if present.
	Specify current severity
___.___	Sleep-Related Hypoventilation (387)
	Specify whether:
G473.34	Idiopathic hypoventilation
G47.35	Congenital central alveolar hypoventilation
G47.36	Comorbid sleep-related hypoventilation
	Specify current severity
___.___	Circadian Rhythm Sleep–Wake Disorders[a] (390)

Continued

	Specify whether:
G47.21	Delayed sleep phase type (391)
	Specify if: Familial, Overlapping with non-24-hour sleep–wake type
G47.22	Advanced sleep phase type (393)
	Specify if: Familial
G47.23	Irregular sleep-wake type (394)
G47.24	Non-24-hour sleep–wake type (396)
G47.26	Shift work type (397)
G47.20	Unspecified type

Parasomnias (399)

—.—	Non–Rapid Eye Movement Sleep Arousal Disorders (399)
	Specify whether:
F51.3	Sleepwalking type
	Specify if: With sleep-related eating, With sleep-related sexual behavior (sexsomnia)
F51.4	Sleep terror type
F51.5	Nightmare Disorder[b,c] (404)
	Specify if: During sleep onset
	Specify if: With associated non–sleep disorder, With associated other medical condition, With associated other sleep disorder
G473.52	Rapid Eye Movement Sleep Behavior Disorder (407)
G25.81	Restless Legs Syndrome (410)
—.—	Substance/Medication-Induced Sleep Disorder (413)
	Note: See the criteria set and corresponding recording procedures for substance-specific codes and ICD-10-CM coding.
	Specify whether: Insomnia type, Daytime sleepiness type, Parasomnia type, Mixed type
	Specify if: With onset during intoxication, With onset during discontinuation/withdrawal
G47.09	Other Specified Insomnia Disorder (420)
G47.00	Unspecified Insomnia Disorder (420)
G47.19	Other Specified Hypersomnolence Disorder (421)
G47.10	Unspecified Hypersomnolence Disorder (421)
G47.8	Other Specified Sleep–Wake Disorder (421)
G47.9	Unspecified Sleep–Wake Disorder (422)

SEXUAL DYSFUNCTIONS (423)

The following specifiers apply to Sexual Dysfunctions where indicated:

F52.32	Delayed Ejaculation[a,b,c] (424)
F52.21	Erectile Disorder[a,b,c] (426)
F52.31	Female Orgasmic Disorder[a,b,c] (429)
	Specify if: Never experienced an orgasm under any situation
F52.22	Female Sexual Interest/Arousal Disorder[a,b,c] (433)
F52.6	Genito-Pelvic Pain/Penetration Disorder[a,c] (437)
F52.0	Male Hypoactive Sexual Desire Disorder[a,b,c] (440)
F52.4	Premature (Early) Ejaculation[a,b,c] (443)
___.___	Substance/Medication-Induced Sexual Dysfunction[c] (446)
	Note: See the criteria and corresponding recording procedures for substance-specific codes ICD-10-CM coding.
	Specify if: With onset during intoxication, With onset during withdrawal, With onset after medication use
F52.8	Other Specified Sexual Dysfunction (450)
F52.9	Unspecified Sexual Dysfunction (450)

[a]Specify whether: Lifelong, Acquired
[b]Specify whether: Generalized, Situational
[c]Specify current severity: Mild, Moderate, Severe

GENDER DYSPHORIA (451)

___.___	Gender Dysphoria (452)
F64.2	Gender Dysphoria in Children
	Specify if: With a disorder of sex development
F64.1	Gender Dysphoria in Adolescents and Adults
	Specify if: With a disorder of sex development
	Specify if: Posttransition
	Note: Code the disorder of sex development if present, in addition to gender dysphoria.
F64.8	Other Specified Gender Dysphoria (459)
F64.9	Unspecified Gender Dysphoria (459)

DISRUPTIVE, IMPULSE-CONTROL, AND CONDUCT DISORDERS (461)

F91.3	Oppositional Defiant Disorder (462)
	Specify current severity: Mild, Moderate, Severe
F63.81	Intermittent Explosive Disorder (466)
—.—	Conduct Disorder (469)
	Specify whether:
F91.1	Childhood-onset type
F91.2	Adolescent-onset type
F91.9	Unspecified onset
	Specify if: With limited prosocial emotions
	Specify current severity: Mild, Moderate, Severe
F60.2	Antisocial Personality Disorder (476)
F63.1	Pyromania (476)
F63.3	Kleptomania (478)
F91.8	Other Specified Disruptive, Impulse-Control, and Conduct Disorder (479)
F91.9	Unspecified Disruptive, Impulse-Control, and Conduct Disorder (480)

SUBSTANCE-RELATED AND ADDICTIVE DISORDERS (481)

The following specifiers and note apply to Substance-Related and Addictive Disorders where indicated:

Substance-Related Disorders (483)

Alcohol-Related Disorders (490)

—.—	Alcohol Use Disorder[a,b] (490)
	Specify current severity:
F10.10	Mild
F10.20	Moderate
F10.20	Severe
—.—	Alcohol Intoxication (497)
F10.129	With use disorder, mild
F10.229	With use disorder, moderate or severe
F10.929	Without use disorder
—.—	Alcohol Withdrawal[c,d] (499)
F10.239	Without perceptual disturbances
F10.232	With perceptual disturbances
—.—	Other Alcohol-Induced Disorder (502)
F10.99	Unspecified Alcohol-Related Disorder (503)

Caffeine-Related Disorders (503)

F15.929	Caffeine Intoxication (503)
F15.93	Caffeine Withdrawal (506)
—.—	Other Caffeine-Induced Disorder (508)
F15.99	Unspecified Caffeine-Related Disorder (509)

Cannabis-Related Disorders (509)

—.—	Cannabis Use Disorder[a,b] (509)
	Specify current severity:
F12.10	Mild
F12.20	Moderate
F12.20	Severe
—.—	Cannabis Intoxication[c] (516)
	Without perceptual disturbances
F12.129	With use disorder, mild
F12.229	With use disorder, moderate or severe
F12.929	Without use disorder
	With perceptual disturbances
F12.122	With use disorder, mild
F12.222	With use disorder, moderate or severe
F12.922	Without use disorder
F12.288	Cannabis Withdrawal[d] (517)
—.—	Other Cannabis-Induced Disorders (519)
F12.99	Unspecified Cannabis-Related Disorder (519)

Hallucinogen-Related Disorders (520)

—.—	Phencyclidine Use Disorder[a,b] (520)
	Specify current severity:
F16.10	Mild
F16.20	Moderate
F16.20	Severe
—.—	Other Hallucinogen Use Disorder[a,b] (523)
	Specify the particular hallucinogen
	Specify current severity:
F16.10	Mild
F16.20	Moderate
F16.20	Severe
—.—	Phencyclidine Intoxication (527)
F16.129	With use disorder, mild
F16.229	With use disorder, moderate or severe
F16.292	Without use disorder
—.—	Other Hallucinogen Intoxication (529)

Continued

F16.129	With use disorder, mild
F16.229	With use disorder, moderate or severe
F16.929	Without use disorder
F16.983	Hallucinogen Persisting Perception Disorder (531)
—.—	Other Phencyclidine-Induced Disorder (532)
—.—	Other Hallucinogen-Induced Disorder (532)
F16.99	Unspecified Phencyclidine-Related Disorder (533)
F16.99	Unspecified Hallucinogen-Related Disorder (533)

Inhalant-Related Disorder (533)

—.—	Inhalant Use Disorder[a,b] (533)
	Specify the particular inhalant
	Specify current severity:
F18.10	Mild
F18.20	Moderate
F18.20	Severe
—.—	Inhalant Intoxication (538)
F18.129	With use disorder, mild
F18.229	With use disorder, moderate or severe
F18.929	Without use disorder
—.—	Other Inhalant-Induced Disorder (540)
F18.99	Unspecified Inhalant-Related Disorder (540)

Opioid-Related Disorders (540)

—.—	Opioid Use Disorder[a] (541)
	Specify if: On maintenance therapy, In a controlled environment
	Specify current severity:
F11.10	Mild
F11.20	Moderate
F11.20	Severe
—.—	Opioid Intoxication[c] (546)
	Without perceptual disturbances
F11.129	With use disorder, mild
F11.229	With use disorder, moderate or severe
F11.929	Without use disorder
	With perceptual disturbances
F11.122	With use disorder, mild
F11.222	With use disorder, moderate or severe
F11.922	Without use disorder
F11.23	Opioid Withdrawal[d] (547)
—.—	Other Opioid-Induced Disorder (549)
F11.99	Unspecified Opioid-Related Disorder (550)

Sedative-, Hynotic-, or Anxiolytic-Related Disorders (550)

—.—	Sedative, Hypnotic, or Anxiolytic Use Disorder[a,b] (550)
	Specify current severity:
F13.10	Mild
F13.20	Moderate
F13.20	Severe
—.—	Sedative, Hypnotic, or Anxiolytic Intoxication (556)
F13.129	With use disorder, mild
F13.229	With use disorder, moderate or severe
F13.929	Without use disorder
—.—	Sedative, Hypnotic, or Anxiolytic Withdrawal[c,d] (557)
F13.229	Without perceptual disturbances
F13.232	With perceptual disturbances
—.—	Other Sedative-, Hypnotic-, or Anxiolytic-Induced Disorder (560)
F13.99	Unspecified Sedative-, Hypnotic-, or Anxiolytic-Related Disorder (560)

Stimulant-Related Disorders (561)

—.—	Stimulant Use Disorder[a,b] (561)
	Specify current severity:
—.—	Mild
F15.10	Amphetamine-type substance
F14.10	Cocaine
F15.10	Other or unspecified stimulant
—.—	Moderate
F15.20	Amphetamine-type substance
F14.20	Cocaine
F15.20	Other or unspecified stimulant
—.—	Severe
F15.20	Amphetamine-type substance
F14.20	Cocaine
F15.20	Other or unspecified stimulant
—.—	Stimulant Intoxication[c] (567)
	Specify the specific intoxicant
—.—	Amphetamine or other stimulant, Without perceptual disturbances
F15.129	With use disorder, mild
F15.229	With use disorder, moderate or severe
F15.929	Without use disorder
—.—	Cocaine, Without perceptual disturbances

Continued

F14.129	With use disorder, mild
F14.229	With use disorder, moderate or severe
F14.929	Without use disorder
—.—	Amphetamine or other stimulant, With perceptual disturbances
F15.122	With use disorder, mild
F15.222	With use disorder, moderate or severe
F15.922	Without use disorder
—.—	Cocaine, With perceptual disturbances
F14.122	With use disorder, mild
F14.222	Without use disorder, moderate or severe
F14.922	Without use disorder
—.—	Stimulant Withdrawal[d] (569)
	Specify the specific substance causing the withdrawal syndrome
F15.23	Amphetamine or other stimulant
F14.23	Cocaine
—.—	Other Stimulant-Induced Disorder (570)
—.—	Unspecified Stimulant-Related Disorder (570)
F15.99	Amphetamine or other stimulant
F14.99	Cocaine

Tobacco-Related Disorders (571)

—.—	Tobacco Use Disorder[a] (571)
	Specify if: On maintenance therapy, In a controlled environment
	Specify current severity:
Z72.0	Mild
F17.200	Moderate
F17.200	Severe
F17.203	Tobacco Withdrawal[d] (575)
—.—	Other Tobacco-Induced Disorder (576)
F17.209	Unspecified Tobacco-Related Disorder (577)

Other (or Unknown) Substance-Related Disorders (577)

—.—	Other (or Unknown) Substance Use Disorder[a,b] (577)
	Specify current severity:
F19.10	Mild
F19.20	Moderate

F19.20	Severe
—.—	Other (or Unknown) Substance Intoxication (581)
F19.129	With use disorder, mild
F19.229	With use disorder, moderate or severe
F19.229	Without use disorder
F19.23	Other (or Unknown) Substance Withdrawal[d] (583)
—.—	Other (or Unknown) Substance-Induced Disorders (584)
F19.99	Unspecified Other (or Unknown) Substance-Related Disorder (585)

Non-Substance-Related Disorders (585)

F63.0	Gambling Disorder[a] (585) Specify if: Episodic, Persistent Specify current severity: Mild, Moderate, Severe

[a]Specify if: In early remission, In sustained remission
[b]Specify if: In a controlled environment
[c]Specify if: With perceptual disturbances
[d]The ICD-10-CM code indicated the comorbid presence of a moderate or severe substance use disorder, which must be present to apply the code for substance withdrawal.

NEUROCOGNITIVE DISORDERS (591)

—.—	Delirium (596) [a]Note: See the criteria set and corresponding recording procedures for substance-specific codes and ICD-10-CM coding. Specify whether:
—.—	Substance intoxication delirium[a]
—.—	Substance withdrawal delirium[a]
—.—	Medication-induced delirium[a]
F05	Delirium due to another medical condition
F05	Delirium due to multiple etiologies Specify if: Acute, Persistent Specify if: Hyperactive, Hypoactive, Mixed level of activity
R41.0	Other Specified Delirium (602)
R41.0	Unspecified Delirium (602)

Major and Mild Neurocognitive Disorders (602)

Specify whether due to: Alzheimer's disease, Frontotemporal lobar degeneration, Lewy body disease, Vascular disease, Traumatic brain injury, Substance/medication use, HIV infection, Prion disease, Parkinson's disease, Huntington's disease, Another medical condition, Multiple etiologies, Unspecified

Major or Mild Neurocognitive Disorder Due to Alzheimer's Disease (611)

—.—	Probable Major Neurocognitive Disorder Due to Alzheimer's Disease[b]
	Note: Code first 331.0 (G30.9) Alzheimer's disease
F02.81	With behavioral disturbance
F02.80	Without behavioral disturbance
G31.9	Possible Major Neurocognitive Disorder Due to Alzheimer's Disease[a,b]
G31.84	Mild Neurocognitive Disorder Due to Alzheimer's Disease[a]

Major or Mild Frontotemporal Neurocognitive Disorder (614)

—.—	Probable Major Neurocognitive Disorder Due to Frontotemporal Labor Degeneration[b]
	Note: Code first 331.19 (G31.09) Frontotemporal disease.
F02.81	With behavioral disturbance
F02.80	Without behavioral disturbance
G31.9	Possible Major Neurocognitive Disorder Due to Frontotemporal Labor Degeneration[a,b]
G31.84	Mild Neurocognitive Disorder Due to Frontotemporal Labor Degeneration[a]

Major or Mild Neurocognitive Disorder With Lewy Bodies (618)

—.—	Probable Major Neurocognitive Disorder With Lewy Bodies[b]
	Note: Code first 331.82 (G31.83) Lewy body disease.
F02.81	With behavioral disturbance
F02.80	Without behavioral disturbance
G31.9	Possible Major Neurocognitive Disorder With Lewy Bodies[a,b]
G31.84	Mild Neurocognitive Disorder With Lewy Bodies[a]

Major or Mild Vascular Neurocognitive Disorder (621)

—.—	Probable Major Vascular Neurocognitive Disorder[b]
	Note: No additional medical code for vascular disease.
F01.51	With behavioral disturbance
F01.50	Without behavioral disturbance
G31.9	Possible Major Vascular Neurocognitive Disorder[a,b]
G31.84	Mild Vascular Neurocognitive Disorder[a]

Major or Mild Neurocognitive Disorder Due to Traumatic Brain Injury (624)

—.—	Major Neurocognitive Disorder Due to Traumatic Brain Injury[b]
	Note: For ICD-10-CM, code first S06.2X9S diffuse traumatic brain injury with loss of consciousness of unspecified duration, sequela.
F02.81	With behavioral disturbance
F02.80	Without behavioral disturbance
G31.84	Mild Neurocognitive Disorder Due to Traumatic Brain Injury[a]

Substance-/Medication-Induced Major or Mild Neurocognitive Disorder[a] (627)

Major or Mild Neurocognitive Disorder Due to HIV Infection (632)

—.—	Major Neurocognitive Disorder Due to HIV Infection[b]
	Note: Code first 042 (B20) HIV infection.
F02.81	With behavioral disturbance
F02.80	Without behavioral disturbance
G31.84	Mild Neurocognitive Disorder Due to HIV Infection[a]

Major or Mild Neurocognitive Disorder Due to Prion Disease (634)

—.—	Major Neurocognitive Disorder Due to Prion Disease[b]
	Note: Code first 046.79 (A81.9) Prion disease.
F02.81	With behavioral disturbance
F02.80	Without behavioral disturbance
G31.84	Mild Neurocognitive Disorder Due to Prion Disease[a]

Major or Mild Neurocognitive Disorder Due to Parkinson's Disease (636)

—.—	Major Neurocognitive Disorder Probably Due to Parkinson's Disease[b]
	Note: Code first 332.0 (G20) Parkinson's disease.
F02.81	With behavioral disturbance
F02.80	Without behavioral disturbance
G31.9	Major Neurocognitive Disorder Possibly Due to Parkinson's Disease[a,b]
G31.84	Mild Neurocognitive Disorder Due to Parkinson's Disease[a]

Major or Mild Neurocognitive Disorder Due to Huntington's Disease (638)

—.—	Major Neurocognitive Disorder Due to Huntington's Disease[b]
	Note: Code first 333.4 (G10) Huntington's disease.
F02.81	With behavioral disturbance
F02.80	Without behavioral disturbance
G31.84	Mild Neurocognitive Disorder Due to Huntington's Disease[a]

Major or Mild Neurocognitive Disorder Due to Another Medical Condition[a] (641)

—.—	Major Neurocognitive Disorder Due to Another Medical Condition[b]
	Note: Code first the other medical condition.
F02.81	With behavioral disturbance
F02.80	Without behavioral disturbance
G31.84	Mild Neurocognitive Disorder Due to Another Medical Condition[a]

Major or Mild Neurocognitive Disorder Due to Multiple Etiologies (642)

—.—	Major Neurocognitive Disorder Due to Multiple Etiologies[b]
	Note: Code first all the etiological medical conditions (with the exception of vascular disease).
F02.81	With behavioral disturbance
F02.80	Without behavioral disturbance
G31.84	Mild Neurocognitive Disorder Due to Multiple Etiologies[a]

Unspecified Neurocognitive Disorder (643)

R41.9	Unspecified Neurocognitive Disorder[a]

[a]Specify: Without behavioral disturbance, With behavioral disturbance. For possible major neurocognitive disorder and for mild neurocognitive disorder, behavioral disturbance cannot be coded but should still be indicated in writing.
[b]Specify current severity: Mild, Moderate, Severe. This specifier applies only to major neurocognitive disorder (including probable and possible).
Note: As indicated for each subtype, an additional medical code is needed for probable major neurocognitive disorder or major neurocognitive disorder. An additional medical code should not be used for possible major neurocognitive disorder or mild neurocognitive disorder.
Note: No additional medical code. See the criteria set and corresponding recording procedures for substance-specific codes and ICD-10-CM coding.
Specify if: Persistent

PERSONALITY DISORDERS (645)

Cluster A Personality Disorders

F60.0	Paranoid Personality Disorder (649)
F60.1	Schizoid Personality Disorder (652)
F21	Schizotypal Personality Disorder (655)

Cluster B Personality Disorders

F60.2	Antisocial Personality Disorder (659)
F60.3	Borderline Personality Disorder (663)
F60.4	Histrionic Personality Disorder (667)
F60.81	Narcissistic Personality Disorder (669)

Cluster C Personality Disorders

F60.6	Avoidant Personality Disorder (672)
F60.7	Dependent Personality Disorder (675)
F60.5	Obsessive–Compulsive Personality Disorder (678)

Other Personality Disorders

F07.0	Personality Change Due to Another Medical Condition (682) Specify whether: Labile type, Disinhibited type, Aggressive type, Apathetic type, Paranoid type, Other type, Combined type, Unspecified type
F60.89	Other Specified Personality Disorder (684)
F60.9	Unspecified Personality Disorder (684)

PARAPHILIC DISORDERS (685)

The following specifier applies to Paraphilic Disorders where indicated:

F65.3	Voyeuristic Disorder[a] (686)
F65.2	Exhibitionistic Disorder[a] (689) Specify whether: Sexually aroused by exposing genitals to prepubertal children, Sexually aroused by exposing genitals to physically mature individuals, Sexually aroused by exposing genitals to prepubertal children and to physically mature individuals
F65.81	Frotteuristic Disorder[a] (691)
F65.51	Sexual Masochism Disorder[a] (694) Specify if: With asphyxiophilia
F65.52	Sexual Sadism Disorder[a] (695)
F65.4	Pedophilic Disorder (697) Specify whether: Exclusive type, Nonexclusive type Specify if: Sexually attracted to males, Sexually attracted to females, Sexually attracted to both Specify if: Limited to incest
F65.0	Fetishistic Disorder[a] (700) Specify: Body part(s), Nonliving object(s), Other
F65.1	Transvestic Disorder[a] (702) Specify if: With fetishism, With autogynephilia
F65.89	Other Specified Paraphilic Disorder (705)
F65.9	Unspecified Paraphilic Disorder (705)

[a]Specify if: In a controlled environment, In full remission

OTHER MENTAL DISORDERS (707)

F06.8	Other Specified Mental Disorder Due to Another Medical Condition (707)
F09	Unspecified Mental Disorder Due to Another Medical Condition (708)
F99	Other Specified Mental Disorder (708)
F99	Unspecified Mental Disorder (708)

MEDICATION-INDUCED MOVEMENT DISORDERS AND OTHER ADVERSE EFFECTS OF MEDICATION (709)

G21.11	Neuroleptic-Induced parkinsonism (709)
G21.19	Other Medication-Induced parkinsonism (709)
G21.0	Neuroleptic Malignant Syndrome (709)
G24.02	Medication-Induced Acute Dystonia (711)
G25.71	Medication-Induced Acute Akathisia (711)
G24.01	Tardive Dyskinesia (712)
G24.09	Tardive Dystonia (712)
G25.71	Tardive Akathisia (712)
G25.1	Medication-Induced Postural Tremor (712)
G25.79	Other Medication-Induced Movement Disorder (712)
—.—	Antidepressant Discontinuation Syndrome (712)
T43.205A	Initial encounter
T43.205D	Subsequent encounter
T43.205S	Sequelae
—.—	Other Adverse Effect of Medication (714)
T50.905A	Initial encounter
T50.905D	Subsequent encounter
T50.905S	Sequelae

OTHER CONDITIONS THAT MAY BE A FOCUS OF CLINICAL ATTENTION (715)

Relational Problems (715)

Problems Related to Family Upbringing (715)

Z62.820	Parent–Child Relational Problem (715)
Z62.891	Sibling Relational Problem (716)
Z62.29	Upbringing Away From Parents (716)
Z62.898	Child Affected by Parental Relationship Distress (716)

Other Problems Related to Primary Support Group (716)

Z63.0	Relationship Distress With Spouse or Intimate Partner (716)
Z63.5	Disruption of Family by Separation or Divorce (716)
Z63.8	High Expressed Emotion Level Within Family (716)
Z63.4	Uncomplicated Bereavement (716)

Abuse and Neglect (717)

Child Maltreatment and Neglect Problems (717)

Child Physical Abuse (717)	
Child Physical Abuse, Confirmed (717)	
T743.12XA	Initial encounter
T74.12XD	Subsequent encounter
Child Physical Abuse, Suspected (717)	
T76.12XA	Initial encounter
T76.12XD	Subsequent encounter
Other Circumstances Related to Child Physical Abuse (718)	
Z69.010	Encounter for mental health services for victim of child abuse by parent
Z69.020	Encounter for mental health services for victim of nonparental child abuse
Z62.810	Personal history (past history) of physical abuse in childhood
Z69.011	Encounter for mental health services for perpetrator of parental child abuse
Z69.021	Encounter for mental health services for perpetrator of nonparental child abuse
Child Sexual Abuse (718)	
Child Sexual Abuse, Confirmed (718)	
T74.22XA	Initial encounter
T74.22XD	Subsequent encounter
Child Sexual Abuse, Suspected (718)	
T76.22XA	Initial encounter
T76.22XD	Subsequent encounter
Other Circumstances Related to Child Sexual Abuse (718)	
Z69.010	Encounter for mental health services for victim of child sexual abuse by parent
Z69.020	Encounter for mental health services for victim of nonparental child sexual abuse
Z62.810	Personal history (past history) of sexual abuse in childhood

Z69.011	Encounter for mental health services for perpetrator of parental child sexual abuse
Z69.021	Encounter for mental health services for perpetrator of nonparental child sexual abuse
Child Neglect (718)	
Child Neglect, Confirmed (718)	
T74.02ZA	Initial encounter
T74.02XD	Subsequent encounter
Child Neglect, Suspected (719)	
T76.02XA	Initial encounter
T76.02XD	Subsequent encounter
Other Circumstances Related to Child Neglect (719)	
Z69.010	Encounter for mental health services for victim of child neglect by parent
Z69.020	Encounter for mental health services for victim of nonparental child neglect
Z62.812	Personal history (past history) of neglect in childhood
Z69.011	Encounter for mental health services for perpetrator of parental child neglect
Z69.021	Encounter for mental health services for perpetrator of nonparental child neglect
Child Psychological Abuse (719)	
Child Psychological Abuse, Confirmed (719)	
T74.32XA	Initial encounter
T74.32XD	Subsequent encounter
Child Psychological Abuse, Suspected (719)	
T76.32XA	Initial encounter
T76.32XD	Subsequent encounter
Other Circumstances Related to Child Psychological Abuse (719)	
Z69.010	Encounter for mental health services for victim of child psychological abuse by parent
Z69.020	Encounter for mental health services for victim of nonparental child psychological abuse
Z62.811	Personal history (past history) of psychological abuse in childhood
Z69.011	Encounter for mental health services for perpetrator of parental child psychological abuse
Z69.021	Encounter for mental health services for perpetrator of nonparental child psychological abuse

Adult Maltreatment and Neglect Problems (720)

Spouse or Partner Violence, Physical (720)
Spouse or Partner Violence, Physical, Confirmed (720)

T74.11XA	Initial encounter
T74.11XD	Subsequent encounter

Spouse or Partner Violence, Physical, Suspected (720)

T76.11XA	Initial encounter
T76.11XD	Subsequent encounter

Other Circumstances Related to Spouse or Partner Violence, Physical (720)

Z96.11	Encounter for mental health services for victim of spouse or partner violence, physical
Z91.410	Personal history (past history) of spouse or partner violence, physical
Z69.12	Encounter for mental health services for perpetrator of spouse or partner violence, physical

Spouse or Partner Violence, Sexual (720)
Spouse or Partner Violence, Sexual, Confirmed (720)

T74.21XA	Initial encounter
T74.21XD	Subsequent encounter

Spouse or Partner Violence, Sexual, Suspected (720)

T76.21XA	Initial encounter
T76.21XD	Subsequent encounter

Other Circumstances Related to Spouse or Partner Violence, Sexual (720)

Z69.81	Encounter for mental health services for victim of spouse or partner violence, sexual
Z91.410	Personal history (past history) of spouse or partner violence, sexual
Z69.12	Encounter for mental health services for perpetrator of spouse or partner violence, sexual

Spouse or Partner Neglect (721)
Spouse or Partner Neglect, Confirmed (721)

T47.01XA	Initial encounter
T74.01XD	Subsequent encounter

Spouse or Partner Neglect, Suspected (721)

T76.01XA	Initial encounter
T76.01XD	Subsequent encounter

Other Circumstances Related to Spouse or Partner Neglect (721)

Z69.11	Encounter for mental health services for victim of spouse or partner neglect

Z91.412	Personal history (past history) of spouse or partner neglect
Z69.12	Encounter for mental health services for perpetrator of spouse or partner neglect
Spouse or Partner Abuse, Psychological (721)	
Spouse or Partner Abuse, Psychological, Confirmed (721)	
T74.31XA	Initial encounter
T74.31XD	Subsequent encounter
Spouse or Partner Abuse, Psychological, Suspected (721)	
T76.31XA	Initial encounter
T76.31XD	Subsequent encounter
Other Circumstances Related to Spouse or Partner Abuse, Psychological (721)	
Z69.11	Encounter for mental health services for victim of spouse or partner psychological abuse
Z91.411	Personal history (past history) of spouse or partner psychological abuse
Z69.12	Encounter for mental health services for perpetrator of spouse or partner psychological abuse
Adult Abuse by Nonspouse or Nonpartner (722)	
Adult Physical Abuse by Nonspouse or Nonpartner, Confirmed (722)	
T74.11XA	Initial encounter
T74.11XD	Subsequent encounter
Adult Physical Abuse by Nonspouse or Nonpartner, Suspected (722)	
T76.11XA	Initial encounter
T76.11XD	Subsequent encounter
Adult Sexual Abuse by Nonspouse or Nonpartner, Confirmed (722)	
T74.21XA	Initial encounter
T74.21XD	Subsequent encounter
Adult Sexual Abuse by Nonspouse or Nonpartner, Suspected (722)	
T76.21XA	Initial encounter
T76.21XD	Subsequent encounter
Adult Psychological Abuse by Nonspouse or Nonpartner, Confirmed (722)	
T74.31XA	Initial encounter
T74.31XD	Subsequent encounter
Adult Psychological Abuse by Nonspouse or Nonpartner, Suspected (722)	
T76.31XA	Initial encounter
T76.31XD	Subsequent encounter
Other Circumstances Related to Adult Abuse by Nonspouse or Nonpartner (722)	

Continued

Z69.81	Encounter for mental health services for victim of nonspousal adult abuse
Z69.82	Encounter for mental health services for perpetrator of nonspousal adult abuse

Educational and Occupational Problems (723)

Educational Problems (723)

Z55.9	Academic or Educational Problem (723)

Occupational Problems (723)

Z56.82	Problem Related to Current Military Deployment Status (723)
Z56.9	Other Problem Related to Employment (723)

Housing and Economic Problems (723)

Housing Problems (723)

Z59.0	Homelessness (723)
Z59.1	Inadequate Housing (723)
Z59.2	Discord With Neighbor, Lodger, or Landlord (723)
Z59.3	Problem Related to Living in a Residential Institution (724)

Economic Problems (724)

Z59.4	Lack of Adequate Food or Safe Drinking Water (724)
Z59.5	Extreme Poverty (724)
Z59.6	Low Income (724)
Z59.7	Insufficient Social Insurance or Welfare Support (724)
Z59.9	Unspecified Housing or Economic Problem (724)

Other Problems Related to the Social Environment (724)

Z60.0	Phase of Life Problem (724)
Z60.2	Problem Related to Living Alone (724)
Z60.3	Acculturation Difficulty (724)
Z60.4	Social Exclusion or Rejection (724)
Z60.5	Target of (Perceived) Adverse Discrimination or Persecution (724)
Z60.9	Unspecified Problem Related to Social Environment (725)

Problems Related to Crime or Interaction With the Legal System (725)

Z65.4	Victim of Crime (725)
Z65.0	Conviction in Civil or Criminal Proceedings Without Imprisonment (725)
Z65.1	Imprisonment or Other Incarceration (725)
Z65.2	Problems Related to Release From Prison (725)
Z65.3	Problems Related to Other Legal Circumstances (725)

Other Health Service Encounters for Counseling and Medical Advice (725)

Z70.9	Sex Counseling (725)
Z71.9	Other Counseling or Consultation (725)

Problems Related to Other Psychosocial, Personal, and Environmental Circumstances (725)

Z65.8	Religious or Spiritual Problem (725)
Z64.0	Problems Related to Unwanted Pregnancy (725)
Z64.1	Problems Related to Multiparity (725)
Z64.4	Discord With Social Service Provider, Including Probation Officer, Case Manager, or Social Service Worker (725)
Z65.4	Victim of Terrorism or Torture (725)
Z65.5	Exposure to Disaster, War, or Other Hostilities (725)
Z65.8	Other Problem Related to Psychosocial Circumstances (725)
Z65.9	Unspecified Problem Related to Unspecified Psychosocial Circumstances (725)

Other Circumstances of Personal History (726)

Z91.49	Other Personal History of Psychological Trauma (726)
Z91.5	Personal History of Self-Harm (726)
Z91.82	Personal History of Military Deployment (726)
Z91.89	Other Personal Risk Factors (726)
Z72.9	Problem Related to Lifestyle (726)
Z72.811	Adult Antisocial Behavior (726)
Z72.810	Child or Adolescent Antisocial Behavior (726)

Problems Related to Access to Medical and Other Health Care (726)

Z75.3	Unavailability or Inaccessibility of Health Care Facilities (726)
Z75.4	Unavailability or Inaccessibility of Other Helping Agencies (726)

Nonadherence to Medical Treatment (726)

Z91.19	Nonadherence to Medical Treatment (726)
E66.9	Overweight or Obesity (726)
Z76.5	Malingering (726)
Z91.83	Wandering Associated With a Mental Disorder (727)
R41.83	Borderline Intellectual Functioning (727)

Index

Page numbers followed by "*f*" indicate figures, "*t*" indicate tables, and "*b*" indicate boxes.

B

D

G

M

N

T

PATIENT PROBLEMS BY CHAPTER